GASTROENTEROLOGY MCQs
for Postgraduate and Superspecialty Medical Entrance Examinations

GASTROENTEROLOGY MCQs
for Postgraduate and Superspecialty Medical Entrance Examinations

Based on 20th Edition of Harrison's Prinicples of Internal Medicine

Dr Ajay Mathur
Senior Professor
Department of Medicine
SMS Medical College and Hospital
Jaipur, Rajasthan, India

Foreword
Ramesh Roop Rai

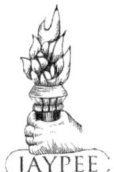

JAYPEE BROTHERS MEDICAL PUBLISHERS
The Health Sciences Publisher
New Delhi | London | Panama

Jaypee Brothers Medical Publishers (P) Ltd.

Headquarters
Jaypee Brothers Medical Publishers (P) Ltd
4838/24, Ansari Road, Daryaganj
New Delhi 110 002, India
Phone: +91-11-43574357
Fax: +91-11-43574314
E-mail: jaypee@jaypeebrothers.com

Overseas Offices

J.P. Medical Ltd
83, Victoria Street, London
SW1H 0HW (UK)
Phone: +44 20 3170 8910
Fax: +44 (0)20 3008 6180
E-mail: info@jpmedpub.com

Jaypee-Highlights Medical Publishers Inc
City of Knowledge, Bld. 235, 2nd Floor, Clayton
Panama City, Panama
Phone: +1 507-301-0496
Fax: +1 507-301-0499
E-mail: cservice@jphmedical.com

Jaypee Brothers Medical Publishers (P) Ltd
Bhotahity, Kathmandu, Nepal
Phone: +977-9741283608
E-mail: kathmandu@jaypeebrothers.com

Website: www.jaypeebrothers.com
Website: www.jaypeedigital.com

© 2019, Jaypee Brothers Medical Publishers

The views and opinions expressed in this book are solely those of the original contributor(s)/author(s) and do not necessarily represent those of editor(s) of the book.

All rights reserved. No part of this publication may be reproduced, stored or transmitted in any form or by any means, electronic, mechanical, photocopying, recording or otherwise, without the prior permission in writing of the publishers.

All brand names and product names used in this book are trade names, service marks, trademarks or registered trademarks of their respective owners. The publisher is not associated with any product or vendor mentioned in this book.

Medical knowledge and practice change constantly. This book is designed to provide accurate, authoritative information about the subject matter in question. However, readers are advised to check the most current information available on procedures included and check information from the manufacturer of each product to be administered, to verify the recommended dose, formula, method and duration of administration, adverse effects and contraindications. It is the responsibility of the practitioner to take all appropriate safety precautions. Neither the publisher nor the author(s)/editor(s) assume any liability for any injury and/or damage to persons or property arising from or related to use of material in this book.

This book is sold on the understanding that the publisher is not engaged in providing professional medical services. If such advice or services are required, the services of a competent medical professional should be sought.

Every effort has been made where necessary to contact holders of copyright to obtain permission to reproduce copyright material. If any have been inadvertently overlooked, the publisher will be pleased to make the necessary arrangements at the first opportunity. The **CD/DVD-ROM** (if any) provided in the sealed envelope with this book is complimentary and free of cost. **Not meant for sale**.

Inquiries for bulk sales may be solicited at: jaypee@jaypeebrothers.com

Gastroenterology MCQs for Postgraduate and Superspecialty Medical Entrance Examinations

First Edition: **2019**

ISBN: 978-93-5270-996-0

Foreword

As a professional who has been practicing medicine for over four decades now, I appreciate the value this book brings to the table in times like today. As we move from a largely descriptive era to the bullet-point generation, this academic initiative appears profoundly relevant.

Dr Mathur is bringing to the students and others, Gastroenterology MCQs in an individual book format. This would be more handy and subject specific. The book has been a reference point for many medical entrance examinations and has left an impact on medical professionals who look for high quality of academic material.

Knowledge is a more processed form of information. Dr Mathur stays true to his pledge by presenting well-digested bytes of knowledge across different fields of medicine. His relying on good old word-of-mouth to make this book a success rather than enthusiastic marketing adds further credibility to his initiative. I recommend this book, without a shadow of doubt, to every medical professional who is looking to continue learning.

Dr Ramesh Roop Rai
Former, Professor and Head
Department of Gastroenterology
SMS Medical College and Hospital, Jaipur
Past President, Indian Society of Gastroenterology (2008)

Preface

Medicine, in all its vastness, needs to be understood in a way that makes most sense to how it is applied today. Memorizing each word is elusive and therefore, testing knowledge of a discipline remains an evergreen challenge.

It is a widely accepted fact that taking a quiz soon after studying helps one retain knowledge better and apply the lessons in practice. Multiple Choice Questions (MCQs) are an effective way of remembering the gist of the matter. This is precisely the reason why most examinations today follow this format. This book is committed to honing your skills to retain knowledge, help diagnose medical conditions, and maximize your impact, as a doctor.

A tremendous volume of questions has been generated over the past ten years. As it stands today, the approach needs to be adjusted according to the knowledge available at hand. This time around, my team has decided that each specialism merits its own edition. This will help you to study existing literature with recent advances in medicine and glean deeper insights into the subject matter. Based on the epic 20th edition of Harrison's Principles of Internal Medicine, published by The McGraw-Hill Companies, Inc., this book is dedicated to the field of Gastroenterology in all its endless scope. This book caters to medical professionals at all levels. Not only can this be used by aspiring doctors to prepare for medical entrance examinations, but also by seasoned physicians to update knowledge long after it has been acquired. The book is sign-posted with references should the reader require elaboration on any given topic.

The book contains 2552 questions and still counting, I continue to keep my promise to continually refine the content of my book and chronicle the advances of medical science.

Dr Ajay Mathur

Contents

1. Dysphagia 1
2. Nausea, Vomiting, and Indigestion 5
3. Diarrhea and Constipation 9
4. Gastrointestinal Bleeding 16
5. Jaundice 19
6. Abdominal Swelling and Ascites 25
7. Diseases of the Esophagus 28
8. Peptic Ulcer Disease and Related Disorders 37
9. Disorders of Absorption 54
10. Inflammatory Bowel Disease 68
11. Irritable Bowel Syndrome 86
12. Mesenteric Vascular Insufficiency 91
13. Approach to the Patient with Liver Disease 93
14. Evaluation of Liver Function 101
15. Hyperbilirubinemias 105
16. Acute Viral Hepatitis 111
17. Toxic and Drug-induced Hepatitis 140
18. Chronic Hepatitis 149
19. Autoimmune Hepatitis 163
20. Alcoholic Liver Disease 166
21. Nonalcoholic Fatty Liver Disease and Nonalcoholic Steatohepatitis 171
22. Cirrhosis and its Complications 173
23. Hepatocellular Carcinoma 190
24. Liver Transplantation 194
25. Diseases of the Gallbladder and Bile Ducts 198
26. Approach to the Patient with Pancreatic Disease 204
27. Acute and Chronic Pancreatitis 207

GASTROENTEROLOGY

Dysphagia

1. Dysphagia is defined as a sensation of "sticking" or obstruction of the passage of food through?
Harrison's 20th Ed. Chapter 40 Page 249

- A. Mouth
- B. Pharynx
- C. Esophagus
- D. All of the above

Dysphagia is defined as a sensation of "sticking" or obstruction of the passage of food through the mouth, pharynx or esophagus.

2. Foreign body sensation localized in the neck is termed as?
Harrison's 20th Ed. Chapter 40 Page 250

- A. Odynophagia
- B. Globus pharyngeus
- C. Transfer dysphagia
- D. Phagophobia

A foreign body sensation localized in the neck that does not interfere with swallowing and is sometimes relieved by swallowing is termed as "Globus pharyngeus" or a "lump in the throat" sensation.

3. Which of the following is characteristic of oropharyngeal dysphagia?
Harrison's 20th Ed. Chapter 40 Page 250

- A. Odynophagia
- B. Globus pharyngeus
- C. Transfer dysphagia
- D. Phagophobia

Transfer dysphagia frequently results in nasal regurgitation and pulmonary aspiration during swallowing and is characteristic of oropharyngeal dysphagia or "high" dysphagia.

4. Which of the following may have a psychogenic cause of dysphagia?
Harrison's 20th Ed. Chapter 40 Page 250

- A. Globus pharyngeus
- B. Transfer dysphagia
- C. Phagophobia
- D. All of the above

Phagophobia refers to fear of swallowing. Refusal to swallow thereby may be psychogenic.

5. Which of the following terms refers to an acute setting of esophageal foreign body impaction?
Harrison's 20th Ed. Chapter 40 Page 250

- A. Globus pharyngeus
- B. Odynophagia
- C. Phagophobia
- D. Aphagia

Aphagia refers to complete esophageal obstruction, most commonly encountered in acute setting of a food bolus or foreign body impaction.

6. "Deglutitive inhibition" best relates to which of the following?
Harrison's 20th Ed. Chapter 40 Page 250

- A. Smell
- B. Mastication
- C. Peristaltic contraction of esophagus
- D. Gastroesophageal reflux

Primary peristalsis refers to peristaltic contractions elicited in response to a swallow. It is an interplay of sequenced inhibition followed by contraction of the entire length of esophageal musculature. The inhibition that precedes peristaltic contraction is called deglutitive inhibition.

7. Deglutitive inhibition refers to?
Harrison's 20th Ed. Chapter 40 Page 250

- A. Complete esophageal obstruction
- B. Difficulty in initiating a swallow
- C. Inhibition that precedes peristaltic contraction
- D. Misdirection of food

Inhibition that precedes the peristaltic contraction is called deglutitive inhibition.

8. Which of the following esophageal contractions is nonperistaltic?
Harrison's 20th Ed. Chapter 40 Page 250

- A. Primary peristalsis
- B. Secondary peristalsis
- C. Tertiary peristalsis
- D. Any of the above

Tertiary esophageal contractions are nonperistaltic, disordered esophageal contractions that occur spontaneously during fluoroscopic observation.

9. Peristalsis that begins at the point of esophageal distention and proceeds distally is called?
Harrison's 20th Ed. Chapter 40 Page 250

- A. Primary peristalsis
- B. Secondary peristalsis
- C. Tertiary peristalsis
- D. Any of the above

Local distention of esophagus activates secondary peristalsis. It begins at the point of distention and proceeds distally as in gastroesophageal reflux.

10. Musculature of which of the following is striated?
Harrison's 20th Ed. Chapter 40 Page 250

- A. Pharynx
- B. Upper esophageal sphincter (UES)
- C. Cervical esophagus
- D. All of the above

The musculature of the oral cavity, pharynx, UES, and cervical esophagus is striated.

11. Lower esophageal sphincter (LES) relaxes when?
Harrison's 20th Ed. Chapter 40 Page 250

- A. As the food enters esophagus
- B. As the food travels through esophagus
- C. As the food bolus is delivered into stomach
- D. All of the above

Lower esophageal sphincter (LES) relaxes as the food enters esophagus and remains relaxed until the peristaltic contraction has delivered the food bolus into the stomach.

12. **Which of the following is physiologically a part of upper esophageal sphincter (UES)?**
    Harrison's 20th Ed. Chapter 40 Page 250
    A. Cricopharyngeus muscle
    B. Inferior pharyngeal constrictor
    C. Proximal portion of cervical esophagus
    D. All of the above

    Physiologically, UES consists of the cricopharyngeus muscle, the adjacent inferior pharyngeal constrictor, and the proximal portion of the cervical esophagus.

13. **Innervation to the musculature acting on UES to facilitate its opening during swallowing comes from?**
    Harrison's 20th Ed. Chapter 40 Page 250
    A. Fifth cranial nerve
    B. Seventh cranial nerve
    C. Twelfth cranial nerve
    D. All of the above

14. **UES innervation is derived from?**
    Harrison's 20th Ed. Chapter 40 Page 250
    A. Fifth cranial nerve
    B. Seventh cranial nerve
    C. Twelfth cranial nerve
    D. Tenth cranial nerve

    UES innervation is derived from vagus nerve, whereas innervation to the musculature acting on UES to facilitate its opening during swallowing comes from fifth, seventh & twelfth cranial nerves.

15. **Which of the following is involved in keeping UES closed at rest?**
    Harrison's 20th Ed. Chapter 40 Page 250
    A. Cricopharyngeus muscle
    B. Inferior pharyngeal constrictor
    C. Proximal portion of cervical esophagus
    D. All of the above

    UES remains closed at rest due to its inherent elastic properties and neurogenically mediated contraction of cricopharyngeus muscle.

16. **Which of the following muscle acts on the upper esophageal sphincter (UES)?**
    Harrison's 20th Ed. Chapter 40 Page 250
    A. Cricopharyngeus muscle
    B. Suprahyoid muscle
    C. Geniohyoid muscle
    D. All of the above

    UES opening during swallowing involves cessation of vagal excitation to cricopharyngeus and simultaneous contraction of suprahyoid and geniohyoid muscles that pull open UES along with upward and forward displacement of larynx.

17. **Which of the following muscle is involved in opening UES during swallowing?**
    Harrison's 20th Ed. Chapter 40 Page 250
    A. Geniohyoid
    B. Mylohyoid
    C. Styloglossus
    D. All of the above

    UES opening during swallowing is due to relaxation of cricopharyngeus muscle (cessation of vagal excitation) and simultaneous contraction of suprahyoid & geniohyoid muscles.

18. **Peristalsis in the proximal esophagus is governed by?**
    Harrison's 20th Ed. Chapter 40 Page 250
    A. Lower motor neurons of the vagus nerve
    B. Vagal motor neurons in the nucleus ambiguus
    C. Neurons within the esophageal myenteric plexus
    D. All of the above

    Striated muscles of cervical esophagus are directly innervated by lower motor neurons of vagus nerve. Peristalsis in proximal esophagus is governed by sequential activation of vagal motor neurons in nucleus ambiguus. Distal esophagus & LES are composed of smooth muscle and are controlled by excitatory & inhibitory neurons within the esophageal myenteric plexus. Medullary preganglionic neurons from dorsal motor nucleus of vagus trigger peristalsis via these ganglionic neurons during primary peristalsis.

19. **Neurotransmitter of the inhibitory ganglionic neurons during primary peristalsis is?**
    Harrison's 20th Ed. Chapter 40 Page 250
    A. Vasoactive intestinal peptide
    B. Acetylcholine
    C. Substance P
    D. All of the above

    For during primary peristalsis, neurotransmitters of excitatory ganglionic neurons are acetylcholine & substance P. Those of inhibitory neurons are vasoactive intestinal peptide & nitric oxide.

20. **Which of the following acts as an external sphincter in the functioning of LES?**
    Harrison's 20th Ed. Chapter 40 Page 250
    A. Muscles of the right diaphragmatic crus
    B. Muscle of the left diaphragmatic crus
    C. Muscle of the central diaphragmatic crus
    D. All of the above

    Function of LES is supplemented by surrounding muscle of the right diaphragmatic crus, which acts as an external sphincter during inspiration, cough or abdominal straining.

21. **Agents that increase LES pressure are all except?**
    Harrison's 20th Ed. Chapter 40 Page 250
    A. Substance P
    B. Prostaglandin $F_{2\alpha}$
    C. Secretin
    D. Gastrin

22. **Agents that reduce LES pressure are all except?**
    Harrison's 20th Ed. Chapter 40 Page 250
    A. Cholecystokinin
    B. Secretin
    C. Dopamine
    D. Gastrin

23. **Agents that reduce LES pressure are all except?**
    Harrison's 20th Ed. Chapter 40 Page 250
    A. VIP
    B. Calcitonin gene-related peptide (CGRP)
    C. Prostaglandin E
    D. Prostaglandin $F_{2\alpha}$

24. Agents that reduce LES pressure are all except?
Harrison's 20th Ed. Chapter 40 Page 250

A. Adenosine
B. Dopamine
C. Substance P
D. Nitrates

Reduction in LES sphincter pressure occurs with phosphodiesterase-5 inhibitors (sildenafil) use, fatty meals, smoking, and beverages with high xanthine content (tea, coffee, cola), nicotine, beta-adrenergic agonists, dopamine, cholecystokinin, secretin, vasoactive intestinal peptide (VIP), calcitonin gene–related peptide, adenosine, prostaglandin E, nitric oxide donors (nitrates). LES contraction occurs with GABA-B agonists (baclofen), muscarinic M_2 and M_3 receptor agonists, alpha-adrenergic agonists, gastrin, substance P & Pg $F_{2\alpha}$.

25. Which of the following statements about upper esophageal sphincter (UES) is false?
Harrison's 20th Ed. Chapter 40 Page 250

A. Formed by cricopharyngeus & inferior pharyngeal constrictor muscles
B. These muscles exhibit myogenic tone
C. These muscles receive no inhibitory innervation
D. Opened by central inhibition of sphincter muscles

The UES remains closed at rest due to its inherent elastic properties and neurogenically mediated contraction of the cricopharyngeus muscle.

26. Which of the following statements about lower esophageal sphincter (LES) is false?
Harrison's 20th Ed. Chapter 40 Page 250

A. Innervated by parallel sets of parasympathetic excitatory & inhibitory pathways
B. Opens in response to activity of inhibitory nerves
C. Neurotransmitters of excitatory nerves are acetylcholine, substance P & nitric oxide
D. Neurotransmitters of inhibitory nerves is VIP

27. Motor dysphagia refers to?
Harrison's 20th Ed. Chapter 40 Page 251

A. Weakness of peristaltic contractions
B. Impaired deglutitive inhibition
C. Impaired sphincter relaxation
D. All of the above

Dysphagia caused by a large bolus or a narrow lumen is called structural dysphagia. Dysphagia due to weakness of peristaltic contractions or to impaired deglutitive inhibition causing nonperistaltic contractions & impaired sphincter relaxation is called propulsive or motor dysphagia.

28. Length of adult esophagus is?
Harrison's 20th Ed. Chapter 40 Page 251

A. 12 – 16 cm
B. 14 – 20 cm
C. 16 – 24 cm
D. 18 – 26 cm

Adult esophagus is 18 – 26 cm in length. Anatomically, it is divided into cervical esophagus (from pharyngoesophageal junction to suprasternal notch) and thoracic esophagus (up to the diaphragmatic hiatus).

29. In an adult, esophageal lumen can distend up to?
Harrison's 20th Ed. Chapter 40 Page 251

A. 2 cm in anteroposterior plane & 3 cm in lateral plane
B. 3 cm in anteroposterior plane & 4 cm in lateral plane
C. 4 cm in anteroposterior plane & 5 cm in lateral plane
D. 5 cm in anteroposterior plane & 6 cm in lateral plane

In adult, esophageal lumen can distend up to 4 cm in diameter or 2 cm in anteroposterior plane & 3 cm in lateral plane. When esophagus cannot dilate beyond 2.5 cm in diameter, dysphagia to normal solid food occurs. Dysphagia is always present when esophagus cannot distend beyond 1.3 cm.

30. Which of the following is a structural cause of dysphagia?
Harrison's 20th Ed. Chapter 40 Page 251

A. Schatzki's rings
B. Eosinophilic esophagitis
C. Peptic strictures
D. All of the above

The most common structural causes of dysphagia are Schatzki's rings, eosinophilic esophagitis and peptic strictures.

31. Hallmark of oropharyngeal dysphagia is?
Harrison's 20th Ed. Chapter 40 Page 251

A. Food impaction
B. Odynophagia
C. Nasal regurgitation
D. Hoarseness

Nasal regurgitation & tracheobronchial aspiration with swallowing are hallmarks of oropharyngeal dysphagia ("high" dysphagia) or a tracheoesophageal fistula.

32. Which of the following is important in medical history of a case of dysphagia?
Harrison's 20th Ed. Chapter 40 Page 252

A. Location
B. Types of foods and/or liquids
C. Progressive or intermittent, duration of symptoms
D. All of the above

In a case of dysphagia, key features to consider in medical history are : location, types of foods and/or liquids, progressive or intermittent and duration of symptoms.

33. Which of the following features suggest structural dysphagia?
Harrison's 20th Ed. Chapter 40 Page 252

A. Dysphagia caused by an oversized bolus or a narrow lumen
B. Intermittent dysphagia that occurs only with solid food
C. Food impaction with a prolonged inability to pass an ingested bolus even with ingestion of liquid
D. All of the above

34. Which of the following features suggest motor dysphagia?
Harrison's 20th Ed. Chapter 40 Page 252

A. Due to abnormalities of peristalsis
B. Due to impaired sphincter relaxation after swallowing
C. Constant dysphagia with both liquids & solids
D. All of the above

35. Malignancy is likely if there is?
Harrison's 20th Ed. Chapter 40 Page 252

A. Short duration (<4 months), disease progression
B. Dysphagia more for solids than for liquids
C. Weight loss
D. All of the above

Malignancy is likely if there is a short duration (<4 months), disease progression, dysphagia more for solids than for liquids and weight loss.

36. **Bird's beak sign best relates to?**
    The American Journal of Medicine. 2015; 128(10):1138.e18
    A. Achalasia
    B. Zenker's diverticulum
    C. Diffuse esophageal spasm (DES)
    D. Schatzki's rings

Achalasia is characterized by dilation & sigmoidization of esophagus with classic bird's beak sign.

37. **Achalasia is more likely if there is?**
    Harrison's 20th Ed. Chapter 40 Page 252
    A. Dysphagia for both solids and liquids
    B. Passive nocturnal regurgitation of mucus or food
    C. Problem that has existed for several months or years
    D. All of the above

Achalasia is more likely if there is dysphagia for both solids & liquids (dysphagia for liquids strongly suggests the diagnosis), there is passive nocturnal regurgitation of mucus or food, has existed for several months or years.

38. **Chest pain frequently accompanies which of the following dysphagias?**
    Harrison's 20th Ed. Chapter 40 Page 252
    A. Motor disorders
    B. Structural disorders
    C. Reflux disease
    D. All of the above

Chest pain frequently accompanies dysphagia whether it is related to motor disorders, structural disorders or reflux disease.

39. **Which of the following skin diseases may involve the esophagus?**
    Harrison's 20th Ed. Chapter 40 Page 252
    A. Scleroderma
    B. Pemphigoid
    C. Epidermolysis bullosa
    D. All of the above

Scleroderma, pemphigoid, lichen planus and epidermolysis bullosa can involve the esophagus.

40. **Oropharyngeal dysphagia may be due to which of the following causes?**
    Harrison's 20th Ed. Chapter 40 Page 251
    A. Neurologic cause
    B. Muscular cause
    C. Metabolic cause
    D. All of the above

Oropharyngeal dysphagia may be due to neurologic (cerebrovascular accidents, Parkinson's disease, amyotrophic lateral sclerosis), muscular, structural (Zenker's diverticulum, cricopharyngeal bar, neoplasia), iatrogenic (surgery and radiation), infectious and metabolic causes.

41. **Oropharyngeal dysphagia most commonly results from?**
    Harrison's 20th Ed. Chapter 40 Page 252
    A. Neurologic cause
    B. Muscular cause
    C. Metabolic cause
    D. All of the above

Oropharyngeal dysphagia most commonly results from functional deficits caused by neurologic disorders.

42. **Zenker's diverticulum is best related to?**
    Harrison's 20th Ed. Chapter 40 Page 251
    A. Glossopharyngeus
    B. Hyoglossus
    C. Cricopharyngeus
    D. Mylohyoid

43. **Zenker's diverticulum is best related to?**
    Harrison's 20th Ed. Chapter 40 Page 251
    A. Diffuse esophageal spasm (DES)
    B. Lower esophageal sphincter (LES)
    C. Killian's dehiscence
    D. Schatzki's rings

Zenker's diverticulum is typically seen in elderly patients. Its pathogenesis is related to stenosis of cricopharyngeus that causes diminished opening of UES leading to increased hypopharyngeal pressure during swallowing. This results in development of a pulsion diverticulum immediately above cricopharyngeus in a region of potential weakness known as Killian's dehiscence. Killian dehiscence is a posterior midline weakness of pharyngoesophageal segment just above cricopharyngeus.

44. **Which of the following about Killian-Jamieson diverticulum is false?**
    Radiology 1983; 146: 117-22
    A. Esophageal diverticulum
    B. In anterolateral wall of cervical esophagus
    C. Inferior to cricopharyngeus
    D. None of the above

Killian-Jamieson diverticulum is a rare esophageal diverticulum protruding through a muscular gap, Killian-Jamieson space, in the anterolateral wall of cervical esophagus inferior to the cricopharyngeus and lateral to the longitudinal tendon of the esophagus.

45. **Dysphagia lusoria is best related to?**
    N Engl J Med. 2016; 375:e4
    A. Right carotid artery
    B. Left carotid artery
    C. Right subclavian artery
    D. Left subclavian artery

Dysphagia lusoria (or Bayford-Autenrieth dysphagia) is an abnormal condition characterized by difficulty in swallowing caused by an aberrant right subclavian artery seen in cases of truncus bicaroticus (a vascular anomaly in which the carotid arteries have a common origin).

46. **Dysphagia aortica is caused by?**
    N Engl J Med. 1941;225:490-94
    A. Thoracic aortic aneurysm
    B. Aortic dissection
    C. Tortuous aorta
    D. All of the above

Dysphagia aortica is caused by extrinsic compression of esophagus due to an ectatic, tortuous, aneurysmatic (true or pseudo) atherosclerotic thoracic aorta or dissection tracts of the aneurysm.

47. **Cricopharyngeal myotomy is useful in?**
    Harrison's 20th Ed. Chapter 40 Page 253
    A. Idiopathic cricopharyngeal bar
    B. Zenker's diverticulum
    C. Oculopharyngeal muscular dystrophy
    D. All of the above

Usually, cricopharyngeal myotomy is not helpful except in the disorders mentioned above.

48. **"Strawberry gums" is a pathognomonic sign of?**
    Harrison's 20th Ed. Chapter 32 Page 220
    A. Granulomatosis with polyangiitis
    B. Acute myelomonocytic leukemia
    C. Down's syndrome
    D. Diabetes mellitus

Pathognomonic sign of Granulomatosis with polyangiitis (Wegener's granulomatosis) is a red-purplish, granular gingivitis called strawberry gums.

Nausea, Vomiting, and Indigestion

49. Which of the following about vomiting is false?
Harrison's 20th Ed. Chapter 41 Page 253

A. No volitional control
B. Oral expulsion of gastrointestinal contents
C. Due to gut & thoracoabdominal wall contractions
D. None of the above

50. Dyspepsia encompasses a range of symptoms thought to originate in?
Harrison's 20th Ed. Chapter 41 Page 253

A. Gastroduodenum
B. Small intestines
C. Large intestines
D. Any of the above

Dyspepsia is a term encompassing symptoms thought to originate in the gastroduodenal region. It usually include nausea, vomiting, heartburn, regurgitation, and dyspepsia.

51. Which of the following coordinate initiation of emesis?
Harrison's 20th Ed. Chapter 41 Page 253

A. Nucleus tractus solitarius
B. Dorsal vagal nuclei
C. Phrenic nuclei
D. All of the above

52. Which of the following coordinate initiation of emesis?
Harrison's 20th Ed. Chapter 41 Page 253

A. Neurokinin NK_1 pathway
B. Serotonin 5-HT_3 pathway
C. Vasopressin pathway
D. All of the above

Brainstem nuclei, including nucleus tractus solitarius, dorsal vagal and phrenic nuclei, medullary nuclei regulating respiration and nuclei that control pharyngeal, facial & tongue movements coordinate initiation of emesis. Pathways involved include neurokinin NK_1, serotonin 5-HT_3, and vasopressin.

53. Chemoreceptor trigger zone best relates to?
Harrison's 20th Ed. Chapter 41 Page 253

A. Area postrema
B. Broca's area
C. Wernicke's area
D. All of the above

Area postrema, termed chemoreceptor trigger zone, is the vomiting center located in floor of IV ventricle.

54. Area postrema in medulla responds to which of the following stimuli?
Harrison's 20th Ed. Chapter 41 Page 253

A. Uremia
B. Hypoxia
C. Ketoacidosis
D. All of the above

Area postrema in medulla, responds to blood borne stimuli like emetogenic drugs, bacterial toxins, uremia, hypoxia, ketoacidosis.

55. Area postrema is served by nerves acting on?
Harrison's 20th Ed. Chapter 41 Page 253

A. 5-HT_3 receptors
B. Muscarinic M_1 receptors
C. Dopamine D_2 receptors
D. All of the above

56. Vagal afferent stimuli activate which of the following receptors?
Harrison's 20th Ed. Chapter 41 Page 253

A. Muscarinic M_1 receptors
B. Histaminergic H_1 receptors
C. Dopamine D_2 receptors
D. 5-HT_3 receptors

Vagal afferent stimuli activate 5-HT_3 receptors.

57. Labyrinthine disorders stimulate which of the following receptors?
Harrison's 20th Ed. Chapter 41 Page 253

A. Muscarinic M_1 receptors
B. Central NK_1 receptors
C. Dopamine D_2 receptors
D. 5-HT_3 receptors

Labyrinthine disorders stimulate vestibular muscarinic M_1 and histaminergic H_1 receptors.

58. Vomiting can be induced via activation of which of the following receptors?
Ther Adv Gastroenterol. 2016;9(1):98-112

A. μ opioid
B. Glucagon peptide 1
C. Vanilloid TRPV1
D. All of the above

Vomiting can be induced via the activation of several cell membrane bound receptors including: serotonergic 5-HT_3 and 5-HT_4; tachykininergic NK_1; dopaminergic D_2 and D_3; muscarinic M_1; histaminergic H_1; μ opioid; cysteinyl leukotriene 1; prostaglandin DP, FP, and EP; thromboxane TP; glucagon peptide 1, and vanilloid TRPV1.

59. In superior mesenteric artery syndrome, which of the following is compressed by the overlying superior mesenteric artery?
Harrison's 20th Ed. Chapter 41 Page 254

A. Stomach
B. Duodenum
C. Jejunum
D. Ileum

In superior mesenteric artery syndrome, duodenum is compressed by overlying superior mesenteric artery.

60. Which of the following causes gastroparesis?
Harrison's 20th Ed. Chapter 41 Page 254

A. Post vagotomy
B. Pancreatic carcinoma
C. Mesenteric vascular insufficiency
D. All of the above

Gastroparesis occurs after vagotomy, with pancreatic carcinoma, mesenteric vascular insufficiency. Also in diabetes, scleroderma, and amyloidosis. Idiopathic gastroparesis is the most common etiology.

61. **Which of the following causes intestinal pseudoobstruction?**
    Harrison's 20th Ed. Chapter 41 Page 254
    A. Scleroderma
    B. Amyloidosis
    C. Paraneoplastic consequence of malignancy
    D. All of the above

62. **Which of the following is a functional gastroduodenal disorder?**
    Harrison's 20th Ed. Chapter 41 Page 254
    A. Chronic nausea vomiting syndrome
    B. Cyclic vomiting syndrome
    C. Cannabinoid hyperemesis syndrome
    D. All of the above

63. **Which of the following is often misdiagnosed as refractory vomiting?**
    Harrison's 20th Ed. Chapter 41 Page 254
    A. Chronic nausea vomiting syndrome
    B. Cyclic vomiting syndrome
    C. Cannabinoid hyperemesis syndrome
    D. Rumination syndrome

Vomiting occurring minutes after meal consumption prompts consideration of rumination syndrome.

64. **Postoperative emesis occurs in what proportion of surgeries?**
    Harrison's 20th Ed. Chapter 41 Page 254
    A. 10%
    B. 25%
    C. 40%
    D. 60%

Postoperative emesis occurs in ~25% of surgeries, most commonly abdominal & orthopedic surgery.

65. **Acute emesis from cisplatin is mediated by?**
    Harrison's 20th Ed. Chapter 41 Page 254
    A. Muscarinic M_1 receptors
    B. Central NK_1 receptors
    C. Dopamine D_2 receptors
    D. $5-HT_3$ receptors

66. **Nausea during first trimester of pregnancy affects what proportion of women?**
    Harrison's 20th Ed. Chapter 41 Page 254
    A. 25%
    B. 50%
    C. 70%
    D. 90%

Pregnancy is the most common endocrinologic cause of nausea. It affects 70% of women in first trimester.

67. **Brainstem dorsal vagal complex (DVC) comprises of?**
    Ther Adv Gastroenterol 2016;9(1):98-112
    A. Area postrema (AP)
    B. Nucleus of the solitary tract (NTS)
    C. Dorsal motor nucleus of the vagus (DMNX)
    D. All of the above

68. **Nucleus tractus solitarius receives inputs from which of the following pathways?**
    Ther Adv Gastroenterol 2016;9(1):98-112
    A. Vestibular and cerebellar
    B. Cerebral cortex and limbic system
    C. Area postrema
    D. All of the above

Afferent information from various stimuli are relayed to nucleus tractus solitarius via four pathways: vestibular & cerebellar, cerebral cortex & limbic system, area postrema and gastrointestinal tract via vagus nerve.

69. **Rise in which of the following hormones precede emesis?**
    Ther Adv Gastroenterol 2016;9(1):98-112
    A. Vasopressin
    B. Estrogen
    C. Melanin
    D. Cortisol

Rise in vasopressin level precedes emesis.

70. **Which of the following evoke emesis via effects on the area postrema?**
    Harrison's 20th Ed. Chapter 41 Page 254
    A. Fulminant liver failure
    B. Exogenous enterotoxins
    C. Ethanol intoxication
    D. All of the above

71. **Which of the following is used in gastric emptying breath test?**
    Harrison's 20th Ed. Chapter 41 Page 255
    A. ^{11}C
    B. ^{12}C
    C. ^{13}C
    D. ^{14}C

72. **Which of the following has antiemetic effects?**
    Harrison's 20th Ed. Chapter 41 Page 255
    A. Mirtazapine
    B. Olanzapine
    C. Gabapentin
    D. All of the above

73. **Which of the following is a NK1 antagonist?**
    Harrison's 20th Ed. Chapter 41 Page 256
    A. Aprepitant
    B. Granisetron
    C. Gabapentin
    D. Dimenhydrinate

74. **Which of the following is a $5-HT_3$ antagonist?**
    Harrison's 20th Ed. Chapter 41 Page 256
    A. Aprepitant
    B. Granisetron
    C. Gabapentin
    D. Dimenhydrinate

75. Which of the following increases gastroduodenal motility by action on receptors for motilin?
    Harrison's 20th Ed. Chapter 41 Page 256
    A. Domperidone
    B. Metoclopramide
    C. Erythromycin
    D. Prucalopride

    Erythromycin increases gastroduodenal motility by action on receptors for motilin. Motilin is a GI peptide released from the duodenum and an endogenous fasting motor stimulant.

76. Which of the following is a combined 5-HT$_4$ agonist and D$_2$ antagonist?
    Harrison's 20th Ed. Chapter 41 Page 256
    A. Domperidone
    B. Prucalopride
    C. Metoclopramide
    D. Octreotide

77. Which of the following is a 5-HT$_4$ agonist?
    Harrison's 20th Ed. Chapter 41 Page 256
    A. Domperidone
    B. Prucalopride
    C. Metoclopramide
    D. Octreotide

78. Which of the following is a D$_2$ antagonist?
    Harrison's 20th Ed. Chapter 41 Page 256
    A. Domperidone
    B. Prucalopride
    C. Metoclopramide
    D. Octreotide

79. Which of the following can induce dangerous cardiac arrhythmias?
    Harrison's 20th Ed. Chapter 41 Page 256
    A. Ondansetron
    B. Domperidone
    C. Erythromycin
    D. All of the above

80. Which of the following is a prokinetic agent?
    Harrison's 20th Ed. Chapter 41 Page 255 Table 41-2
    A. Pyridostigmine
    B. Octreotide
    C. Erythromycin
    D. All of the above

81. Which of the following is useful in anticipatory nausea and vomiting with chemotherapy?
    Harrison's 20th Ed. Chapter 41 Page 255 Table 41-2
    A. Lorazepam
    B. Olanzapine
    C. Pyridostigmine
    D. Dexamethasone

82. Gastric fundus relaxation after eating is called?
    Harrison's 20th Ed. Chapter 41 Page 256
    A. Accommodation
    B. Appetation
    C. Rumination
    D. Gastration

83. Which of the following promote gastroesophageal reflux?
    Harrison's 20th Ed. Chapter 41 Page 256
    A. Theophylline
    B. Progesterone
    C. Calcium channel blockers
    D. All of the above

84. Which of the following promote LES relaxation?
    Harrison's 20th Ed. Chapter 41 Page 256
    A. Ethanol
    B. Tobacco
    C. Caffeine
    D. All of the above

85. Alkaline reflux esophagitis produces GERD-like symptoms most often in?
    Harrison's 20th Ed. Chapter 41 Page 257
    A. Pregnancy
    B. Patients who underwent surgery for peptic ulcer disease
    C. Achalasia
    D. All of the above

    Alkaline reflux esophagitis produces GERD-like symptoms most often in patients who underwent surgery for peptic ulcer disease.

86. Epigastric pain syndrome is best related to?
    Harrison's 20th Ed. Chapter 41 Page 257
    A. Gastroesophageal reflux disease (GERD)
    B. Functional dyspepsia
    C. Peptic ulcer disease
    D. Zollinger-Ellison syndrome

    Functional dyspepsia is subdivided into postprandial distress syndrome and epigastric pain syndrome.

87. Barrett's metaplasia predisposes to?
    Harrison's 20th Ed. Chapter 41 Page 257
    A. Esophageal squamous cell carcinoma
    B. Esophageal adenocarcinoma
    C. Lymphoma
    D. All of the above

    8–20% of GERD patients exhibit esophageal intestinal metaplasia, termed Barrett's metaplasia, which predisposes to esophageal adenocarcinoma.

88. GERD classically produces which of the following?
    Harrison's 20th Ed. Chapter 41 Page 257
    A. Water brash
    B. Heartburn
    C. Hoarseness
    D. Chest pain

    GERD classically produces heartburn, a substernal warmth that moves up toward the neck.

89. Functional dyspepsia overlaps with which of the following disorders?
Harrison's 20th Ed. Chapter 41 Page 257

- A. GERD
- B. IBS
- C. Idiopathic gastroparesis
- D. All of the above

90. Odynophagia suggests which of the following?
Harrison's 20th Ed. Chapter 41 Page 257

- A. Food bolus impaction
- B. Esophageal infection
- C. Zenker's diverticulum
- D. Achalasia

Odynophagia suggests esophageal infection.

91. Alarm feature for malignant esophageal blockage is?
Harrison's 20th Ed. Chapter 41 Page 257

- A. Recurrent vomiting
- B. Occult or gross bleeding
- C. Jaundice
- D. All of the above

Malignant esophageal blockage leading to dysphagia is suggested by unexplained weight loss, recurrent vomiting, occult or gross bleeding, jaundice, palpable mass or adenopathy, and a family history of gastrointestinal neoplasm.

92. Which of the following about "Steakhouse syndrome" is true?
World J Gastrointest Endosc. 2011;3(5):101-104

- A. Food impaction of the esophagus
- B. Esophageal tear
- C. Esophageal agenesis
- D. Any of the above

Acute esophageal obstruction caused by the impaction of a large bolus of food is called the 'steakhouse syndrome'. It was first reported by Norton in 1963.

93. Complication of long-term PPI therapy is?
Harrison's 20th Ed. Chapter 41 Page 258

- A. Hypomagnesemia
- B. Interstitial nephritis
- C. Impaired absorption of clopidogrel
- D. All of the above

Complications of long-term PPI therapy include diarrhea (from Clostridium difficile infection or microscopic colitis), small-intestinal bacterial overgrowth, nutrient deficiency (vitamin B_{12}, iron, calcium), hypomagnesemia, bone demineralization, interstitial nephritis & impaired medication absorption (clopidogrel).

94. Which of the following is useful for functional dyspepsia?
Harrison's 20th Ed. Chapter 41 Page 258

- A. Buspirone
- B. Acotiamide
- C. Tandospirone
- D. All of the above

95. Which of the following reduces esophageal exposure to acid and nonacidic fluids by reducing TLESRs?
Harrison's 20th Ed. Chapter 41 Page 258

- A. Buspirone
- B. Acotiamide
- C. Tandospirone
- D. Baclofen

Baclofen is a γ-aminobutyric acid B (GABA-B) agonist.

96. Which of the following is a long-term complication of fundoplication?
Harrison's 20th Ed. Chapter 41 Page 258

- A. Dysphagia
- B. Gas-bloat syndrome
- C. Gastroparesis
- D. All of the above

Diarrhea and Constipation

97. Which of the following names is associated with neuro-gastroenterology?
Gut 1999;45(Suppl II):II6–II16

A. Rice
B. Bayliss and Starling
C. Edith Bülbring
D. Langley

English investigators William M. Bayliss & Ernest H. Starling demonstrated that application of pressure to intestinal lumen of anesthetized dogs resulted in oral contraction & anal relaxation, followed by a propulsive wave ("law of the intestine" and now called the peristaltic reflex).

98. Which of the following is false about myenteric (or Auerbach's plexus)?
Harrison's 20th Ed. Chapter 42 Page 259

A. Ganglionated plexus
B. Lies between longitudinal & circular muscle layers
C. Control activity of smooth muscle of the gut
D. None of the above

99. Which of the following is false about submucosal (or Meissner's plexus)?
Harrison's 20th Ed. Chapter 42 Page 259

A. Ganglionated plexus
B. Lies between circular muscle layer and the mucosa
C. Regulates mucosal secretion & blood flow
D. None of the above

The ENS is organized in two ganglionated plexuses, myenteric (or Auerbach's plexus) and submucosal (or Meissner's plexus), composed of neurons and enteric glial cells. myenteric (or Auerbach's plexus) lies between the external longitudinal & internal circular muscle layers.

100. Enteric nervous system comprises of which of the following?
Harrison's 20th Ed. Chapter 42 Page 259

A. Myenteric layer
B. Submucosal layer
C. Mucosal neuronal layer
D. All of the above

Small intestine & colon have intrinsic & extrinsic innervation. Intrinsic innervation or the enteric nervous system comprises myenteric, submucosal, and mucosal neuronal layers.

101. Which of the following is a neurotransmitter in the enteric nervous system?
Harrison's 20th Ed. Chapter 42 Page 259

A. Acetylcholine
B. Vasoactive intestinal peptide (VIP)
C. Norepinephrine
D. All of the above

102. Which of the following is a neurotransmitter in the enteric nervous system?
Harrison's 20th Ed. Chapter 42 Page 259

A. Serotonin
B. Adenosine triphosphate (ATP)
C. Nitric oxide (NO)
D. All of the above

The function of layers of enteric nervous system are modulated by "interneurons" through actions of neurotransmitter amines or peptides that include acetylcholine, vasoactive intestinal peptide (VIP), opioids, norepinephrine, serotonin, adenosine triphosphate (ATP), and nitric oxide (NO).

103. Interstitial cells of Cajal are best related to?
Harrison's 20th Ed. Chapter 42 Page 259

A. Myenteric layer
B. Submucosal layer
C. Mucosal neuronal layer
D. All of the above

104. Which of the following is called pacemakers in gastrointestinal muscles?
Harrison's 20th Ed. Chapter 42 Page 259

A. Auerbach's plexus
B. Meissner's plexus
C. Interstitial cells of Cajal
D. All of the above

Interstitial cells of Cajal (ICC) are distinctive populations of muscle-like cells. They make contact with each other & with muscle cells & nerve terminals & function as pacemakers in gastrointestinal muscles by initiating rhythmic electrical activity.

105. Which of the following affects secretion, absorption, and mucosal blood flow?
Harrison's 20th Ed. Chapter 42 Page 259

A. Myenteric layer
B. Submucosal layer
C. Mucosal neuronal layer
D. All of the above

Myenteric plexus regulates smooth-muscle function through intermediary pacemaker-like cells called "interstitial cells of Cajal". Submucosal plexus affects secretion, absorption, and mucosal blood flow.

106. Which of the following statements is false?
Harrison's 20th Ed. Chapter 42 Page 259

A. Parasympathetic nerves convey visceral sensations from small intestine & colon
B. Parasympathetic nerves convey excitatory motor impulses to small intestine & colon
C. Parasympathetic fibers reach small intestine & proximal colon along branches of superior mesenteric artery
D. None of the above

107. Which of the following statements is false?
Harrison's 20th Ed. Chapter 42 Page 259

A. Sympathetic nerve supply to gut modulates motor functions
B. Sympathetic input to gut is excitatory to sphincters
C. Sympathetic input to gut is inhibitory to non-sphincteric muscle
D. None of the above

108. On an average day, how much fluid enter the GI tract?
Harrison's 20th Ed. Chapter 42 Page 260

A. 6 liters
B. 9 liters
C. 12 liters
D. 15 liters

On an average day, 9 liters of fluid enter GI tract. About 1 liter of residual fluid reaches colon, and stool excretion of fluid constitutes about 0.2 liters/day.

109. Migrating motor complex (MMC) best relates to?
Harrison's 20th Ed. Chapter 42 Page 260

A. Motility of the stomach
B. Motility of the small intestine
C. Motility of the large intestine
D. All of the above

During fasting period, in order to clear nondigestible residue from small intestine, motility of small intestine is characterized by a cyclical event. This is referred to as migrating motor complex (MMC) or intestinal "housekeeper".

110. Which of the following about migrating motor complex (MMC) is false?
Harrison's 20th Ed. Chapter 42 Page 260

A. Organized, propagated series of contractions
B. Lasts for ~4 minutes & occurs every 60–90 minutes
C. Involves the entire small intestine
D. None of the above

111. Which of the following is true for distal ileum?
Harrison's 20th Ed. Chapter 42 Page 260

A. Acts as a reservoir
B. Empties intermittently by powerful contractions
C. MMC rarely continues into the colon
D. All of the above

112. Which of the following statements is false?
Harrison's 20th Ed. Chapter 42 Page 260

A. Ascending & transverse colons function as reservoirs
B. Descending colon acts as a conduit
C. Transit time in ascending & transverse colons is 15 hours
D. Transit time in descending colon is 8 hours

Ascending & transverse colons function as reservoirs and average transit time is 15 hours. The descending colon acts as a conduit and average transit time is 3 hours.

113. High-amplitude propagated contractions (HAPCs) with mass movements in colon occur how many times per day?
Harrison's 20th Ed. Chapter 42 Page 260

A. Four times
B. Five times
C. Six times
D. Eight times

High-amplitude (>75 mm Hg) propagated contractions (HAPCs) associated with mass movements of colon and normally occur ~five times per day, usually on awakening in morning & postprandially.

114. After meal ingestion, colonic phasic & tonic contractility increases for a period of?
Harrison's 20th Ed. Chapter 42 Page 260

A. ~30 minutes
B. ~1 hour
C. ~2 hours
D. ~3 hours

After meal ingestion, colonic phasic & tonic contractility increases for a period of ~2 hours. Initial phase (~10 minutes) is mediated by vagus nerve in response to mechanical distention of "stomach". Subsequent response of colon is by caloric stimulation (intake of at least 500 kcal) and is partly mediated by hormones like gastrin & serotonin.

115. Sling around the rectoanal junction is formed by?
Harrison's 20th Ed. Chapter 42 Page 260

A. Ischiocavernosus muscle
B. External anal sphincter muscle
C. Puborectalis muscle
D. All of the above

Puborectalis muscle forms a sling around the rectoanal junction to maintain continence by tonic contraction.

116. Continence is maintained by?
Harrison's 20th Ed. Chapter 42 Page 260 Figure 42-1

A. Normal rectal sensation
B. Tonic contraction of internal anal sphincter
C. Tonic contraction of puborectalis muscle
D. All of the above

117. Puborectalis muscle wraps around anorectum to maintain an anorectal angle between?
Harrison's 20th Ed. Chapter 42 Page 260 Figure 42-1

A. 35° and 60°
B. 60° and 90°
C. 80° and 110°
D. 100° and 140°

Puborectalis muscle wraps around anorectum to maintain an anorectal angle between 80° and 110°.

118. During defecation, the anorectal angle to straighten by at least?
Harrison's 20th Ed. Chapter 42 Page 260 Figure 42-1

A. 5°
B. 10°
C. 15°
D. 20°

During defecation, the anorectal angle straightens by at least 15°, perineum descends by 1–3.5 cm. and the external anal sphincter relaxes and reduces pressure on anal canal.

119. What weight of stool for adults on a typical Western diet is considered diarrheal?
Harrison's 20th Ed. Chapter 42 Page 261

A. >75 grams/day
B. >100 grams/day
C. >150 grams/day
D. >200 grams/day

>200 grams/day of stool for adults on a typical Western diet is considered diarrheal. Diarrhea is defined as acute if <2 weeks, persistent if 2–4 weeks, and chronic if >4 weeks in duration.

120. **Which of the following may be confused with true diarrhea?**
Harrison's 20th Ed. Chapter 42 Page 261
    A. Pseudodiarrhea
    B. Fecal incontinence
    C. Overflow diarrhea
    D. All of the above

Pseudodiarrhea is frequent passage of small volumes of stool. It is associated with rectal urgency, tenesmus, or a feeling of incomplete evacuation, and accompanies IBS or proctitis. Fecal incontinence is involuntary discharge of rectal contents and is caused by neuromuscular disorders or structural anorectal problems. Overflow diarrhea occurs due to fecal impaction.

121. **Persons with hemochromatosis are especially prone to?**
Harrison's 20th Ed. Chapter 42 Page 261
    A. Yersinia infections
    B. Chlamydia infections
    C. Salmonella infections
    D. Staphylococcus aureus infections

Persons with hemochromatosis are prone to enteric infections with Vibrio species and Yersinia infections and should avoid raw fish.

122. **Profuse, watery diarrhea secondary to small-bowel hypersecretion occurs with?**
Harrison's 20th Ed. Chapter 42 Page 261
    A. Ingestion of preformed bacterial toxins
    B. Ingestion of enterotoxin-producing bacteria
    C. Ingestion of enteroadherent pathogens
    D. All of the above

Profuse, watery diarrhea secondary to small-bowel hypersecretion occurs with ingestion of preformed bacterial toxins, enterotoxin-producing bacteria & enteroadherent pathogens.

123. **Infection with which of the following can cause severe abdominal pain with tenderness mimicking acute appendicitis?**
Harrison's 20th Ed. Chapter 42 Page 261
    A. Yersinia infections
    B. E. coli infections
    C. Salmonella infections
    D. Staphylococcus aureus infections

Yersinia invades terminal ileal & proximal colon mucosa. It may cause severe abdominal pain with tenderness mimicking acute appendicitis.

124. **Reactive arthritis (Reiter's syndrome) may accompany or follow infections by?**
Harrison's 20th Ed. Chapter 42 Page 261
    A. Salmonella
    B. Campylobacter
    C. Shigella
    D. All of the above

Reactive arthritis (Reiter's syndrome), may accompany or follow infections by Salmonella, Campylobacter, Shigella & Yersinia.

125. **Yersiniosis may lead to?**
Harrison's 20th Ed. Chapter 42 Page 261
    A. Autoimmune-type thyroiditis
    B. Pericarditis
    C. Glomerulonephritis
    D. All of the above

Yersiniosis may lead to autoimmune-type thyroiditis, pericarditis & glomerulonephritis.

126. **Infection with which of the following can cause hemolytic-uremic syndrome?**
Harrison's 20th Ed. Chapter 42 Page 261
    A. E. coli (O113:H7)
    B. E. coli (O121:H7)
    C. E. coli (O145:H7)
    D. E. coli (O157:H7)

127. **Infection with which of the following can cause hemolytic-uremic syndrome?**
Harrison's 20th Ed. Chapter 42 Page 261
    A. Enterohemorrhagic E. coli (O157:H7)
    B. Campylobacter
    C. Salmonella
    D. All of the above

Enterohemorrhagic E. coli (O157:H7) and Shigella can lead to the hemolytic-uremic syndrome with an attendant high mortality rate.

128. **Which of the following pathotypes of intestinal pathogenic E. coli does not cause acute diarrheal disease?**
Harrison's 20th Ed. Chapter 156 Page 1152
    A. Shiga toxin–producing E. coli (STEC)
    B. Enteroinvasive E. coli (EIEC)
    C. Adherent invasive E. coli (AIEC)
    D. Diffusely adherent E. coli (DAEC)

Pathotypes of intestinal pathogenic E. coli include Shiga toxin–producing E. coli (STEC), enterohemorrhagic E. coli (EHEC), Shiga toxin-producing enteroaggregative E. coli (ST-EAEC); enterotoxigenic E. coli (ETEC); enteropathogenic E. coli (EPEC); enteroinvasive E. coli (EIEC); enteroaggregative E. coli (EAEC); Diffusely adherent E. coli (DAEC); cytodetaching E. coli and adherent invasive E. coli (AIEC). AIEC is associated with Crohn's disease but does not cause acute diarrheal disease.

129. **Acute diarrhea can be a major symptom of?**
Harrison's 20th Ed. Chapter 42 Page 261
    A. Viral hepatitis
    B. Listeriosis
    C. Legionellosis
    D. All of the above

Acute diarrhea can be a major symptom of viral hepatitis, listeriosis, legionellosis & toxic shock syndrome.

130. **Increased levels of which of the following signal intestinal inflammation?**
Harrison's 20th Ed. Chapter 42 Page 261
    A. Fecal hemoglobin
    B. Lactoferrin
    C. Neopterin
    D. All of the above

131. **Increased levels of which of the following signal intestinal inflammation?**
Harrison's 20th Ed. Chapter 42 Page 261
    A. Calprotectin
    B. Protectin
    C. Resolvin
    D. All of the above

132. Which of the following is an abrupt onset diarrhea that persists for at least 4 weeks or longer?
Harrison's 20th Ed. Chapter 42 Page 263

   A. Runner's diarrhea
   B. Brainerd diarrhea
   C. Traveler's diarrhea
   D. Factitious diarrhea

Brainerd diarrhea was first described in Brainerd, Minnesota in 1983.

133. Nitazoxanide is active against?
Harrison's 20th Ed. Chapter 42 Page 263

   A. Giardia
   B. Cryptosporidium
   C. E. histolytica
   D. All of the above

Nitazoxanide is used for the treatment of cryptosporidiosis and giardiasis. It is active against other intestinal protozoa also.

134. Which of the following about Nitazoxanide is false?
Harrison's 20th Ed. Chapter 217 Page 1566

   A. 1-nitrothiazole compound
   B. 3-nitrothiazole compound
   C. 5-nitrothiazole compound
   D. 7-nitrothiazole compound

Nitazoxanide is a 5-nitrothiazole compound.

135. Which of the following is an active metabolite of Nitazoxanide?
Harrison's 20th Ed. Chapter 217 Page 1566

   A. Dizoxanide
   B. Tizoxanide
   C. Nizoxanide
   D. Rizoxanide

Nitazoxanide is hydrolyzed to an active metabolite, tizoxanide (desacetylnitazoxanide) which then undergoes conjugation, primarily by glucuronidation. It is is highly bound to plasma protein.

136. Mechanism of action of Nitazoxanide is related to which of the following?
Harrison's 20th Ed. Chapter 217 Page 1566

   A. Pyruvate-ferredoxin oxidoreductase (PFOR)
   B. P450 oxidoreductase (POR)
   C. Ubiquinone oxidoreductase
   D. All of the above

Antiprotozoal activity of nitazoxanide is due to interference with the pyruvate-ferredoxin oxidoreductase (PFOR) enzyme–dependent electron transfer reaction that is essential to anaerobic energy metabolism.

137. Which of the following is an active metabolite of Nitazoxanide?
Harrison's 20th Ed. Chapter 217 Page 1566

   A. Approved for use in children between 1–11 years of age
   B. Tizoxanide glucuronide is excreted in urine & bile
   C. Tizoxanide is highly bound to plasma protein
   D. None of the above

138. Which of the following is false about secretory diarrheas?
Harrison's 20th Ed. Chapter 42 Page 263

   A. Due to derangements across enterocolonic mucosa
   B. Watery, large-volume fecal outputs
   C. Painless and respond to fasting
   D. No fecal osmotic gap

Secretory diarrheas are due to derangements in fluid & electrolyte transport across enterocolonic mucosa, characterized by painless, watery, large-volume fecal outputs that persist with fasting. There is no fecal osmotic gap.

139. Which of the following is an endogenous laxative?
Harrison's 20th Ed. Chapter 42 Page 263 Table 42-3

   A. Dihydroxy bile acids
   B. Oxidized bile acids
   C. Hydrolized bile acids
   D. Dimethyl bile acids

140. Which of the following angiotensin-receptor blocker is associated with diarrhea?
Harrison's 20th Ed. Chapter 42 Page 264

   A. Irbesartan
   B. Losartan
   C. Olmesartan
   D. All of the above

Angiotensin-receptor blocker, olmesartan, is associated with diarrhea due to sprue-like enteropathy.

141. Which of the following is not a cause of secretory chronic diarrhea?
Harrison's 20th Ed. Chapter 42 Page 263 Table 42-3

   A. Addison's disease
   B. VIPoma
   C. Lactase and other disaccharide deficiencies
   D. Carcinoid syndrome

142. Mucosal malabsorption can be due to?
Harrison's 20th Ed. Chapter 42 Page 263 Table 42-3

   A. Celiac sprue
   B. Whipple's disease
   C. Abetalipoproteinemia
   D. All of the above

143. Which of the following does not cause diarrhea?
Harrison's 20th Ed. Chapter 42 Page 264

   A. Ca^{2+} blockers
   B. Chronic ethanol consumption
   C. Olmesartan
   D. Arsenic

Ca^{2+} blockers and antidepressants cause constipation in adults.

144. Which of the following is a negative regulator of bile acid synthesis?
Harrison's 20th Ed. Chapter 42 Page 264

   A. FGF-7
   B. FGF-11
   C. FGF-13
   D. FGF-19

Fibroblast growth factor 19 (FGF-19) is produced by ileal enterocytes and serves as a negative feedback of bile acid synthesis in hepatocytes.

145. Which of the following mediates the effect of FGF-19 on the hepatocyte?
   Harrison's 20th Ed. Chapter 42 Page 264
   A. α-klotho
   B. β-klotho
   C. γ-klotho
   D. δ-klotho

146. Which of the following is the most common cause of unexplained chronic diarrhea?
   Harrison's 20th Ed. Chapter 42 Page 264
   A. Cystic fibrosis
   B. Idiopathic bile acid malabsorption (BAM)
   C. Metastatic gastrointestinal carcinoid tumors
   D. Pancreatic cholera

147. Which of the following is an intestinal secretagogue?
   Harrison's 20th Ed. Chapter 42 Page 264
   A. Serotonin
   B. Histamine
   C. Prostaglandins
   D. All of the above

148. Glucose-dependent insulinotropic peptide is also called?
   Harrison's 20th Ed. Chapter 42 Page 264
   A. Secretin
   B. Gastrin-inhibitory polypeptide
   C. Neurotensin
   D. Calcitonin

149. Non-β cell pancreatic adenoma best relates to?
   Harrison's 20th Ed. Chapter 42 Page 264
   A. Watery diarrhea hypokalemia achlorhydria syndrome
   B. Pancreatic cholera
   C. VIPoma
   D. All of the above

150. Mutation in NHE3 gene leads to?
   Harrison's 20th Ed. Chapter 42 Page 264
   A. Congenital chloridorrhea
   B. Congenital sodium diarrhea
   C. Addison's disease
   D. All of the above

In congenital sodium diarrhea, mutation in NHE3 (sodium-hydrogen exchanger) gene causes defective Na+/H+ exchange resulting in diarrhea and acidosis.

151. One of the most common causes of chronic diarrhea in adults is?
   Harrison's 20th Ed. Chapter 42 Page 264
   A. Lactase deficiency
   B. Ingestion of magnesium-containing antacids
   C. Gastrinoma
   D. Chronic ethanol consumption

152. In the acronym FODMAP, F stands for?
   Harrison's 20th Ed. Chapter 42 Page 264
   A. Fermentable
   B. Food
   C. Fecal
   D. Free

153. In the acronym FODMAP, P stands for?
   Harrison's 20th Ed. Chapter 42 Page 264
   A. Polyol
   B. Polysaccharide
   C. Phenyl
   D. Phenol

FODMAP stands for fermentable oligosaccharides, disaccharides, monosaccharides, and polyols.

154. Steatorrhea is defined as stool fat exceeding?
   Harrison's 20th Ed. Chapter 42 Page 264
   A. 3 grams/day
   B. 4 grams/day
   C. 6 grams/day
   D. 7 grams/day

Steatorrhea is defined as stool fat exceeding the normal 7 grams/day.

155. Of the following, fecal fat excretion is most in?
   Harrison's 20th Ed. Chapter 42 Page 264
   A. Rapid-transit diarrhea
   B. Small-intestinal diseases
   C. Pancreatic exocrine insufficiency
   D. Postmucosal lymphatic obstruction

156. Pancreatic exocrine insufficiency occurs when what percentage of pancreatic secretory function is lost?
   Harrison's 20th Ed. Chapter 42 Page 264
   A. > 30%
   B. > 50%
   C. > 75%
   D. > 90%

Pancreatic exocrine insufficiency occurs when >90% of pancreatic secretory function is lost.

157. Most frequent cause of pancreatic insufficiency is?
   Harrison's 20th Ed. Chapter 42 Page 264
   A. Chronic pancreatitis
   B. Cystic fibrosis
   C. Pancreatic duct obstruction
   D. Somatostatinoma

Ethanol abuse is the most common cause of chronic pancreatitis.

158. Mucosal malabsorption most commonly occurs from?
   Harrison's 20th Ed. Chapter 42 Page 265
   A. Giardiasis
   B. Whipple's disease
   C. Celiac disease
   D. Tropical sprue

Mucosal malabsorption most commonly occurs from celiac disease.

159. Which of the following is associated with acanthocytic erythrocytes, ataxia & retinitis pigmentosa?

Harrison's 20th Ed. Chapter 42 Page 265

A. Abetalipoproteinemia
B. Whipple's disease
C. Celiac disease
D. Tropical sprue

Abetalipoproteinemia is a defect of chylomicron formation & fat malabsorption in children. It is associated with acanthocytic erythrocytes, ataxia & retinitis pigmentosa.

160. Which of the following medication may cause mucosal malabsorption?

Harrison's 20th Ed. Chapter 42 Page 265

A. Olmesartan
B. Mycophenolate mofetil
C. Cholestyramine
D. All of the above

161. Which of the following about postmucosal lymphatic obstruction is false?

Harrison's 20th Ed. Chapter 42 Page 265

A. Fat malabsorption with enteric losses of protein
B. Lymphocytopenia
C. Carbohydrate and amino acid absorption preserved
D. None of the above

162. Which of the following is a polyposis colonic syndrome?

Gastroenterol Hepatol (NY) 2012;8:197-201

A. Cowden syndrome
B. Peutz-Jeghers syndrome
C. Cronkhite-Canada syndrome
D. All of the above

163. Which of the following is a feature of Cronkhite-Canada syndrome (CCS)?

Gastroenterol Hepatol (NY) 2012;8:197-201

A. Gastrointestinal hamartomatous polyposis
B. Alopecia & onychodystrophy
C. Hyperpigmentation
D. All of the above

Cronkhite-Canada syndrome (CCS) is a noninherited condition characterized by gastrointestinal hamartomatous polyposis, alopecia, onychodystrophy, hyperpigmentation & diarrhea.

164. Which of the following is not a feature of irritable bowel syndrome (IBS)?

Harrison's 20th Ed. Chapter 42 Page 265

A. Stool frequency ceases at night
B. Abdominal pain relieved with defecation
C. Weight loss
D. Diarrhea alternating with periods of constipation

Irritable bowel syndrome (IBS) is characterized by stool frequency that ceases at night, alternates with periods of constipation, abdominal pain relieved with defecation, no weight loss.

165. Which of the following is recommended for the control of diabetic diarrhea?

Harrison's 20th Ed. Chapter 42 Page 267

A. Diphenoxylate
B. Codeine
C. Clonidine
D. Rifaximin

α_2-adrenergic agonist clonidine may be of use for the control of diabetic diarrhea.

166. Which of the following is useful for the treatment of diarrhea associated with IBS?

Harrison's 20th Ed. Chapter 42 Page 267

A. Alosetron
B. Rifaximin
C. Eluxadoline
D. All of the above

167. Which of the following may induce sphincter of Oddi spasm?

Harrison's 20th Ed. Chapter 42 Page 267

A. Alosetron
B. Rifaximin
C. Eluxadoline
D. All of the above

Eluxadoline may induce sphincter of Oddi spasm and lead to acute pancreatitis, mostly in patients with past h/o cholecystectomy.

168. Eluxadoline is an antagonist of which of the following opioid receptor?

Harrison's 20th Ed. Chapter 42 Page 267

A. μ
B. κ
C. δ
D. All of the above

Eluxadoline is an oral agent with mixed opioid effects i.e. μ- and κ-opioid receptor agonist and δ-opioid receptor (OR) antagonist.

169. In constipation, recommended quantity of dietary fiber as a supplement is?

Harrison's 20th Ed. Chapter 42 Page 268

A. 5 – 15 grams/day
B. 15 – 25 grams/day
C. 30 – 50 grams/day
D. 50 – 60 grams/day

170. Melanosis coli is best related to?

Harrison's 20th Ed. Chapter 42 Page 268

A. Anthraquinone
B. Benzoquinone
C. Naphthoquinone
D. Parietin

Plants with high levels of anthraquinones include aloe, cascara, sagrada, frangula (buckthorn), rhubarb, senna.

171. The dark pigment seen in melanosis coli is?
N Engl J Med. 2013; 368:2303

A. Melanin
B. Lipofuscin
C. Hemosiderin
D. Alizarin

Anthraquinone use causes injury to colonic epithelial cells resulting in the production of lipofuscin, the dark pigment seen in melanosis coli.

172. Which of the following about melanosis coli is false?
Harrison's 20th Ed. Chapter 42 Page 268

A. Due to use of anthraquinone laxatives
B. Pigmentation of colon mucosa
C. Benign and reversible
D. None of the above

173. Which of the following is not a osmotic laxative?
Harrison's 20th Ed. Chapter 42 Page 268

A. Lactulose
B. Sorbitol
C. Glycerin
D. Polyethylene glycol

174. Which of the following is a cause of constipation?
Harrison's 20th Ed. Chapter 42 Page 268

A. Descending perineum syndrome
B. Paradoxical contraction of puborectalis muscle
C. Rectocele
D. All of the above

175. Lubiprostone is best related to?
Harrison's 20th Ed. Chapter 42 Page 268

A. Guanylate cyclase C agonist
B. Chloride channel activator
C. µ-opioid receptor (OR) agonist
D. κ-opioid receptor (OR) agonist

Lubiprostone is a locally acting, bicyclic functional fatty acid derived from prostaglandin E1 that acts by specifically activating ClC-2 chloride channels on the apical aspect of enterocytes, thereby eliciting a chloride-rich fluid secretion. CIC refers to chronic idiopathic constipation.

176. Linaclotide is best related to?
Harrison's 20th Ed. Chapter 42 Page 268

A. Guanylate cyclase C agonist
B. Chloride channel activator
C. µ-opioid receptor (OR) agonist
D. κ-opioid receptor (OR) agonist

Linaclotide is a guanylate cyclase C agonist that activates chloride secretion. Plecanatide is also an oral, locally acting guanylate cyclase agonist.

177. Which of the following is a 5-HT4 agonist?
Harrison's 20th Ed. Chapter 42 Page 269

A. Lubiprostone
B. Linaclotide
C. Bisacodyl
D. Prucalopride

Gastrointestinal Bleeding

178. Risk-assessment score for upper gastrointestinal bleeding is done by?

N Engl J Med. 2016;374:2367-76

A. Glasgow - Barkun Score
B. Glasgow - Blatchford Score
C. Glasgow - Cooper Score
D. Glasgow - Hearnshaw Score

Risk assessment is performed to determine the severity of upper gastrointestinal bleeding by Glasgow - Blatchford Score.

179. Variables used in Glasgow - Blatchford Score include all except?

N Engl J Med. 2016;374:2367-76

A. Blood urea nitrogen
B. Serum creatinine
C. Melena
D. Syncope

Variables used in Glasgow - Blatchford Score include Blood urea nitrogen, Hemoglobin, Systolic blood pressure, Heart rate, Melena, Syncope, Hepatic disease and Cardiac failure. Glasgow–Blatchford scores range from 0 to 23, with higher scores indicating higher risk. High clinical risk is when Glasgow–Blatchford score is ≥12.

180. Risk-assessment score for upper gastrointestinal bleeding is done by?

Tropical Gastroenterology 2016;37(4):276-282

A. AIMS65 scoring system
B. Rockall score
C. Glasgow - Blatchford Score
D. All of the above

Rockall score (described in 1996) is more useful in non-variceal bleeding. It is used to predict mortality and consists of a pre-endoscopic clinical score and a complete endoscopic score after endoscopy. AIMS65 helps in predicting mortality using five factors including albumin levels, deranged INR, impaired mental status, SBP of 90 or less, age of 65 or more.

181. Risk-assessment score for upper gastrointestinal bleeding is done by?

World J Gastroenterol. 2013;19(22):3466-72

A. Rockall score
B. Baylor bleeding score
C. Cedars-Sinai Medical Centre Predictive Index
D. All of the above

182. Endoscopic findings in bleeding peptic ulcers are classified by?

Lancet. 1974;2:394.

A. Pateron classification
B. Forrest classification
C. Laursen classification
D. Barth classification

Endoscopic findings in patients with bleeding peptic ulcers are described using Forrest classification. Findings include spurting hemorrhage (class Ia), oozing hemorrhage (class Ib), a nonbleeding visible vessel (class IIa), an adherent clot (class IIb), a flat pigmented spot (class IIc), and a clean ulcer base (class III). The endoscopic appearance helps determine which lesions require endoscopic therapy.

183. Overt Gastrointestinal bleeding (GIB) is manifested by?

Harrison's 20th Ed. Chapter 44 Page 272

A. Hematemesis
B. Melena
C. Hematochezia
D. All of the above

184. Upper gastrointestinal bleeding (UGIB) is said to occur when the site of bleeding is from?

Harrison's 20th Ed. Chapter 44 Page 272, N Engl J Med. 2018;378:2506-16

A. Esophagus
B. Stomach
C. Duodenum
D. All of the above

Hemorrhage from upper gastrointestinal tract (esophagus, stomach, or duodenum) is defined as primary when it is the cause of hospital admission and is defined as secondary when it complicates the hospital course for patients who have been admitted for other reasons.

185. Lower gastrointestinal bleeding (LGIB) is said to occur when the site of bleeding is from?

Harrison's 20th Ed. Chapter 44 Page 272

A. Small intestine
B. Colon
C. Obscure
D. All of the above

186. Upper gastrointestinal tract is up to?

Harrison's 20 Ed. Chapter 322 Page 2293

A. Pylorus
B. Ampulla of Vater
C. Ligament of Treitz
D. End of jejunum

Upper GI is above the ligament of Treitz. Over 90% of patients with melena are bleeding proximal to the ligament of Treitz, and about 90% of patients with hematochezia are bleeding from the colon.

187. Most common cause of upper GI bleeding (UGIB) is?

Harrison's 20th Ed. Chapter 44 Page 272

A. Esophageal varices
B. Peptic ulcers
C. Gastroduodenal erosions
D. Erosive esophagitis

Peptic ulcers are the most common cause of UGIB, accounting for up to ~50% of cases of UGIB hospitalizations.

188. High-risk peptic ulcer refers to?

Harrison's 20th Ed. Chapter 44 Page 272

A. Active bleeding
B. Nonbleeding visible vessel
C. Adherent clot
D. All of the above

189. **High-dose, constant-infusion IV proton pump inhibitor (PPI) applies to?**
Harrison's 20th Ed. Chapter 44 Page 272

   A. 40 mg bolus & 4 mg/hour infusion
   B. 60 mg bolus & 6 mg/hour infusion
   C. 80 mg bolus & 8 mg/hour infusion
   D. 100 mg bolus & 10 mg/hour infusion

High-dose, constant-infusion IV proton pump inhibitor (PPI) means 80 mg bolus & 8 mg/hour infusion.

190. **Objective of high-dose, constant IV infusion of proton pump inhibitor is to sustain intragastric pH at?**
Harrison's 20th Ed. Chapter 44 Page 272

   A. > 4
   B. > 5
   C. > 6
   D. > 7

191. **Prevention of recurrent bleeding focuses on?**
Harrison's 20th Ed. Chapter 44 Page 272

   A. Helicobacter pylori
   B. Nonsteroidal anti-inflammatory drugs (NSAIDs)
   C. Gastric acid
   D. All of the above

192. **Portal hypertension is responsible for bleeding from?**
Harrison's 20th Ed. Chapter 44 Page 272

   A. Varices in the small & large intestine
   B. Portal hypertensive gastropathy
   C. Enterocolopathy
   D. All of the above

Portal hypertension is responsible for bleeding from gastric varices, varices in small & large intestine, portal hypertensive gastropathy and enterocolopathy. Endoscopic appearance of Gastric antral vascular ectasia (GAVE) syndrome resembles that in portal hypertensive gastropathy (PHG) or antral gastritis. PHG causes predominant changes in the fundus and corpus.

193. **Watermelon stomach best relates to?**
Harrison's 20th Ed. Chapter 44 Page 273

   A. Gastric antral vascular ectasia (GAVE)
   B. Hereditary hemorrhagic telangiectasias
   C. Prolapse gastropathy
   D. Hemosuccus pancreaticus

Gastric antral vascular ectasia (GAVE) was first described by Rider as "fiery red changes with marked hypertrophic mucosal changes, and scattered profuse bleeding" and later as columns of red tortuous ectatic vessels along longitudinal folds of the antrum resembling watermelon stripes.

194. **Dieulafoy's lesion is also termed as?**
Ann R Coll Surg Engl. 2010;92(7):548-554

   A. Caliber persistent artery
   B. Exulceratio simplex
   C. Miliary aneurysms of the stomach
   D. All of the above

Dieulafoy's lesion refers to an aberrant vessel in the mucosa that bleeds from a pinpoint mucosal defect.

195. **The most common cause of LGIB in adults is?**
Harrison's 20th Ed. Chapter 44 Page 273

   A. NSAID-induced colitis
   B. Diverticulosis
   C. Ulcerative colitis
   D. Crohn's disease

The most common cause of LGIB in adults is diverticulosis.

196. **Which of the following is false about diverticular bleeding?**
Harrison's 20th Ed. Chapter 44 Page 273

   A. Abrupt in onset, usually painless
   B. Commonly from right colon
   C. Bleeding stops spontaneously
   D. None of the above

197. **In Heyde's syndrome, which of the following is a feature besides bleeding vascular ectasias?**
Harrison's 20th Ed. Chapter 44 Page 273

   A. Aortic stenosis
   B. Mitral stenosis
   C. Aortic regurgitation
   D. Mitral regurgitation

Heyde's syndrome refers to bleeding vascular ectasias & aortic stenosis.

198. **Blood transfusion is recommended in acute GIB when the hemoglobin drops below?**
Harrison's 20th Ed. Chapter 44 Page 273

   A. 5 grams/dL
   B. 6 grams/dL
   C. 7 grams/dL
   D. 8 grams/dL

199. **For melena, blood should be present in GI tract for what duration?**
Harrison's 20th Ed. Chapter 44 Page 273

   A. 3 hours
   B. 7 hours
   C. 14 hours
   D. 22 hours

Melena indicates that blood has been present in the GI tract for at least 14 hours and as long as 3–5 days.

200. **Clues to upper gastrointestinal bleed include?**
Harrison's 20th Ed. Chapter 44 Page 273

   A. Hyperactive bowel sounds
   B. Melena
   C. Elevated blood urea nitrogen
   D. All of the above

Clues to UGIB include melena, hyperactive bowel sounds & elevated BUN level (due to volume depletion and blood proteins absorbed in the small intestine).

201. **Rectal ulcer is found in what proportion of patients of solitary rectal ulcer syndrome?**
World J Gastroenterol. 2014;20(3):738-744

A. 40%
B. 60%
C. 80%
D. 100%

Solitary rectal ulcer syndrome is a misnomer because ulcers are found in 40% of patients. Passage of blood during defecation is the hallmark.

202. **Cirrhotic patients presenting with UGIB should be placed on?**
Harrison's 20th Ed. Chapter 44 Page 274

A. Antibiotics
B. Tranquillizers
C. Lactulose
D. Domperidone

Cirrhotic patients presenting with UGIB should be placed on antibiotics (quinolone, ceftriaxone) and started on a vasoactive medication (octreotide, terlipressin, somatostatin, vapreotide) upon presentation, even before endoscopy. Antibiotics decrease bacterial infections, rebleeding, and mortality in this population, and vasoactive medications improve control of bleeding in the first 12 hours after presentation.

203. **Which of the following is not a low-risk endoscopic lesion?**
Harrison's 20th Ed. Chapter 44 Page 274, N Engl J Med. 2016;374:2367-76

A. Visible vessel
B. Clean-based ulcers
C. Erosions
D. Nonbleeding Mallory-Weiss tears

An adherent clot is also a high-risk endoscopic finding.

204. **Which of the following statements is false?**
N Engl J Med. 2016;374:2367-76

A. No advantage of nasogastric lavage in upper GI bleed
B. BUN / creatinine ratio helpful to identify upper GI bleed
C. Restrictive transfusion strategy is beneficial
D. None of the above

205. **Tissue deposition of bilirubin occurs in?**
Harrison's 20th Ed. Chapter 45 Page 276

A. Serum hyperbilirubinemia
B. Hemolytic disorder
C. Disorder of bilirubin metabolism
D. All of the above

Jaundice

206. Sclerae have affinity for bilirubin due to its?
Harrison's 20th Ed. Chapter 45 Page 276

- A. High collagen content
- B. High elastin content
- C. High mucopolysaccharide content
- D. All of the above

Sclerae have affinity for bilirubin due to its high elastin content.

207. Presence of scleral icterus indicates a serum bilirubin level of at least?
Harrison's 20th Ed. Chapter 45 Page 276

- A. 1.5 mg/dL
- B. 2 mg/dL
- C. 2.5 mg/dL
- D. 3 mg/dL

Presence of scleral icterus indicates a serum bilirubin level of at least 3 mg/dL (51 μmol/L). Jaundice is rarely detectable if the serum bilirubin level is <2.5 mg/dL but may remain detectable below this level during recovery from jaundice (because of protein and tissue binding of conjugated bilirubin).

208. A second site to detect icterus is?
Harrison's 20th Ed. Chapter 45 Page 276

- A. Uvula
- B. Hard palate
- C. Nails
- D. Underneath the tongue

A second site to detect icterus is underneath the tongue.

209. In long-standing deep jaundice, skin color may become?
Harrison's 20th Ed. Chapter 45 Page 276

- A. Gray
- B. Brown
- C. Green
- D. Orange

As serum bilirubin levels rises and the process is long-standing, skin becomes green due to oxidation of bilirubin to biliverdin.

210. Yellowing of the skin may occur in?
Harrison's 20th Ed. Chapter 45 Page 276

- A. Carotenoderma
- B. Quinacrine use
- C. Excessive exposure to phenols
- D. All of the above

211. Carotenoderma develops with ingestion of excessive amounts of?
Harrison's 20th Ed. Chapter 45 Page 276

- A. Carrots
- B. Leafy vegetables
- C. Oranges
- D. All of the above

Carotenoderma develops in healthy individuals who ingest excessive amounts of vegetables and fruits that contain carotene, such as carrots, leafy vegetables, squash, peaches, and oranges.

212. In carotenoderma, the pigment is concentrated on?
Harrison's 20th Ed. Chapter 45 Page 276

- A. Palms & soles
- B. Forehead
- C. Nasolabial folds
- D. All of the above

In carotenoderma, the pigment is concentrated on palms, soles, forehead & nasolabial folds but spares the sclerae ("pseudo-jaundice").

213. Pruritis may be seen when the bilirubin reaches?
Harrison's 20th Ed. Chapter 79 Page 593

- A. 4 - 6 mg/dL
- B. 6 - 8 mg/dL
- C. 8 - 10 mg/dL
- D. 10 - 12 mg/dL

Pruritis may be seen when the bilirubin reaches 6 - 8 mg/dL.

214. Which of the following is true for bilirubin?
Harrison's 20th Ed. Chapter 45 Page 276

- A. Bipyrrole pigment
- B. Tripyrrole pigment
- C. Tetrapyrrole pigment
- D. Pentapyrrole pigment

Bilirubin is a tetrapyrrole pigment. Heme is an iron-chelated tetrapyrrole or porphyrin.

215. What amount of bilirubin is produced each day?
Harrison's 20th Ed. Chapter 45 Page 276

- A. 1 mg/kg body weight
- B. 2 mg/kg body weight
- C. 3 mg/kg body weight
- D. 4 mg/kg body weight

216. Which of the following is a hemoprotein?
Harrison's 20th Ed. Chapter 45 Page 276

- A. Heme
- B. Myoglobin
- C. Cytochrome
- D. All of the above

217. Formation of bilirubin occurs in?
Harrison's 20th Ed. Chapter 45 Page 276

- A. Bone marrow
- B. Spleen
- C. Kidneys
- D. Intestine

Formation of bilirubin occurs in reticuloendothelial cells, primarily in spleen & liver.

218. Oxidative cleavage of α bridge of porphyrin group and opening of heme ring is catalyzed by?
Harrison's 20th Ed. Chapter 45 Page 276
   A. Heme oxygenase
   B. ALA-dehydratase
   C. Hydroxymethylbilane synthase
   D. PROTO-oxidase

Oxidative cleavage of α bridge of porphyrin group and opening of heme ring is catalyzed by heme oxygenase.

219. The end product of reaction catalyzed by heme oxygenase is?
Harrison's 20th Ed. Chapter 45 Page 276
   A. Biliverdin
   B. Carbon monoxide
   C. Iron
   D. All of the above

220. Which of the following about biliverdin reductase is false?
Harrison's 20th Ed. Chapter 45 Page 276
   A. Cytosolic enzyme
   B. Microsomal enzyme
   C. Reduces central methylene bridge of biliverdin
   D. Converts biliverdin to bilirubin

Biliverdin reductase is a cytosolic enzyme. Heme oxygenase is a microsomal enzyme.

221. Which of the following is a moiety of bilirubin?
Harrison's 20th Ed. Chapter 45 Page 276
   A. Propionic acid carboxyl groups
   B. Imino group
   C. Lactam group
   D. All of the above

222. Solubilization is accomplished by reversible, noncovalent binding of bilirubin to?
Harrison's 20th Ed. Chapter 45 Page 276
   A. Albumin
   B. Globulin
   C. Biliverdin
   D. All of the above

Solubilization is accomplished by the reversible, noncovalent binding of bilirubin to albumin.

223. Unconjugated bilirubin is bound in cytosol to proteins in?
Harrison's 20th Ed. Chapter 45 Page 276
   A. Glutathione-S-transferase superfamily
   B. Cystatin superfamily
   C. Cytochrome P450 (CYP) monooxygenase superfamily
   D. GPCR superfamily

Unconjugated bilirubin is bound in cytosol to proteins in the glutathione-S-transferase superfamily.

224. Bilirubin is made aqueous soluble by conjugation to glucuronic acid in?
Harrison's 20th Ed. Chapter 45 Page 276
   A. Golgi apparatus
   B. Endoplasmic reticulum
   C. Mitochondria
   D. Lysosome

In endoplasmic reticulum (ER), bilirubin is made aqueous soluble by conjugation to glucuronic acid by disrupting hydrophobic internal hydrogen bonds & formation of bilirubin monoglucuronide & diglucuronide.

225. Conjugation of glucuronic acid to bilirubin is catalyzed by?
Harrison's 20th Ed. Chapter 45 Page 276
   A. Bilirubin uridine diphosphate-glucuronyl transferase
   B. Bilirubin uridine diphosphate-glucuronosyl transferase
   C. Bilirubin uridine diphosphate-glucuronidase transferase
   D. Bilirubin uridine diphosphate-glucuronide transferase

Conjugation of glucuronic acid to bilirubin is catalyzed by bilirubin uridine diphosphate-glucuronosyl transferase (UDPGT).

226. Bilirubin monoglucuronide & diglucuronide are actively transported into canalicular bile by?
Harrison's 20th Ed. Chapter 45 Page 276
   A. Macrophage associated protein type 2
   B. Contactin-associated protein-like 2 (Caspr2)
   C. Hemidesmosome-associated protein
   D. Multidrug resistance-associated protein 2 (MRP2)

Bilirubin monoglucuronide & diglucuronide are actively transported into canalicular bile by multidrug resistance-associated protein 2 (MRP2).

227. Sinusoidal organic anion transport protein 1B1 and 1B3 best relate to?
Harrison's 20th Ed. Chapter 45 Page 276
   A. Transportation of unconjugated bilirubin into hepatocytes
   B. Transportation of bilirubin glucuronides into canalicular bile
   C. Reuptake of bilirubin glucuronides into hepatocyte
   D. Efflux of bilirubin back into serum

A portion of bilirubin glucuronides is transported into sinusoids & portal circulation by MRP3 from where reuptake into hepatocyte occurs by sinusoidal organic anion transport protein 1B1 (OATP1B1) & OATP1B3.

228. Which of the following statements is false?
Harrison's 20th Ed. Chapter 45 Page 276
   A. Conjugated bilirubin is not reabsorbed by intestinal mucosa
   B. Conjugated bilirubin is hydrolyzed to unconjugated bilirubin in distal ileum & colon
   C. Conjugated bilirubin is hydrolyzed to unconjugated bilirubin by bacterial β-glucuronidases
   D. None of the above

229. Which of the following about urobilinogen is false?
Harrison's 20th Ed. Chapter 45 Page 276
   A. Colorless tetrapyrrole
   B. Formed from conjugated bilirubin
   C. Most of it is excreted in feces
   D. Urobilins are oxidized urobilinogen

The "unconjugated" bilirubin is reduced by normal gut bacteria to colorless tetrapyrroles called urobilinogens, ~80 – 90% are excreted in feces, either unchanged or oxidized to orange derivatives called urobilins.

230. What percentage of urobilinogens undergo enterohepatic cycling?
Harrison's 20th Ed. Chapter 45 Page 276
   A. 10 – 20%
   B. 20 – 30%
   C. 30 – 40%
   D. 40 – 50%

10 - 20% of urobilinogens undergo enterohepatic cycling.

231. Increased urinary excretion of urobilinogen can be due to?
Harrison's 20th Ed. Chapter 45 Page 276

A. Increased bilirubin production
B. Increased hepatic reabsorption of urobilinogen from colon
C. Decreased hepatic clearance of urobilinogen
D. All of the above

232. Nationality of Abraham Albert Hijmans van den Bergh was?

A. Russian
B. Dutch
C. German
D. Spanish

Abraham Albert Hijmans van den Bergh (1869 - 1943) was a Dutch physician.

233. Serum bilirubin assay is best related to?
Harrison's 20th Ed. Chapter 45 Page 276

A. Azo pigment
B. Phthalocyanine pigment
C. Quinacridone pigment
D. Arylide yellow

In serum bilirubin assay, bilirubin is exposed to diazotized sulfanilic acid. It splits into two stable dipyrromethene azo pigments that allows photometric analysis at 540 nm.

234. Accelerator substance in van den Bergh reaction is?
Harrison's 20th Ed. Chapter 45 Page 276

A. Alcohol
B. HCl
C. H_2SO_4
D. HNO_3

In van den Bergh reaction, direct fraction is that which reacts with diazotized sulfanilic acid in absence of accelerator substance (alcohol). Direct fraction correlates with the conjugated bilirubin level in serum. Total serum bilirubin is the amount that reacts after addition of alcohol.

235. Unconjugated hyperbilirubinemia is present when direct fraction is what percentage of total serum bilirubin?
Harrison's 20th Ed. Chapter 45 Page 277

A. < 10%
B. < 15%
C. < 20%
D. < 25%

Unconjugated hyperbilirubinemia is said to be present when direct fraction is <15% of total serum bilirubin.

236. Which of the following statements about calculated indirect bilirubin is true?
Harrison's 20th Ed. Chapter 45 Page 277

A. Under estimates true amount of unconjugated bilirubin
B. Over estimates true amount of unconjugated bilirubin
C. Same as true amount of unconjugated bilirubin
D. Any of the above

Unconjugated bilirubin slowly reacts with diazo reagents, even without the accelerator. Thus, calculated indirect bilirubin is an underestimate of the true amount of unconjugated bilirubin in circulation.

237. In 95% of a normal population, total serum bilirubin concentrations are between?
Harrison's 20th Ed. Chapter 45 Page 277

A. 0.1 and 0.5 mg/dL
B. 0.2 and 0.9 mg/dL
C. 0.3 and 1.0 mg/dL
D. 0.4 and 1.1 mg/dL

With the van den Bergh method, the normal serum bilirubin concentration usually is between 1 and 1.5 mg/dL. Total serum bilirubin concentrations are between 0.2 and 0.9 mg/dL in 95% of a normal population.

238. Albumin-linked fraction of conjugated bilirubin is called?
Harrison's 20th Ed. Chapter 45 Page 277

A. Delta fraction
B. Delta bilirubin
C. Biliprotein
D. All of the above

239. Clearance rate of delta bilirubin is?
Harrison's 20th Ed. Chapter 45 Page 277

A. 1 – 4 days
B. 4 – 7 days
C. 7 – 10 days
D. 12 – 14 days

Because of the tight binding between bilirubin and albumin, the clearance rate of delta bilirubin from serum approximates half-life of albumin (12 - 14 days) rather than the short half-life of bilirubin (about 4 hours).

240. Biliprotein was undetectable in?
N Engl J Med. 1983; 309:1654-1655

A. Serum from horses
B. Icteric human fluids (cyst fluid, pleural exudate)
C. Serum from patients with hemolytic jaundice
D. All of the above

Biliprotein is undetectable in serum from horses (the animal model of Gilbert's syndrome) and in icteric human fluids (cyst fluid, pleural exudate, or serum from patients with hemolytic jaundice).

241. Which of the following about bilirubin is false?
Am J Physiol Endocrinol Metab. 2017;312(4):E244-E252

A. Antioxidant and anti-inflammatory molecule
B. Activates PPARα
C. Suppressor of PPARγ activity
D. None of the above

Bilirubin reduces lipid accumulation by PPARα activation and a reduction in PPARγ transcriptional activity. Patients with Gilbert's syndrome are protected from development of cardiovascular disease.

242. Which of the following statements is false?
Harrison's 20th Ed. Chapter 45 Page 277

A. Unconjugated bilirubin is always bound to albumin in serum
B. Unconjugated bilirubin is not found in urine
C. Most of conjugated bilirubin is reabsorbed by proximal tubules
D. None of the above

243. Hyperbilirubinemia may result from?
Harrison's 20th Ed. Chapter 45 Page 277

A. Overproduction of bilirubin
B. Impaired uptake, conjugation, or excretion of bilirubin
C. Regurgitation of unconjugated or conjugated bilirubin from damaged hepatocytes or bile ducts
D. All of the above

244. Increase in unconjugated bilirubin in serum results from?
Harrison's 20th Ed. Chapter 45 Page 277

A. Overproduction
B. Impaired uptake
C. Impaired conjugation of bilirubin
D. All of the above

245. An increase in conjugated bilirubin in serum is due to?
Harrison's 20th Ed. Chapter 45 Page 277

A. Overproduction
B. Impaired uptake
C. Impaired conjugation of bilirubin
D. Decreased excretion into bile ductules

An increase in conjugated bilirubin is due to decreased excretion into bile ductules or backward leakage of the pigment.

246. Ineffective erythropoiesis occurs in?
Harrison's 20th Ed. Chapter 45 Page 277

A. Cobalamin deficiency
B. Folate deficiency
C. Iron deficiency
D. All of the above

247. Impaired bilirubin conjugation occurs in?
Harrison's 20th Ed. Chapter 45 Page 277

A. Crigler-Najjar syndrome type I
B. Crigler-Najjar syndrome type II
C. Gilbert's syndrome
D. All of the above

248. In Crigler-Najjar type II, bilirubin UDPGT activity is reduced to?
Harrison's 20th Ed. Chapter 45 Page 278

A. < 10%
B. < 20%
C. < 30%
D. < 40%

Because of mutations in bilirubin UDPGT gene, there occurs reduction in enzyme's activity to ≤10% in patients of Crigler-Najjar type II.

249. In Gilbert's syndrome, bilirubin UDPGT activity is reduced to?
Harrison's 20th Ed. Chapter 45 Page 278

A. 2 – 10% of normal
B. 10 – 35% of normal
C. 35 – 50% of normal
D. 50 – 75% of normal

Gilbert's syndrome is marked by impaired conjugation of bilirubin due to reduced bilirubin UDPGT activity - typically 10 - 35% of normal.

250. Serum bilirubin level in patients with Gilbert's syndrome is almost always?
Harrison's 20th Ed. Chapter 45 Page 278

A. < 3 mg/dL
B. < 4 mg/dL
C. < 5 mg/dL
D. < 6 mg/dL

Patients with Gilbert's syndrome have mild unconjugated hyperbilirubinemia, with serum bilirubin levels almost always < 6 mg/dL (103 µmol/L).

251. In Gilbert's syndrome, serum bilirubin levels worsen with?
Harrison's 20th Ed. Chapter 45 Page 278

A. Stress, concurrent illness
B. Alcohol use
C. Fasting
D. All of the above

In Gilbert's syndrome, serum bilirubin levels worsen during periods of stress, concurrent illness, alcohol use, or fasting.

252. The reported incidence of Gilbert's syndrome is?
Harrison's 20th Ed. Chapter 45 Page 278

A. 0.3 – 0.7% of the population
B. 0.7 – 1.5% of the population
C. 1.5 – 3% of the population
D. 3 – 7% of the population

Reported incidence of Gilbert's syndrome is 3 - 7% of the population, with males predominating over females by a ratio of 1.5 - 7:1.

253. Which of the following is a more common condition?
Harrison's 20th Ed. Chapter 45 Page 278

A. Dubin-Johnson syndrome
B. Rotor syndrome
C. Gilbert's syndrome
D. Crigler-Najjar type II

254. Mutations in the gene for MRP2 best relates to?
Harrison's 20th Ed. Chapter 45 Page 278

A. Dubin-Johnson syndrome
B. Rotor syndrome
C. Gilbert's syndrome
D. All of the above

255. Deficiency of hepatic drug reuptake transporters OATP1B1 & OATP1B3 best relates to?
Harrison's 20th Ed. Chapter 45 Page 278

A. Dubin-Johnson syndrome
B. Rotor syndrome
C. Gilbert's syndrome
D. All of the above

256. Which of the following has a benign nature?
Harrison's 20th Ed. Chapter 45 Page 278

A. Dubin-Johnson syndrome
B. Rotor syndrome
C. Gilbert's syndrome
D. All of the above

257. Which of the following is true for Virchow's node?
Harrison's 20th Ed. Chapter 45 Page 279, 412

A. Enlarged right supraclavicular node
B. Enlarged left supraclavicular node
C. Enlarged right infraclavicular node
D. Enlarged left infraclavicular node

Virchow's node refers to an enlarged left supraclavicular node which is infiltrated with metastatic cancer from a gastrointestinal primary. Metastases to supraclavicular nodes also occur from lung, breast, testis, or ovarian cancers. Tuberculosis, sarcoidosis, and toxoplasmosis are nonneoplastic causes of supraclavicular adenopathy.

258. Location of Sister Mary Joseph's nodule is?
Harrison's 20th Ed. Chapter 45 Page 279

A. Neck
B. Chest
C. Abdomen
D. Lower limbs

Sister Mary Joseph's nodule refers to a periumbilical nodule & suggests an abdominal malignancy.

259. Murphy's sign best relates to?
Harrison's 20th Ed. Chapter 45 Page 279

A. Cholecystitis
B. Alcoholic hepatitis
C. Pancreatic cancer
D. Cirrhosis liver

Murphy's sign refers to severe right-upper-quadrant abdominal tenderness ("liver pain") with respiratory arrest on inspiration. It suggests cholecystitis.

260. Which of the following is a feature of cirrhosis liver?
Harrison's 20th Ed. Chapter 45 Page 279

A. Ascites in the presence of jaundice
B. Enlarged left lobe of the liver
C. Temporal and proximal muscle wasting
D. All of the above

261. Which of the following is not an enzyme test?
Harrison's 20th Ed. Chapter 45 Page 279

A. Serum bilirubin
B. Serum alanine aminotransferase (ALT)
C. Serum aspartate aminotransferase (AST)
D. Serum alkaline phosphatase (ALP)

262. Elevated prothrombin time indicates which of the following?
Harrison's 20th Ed. Chapter 45 Page 279

A. Vitamin K deficiency due to prolonged jaundice
B. Malabsorption of vitamin K
C. Significant hepatocellular dysfunction
D. All of the above

Failure of PT to correct with parenteral administration of vitamin K indicates severe hepatocellular injury.

263. In alcoholic hepatitis, AST-to-ALT ratio is at least?
Harrison's 20th Ed. Chapter 45 Page 279

A. 1:1.5
B. 1:2
C. 1.5:1
D. 2:1

In alcoholic hepatitis, AST-to-ALT ratio is at least 2:1. AST level rarely is > 300 U/L.

264. In acute hepatocellular disease, ALT & AST values are how many times higher than normal?
Harrison's 20th Ed. Chapter 45 Page 279

A. 5 times
B. 15 times
C. 25 times
D. 35 times

265. In cholestatic liver disease, ALT & AST values are how many times higher than normal?
Harrison's 20th Ed. Chapter 45 Page 279

A. < 8 times
B. < 12 times
C. < 16 times
D. < 20 times

266. Which of the following mushroom causes hepatotoxicity?
Harrison's 20th Ed. Chapter 45 Page 280

A. Amanita muscaria
B. Amanita pantherina
C. Amanita phalloides
D. All of the above

Mushrooms Amanita phalloides and A. verna contain highly hepatotoxic amatoxins and produces massive hepatic necrosis. The lethal dose of the toxin is ~10 mg,

267. Which of the following can cause cholestatic hepatitis?
Harrison's 20th Ed. Chapter 45 Page 280

A. Hepatitis A and E
B. Hepatitis B
C. Hepatitis C
D. All of the above

268. Which of the following can cause cholestatic hepatitis?
Harrison's 20th Ed. Chapter 45 Page 280

A. Alcoholic hepatitis
B. EBV infection
C. CMV infection
D. All of the above

269. Chronic cholestasis is associated with?
Harrison's 20th Ed. Chapter 45 Page 280

A. Chlorpromazine
B. Imipramine
C. Tolbutamide
D. Erythromycin estolate

Chronic cholestasis has been associated with chlorpromazine and prochlorperazine.

270. About 75% of patients with primary sclerosing cholangitis (PSC) have?
Harrison's 20th Ed. Chapter 45 Page 280

A. Diabetes mellitus
B. Retroperitoneal fibrosis
C. Budd-Chiari syndrome
D. Inflammatory bowel disease

Also, cholangiocarcinoma is most commonly associated with PSC.

271. Vanishing bile duct syndrome is seen in?
Harrison's 20th Ed. Chapter 45 Page 281

A. Graft-versus-host disease
B. Sarcoidosis
C. Chlorpromazine
D. All of the above

272. Which of the following is not a feature of benign recurrent intrahepatic cholestasis (BRIC)?
Harrison's 20th Ed. Chapter 45 Page 281

A. Episodic attacks of pruritus
B. Cholestasis
C. Jaundice beginning at any age
D. Chronic liver disease

Benign recurrent intrahepatic cholestasis (BRIC) types 1 and 2 are a familial form of intrahepatic cholestasis that does not lead to chronic liver disease. Serum bile acids are elevated during episodes, but serum γ-glutamyltransferase (γ-GT) activity is normal.

273. **High levels of serum γ-glutamyltransferase are found in?**
    Harrison's 20th Ed. Chapter 45 Page 281
    A. Benign recurrent intrahepatic cholestasis (BRIC)
    B. Progressive familial intrahepatic cholestasis (PFIC) types 1
    C. Progressive familial intrahepatic cholestasis (PFIC) types 2
    D. Progressive familial intrahepatic cholestasis (PFIC) types 3

274. **Which of the following is false about cholestasis of pregnancy?**
    Harrison's 20th Ed. Chapter 45 Page 281
    A. Occurs in II & III trimesters, resolves after delivery
    B. Probably inherited
    C. Cholestasis can be triggered by estrogen administration
    D. None of the above

275. **Stauffer's syndrome best relates to?**
    Harrison's 20th Ed. Chapter 45 Page 281
    A. Hodgkin's disease
    B. Medullary thyroid cancer
    C. Renal cell cancer
    D. Prostate cancer

Stauffer's syndrome refers to intrahepatic cholestasis specifically associated with renal cell cancer.

276. **"Shock liver" best relates to?**
    Harrison's 20th Ed. Chapter 45 Page 281
    A. Ischemic hepatitis
    B. Graft-versus-host disease
    C. Heart failure
    D. Sepsis

Ischemic hepatitis is a distinct entity of acute hypoperfusion characterized by acute (dramatic) elevation in serum aminotransferases followed by a gradual peak in serum bilirubin.

277. **In severe cases of Plasmodium falciparum malaria, jaundice is due to?**
    Harrison's 20th Ed. Chapter 45 Page 281
    A. Hemolysis
    B. Cholestasis
    C. Hepatocellular damage
    D. All of the above

278. **Weil's syndrome consists of?**
    Harrison's 20th Ed. Chapter 45 Page 281, 1290
    A. Jaundice
    B. Renal dysfunction
    C. Hemorrhagic diathesis
    D. All of the above

With or without jaundice, severe pulmonary hemorrhage is increasingly recognized as an important presentation of severe Weil's disease.

279. **Which of the following malignancies has the highest surgical cure rate?**
    Harrison's 20th Ed. Chapter 45 Page 281
    A. Ampullary carcinoma
    B. Pancreatic tumor
    C. Gallbladder tumor
    D. Cholangiocarcinoma

Ampullary carcinoma has the highest surgical cure rate of all the tumors that present as painless jaundice.

280. **Findings of which of the following is often identical to that of PSC?**
    Harrison's 20th Ed. Chapter 45 Page 281
    A. Cholangiocarcinoma
    B. AIDS cholangiopathy due to CMV
    C. AIDS cholangiopathy due to cryptosporidia
    D. All of the above

281. **Which of the following is a cause of benign extrahepatic cholestatic conditions that may produce jaundice?**
    Harrison's 20th Ed. Chapter 45 Page 280 Table 45-3
    A. Mirizzi's syndrome
    B. AIDS cholangiopathy
    C. Primary sclerosing cholangitis
    D. All of the above

Mirizzi's syndrome is a rare complication in which a gallstone becomes impacted in cystic duct or neck of gallbladder compressing CBD, resulting in CBD obstruction & jaundice.

282. **Jaundice is a feature of?**
    Harrison's 20th Ed. Chapter 45 Page 281
    A. Babesiosis
    B. Typhoid fever
    C. Dengue hemorrhagic fever
    D. All of the above

283. **Charcot's triad in patients with ascending cholangitis & biliary sepsis consists of all except?**
    Harrison's 20th Ed. Chapter 315 Page 2200
    A. Nausea, vomiting
    B. Jaundice
    C. Abdominal pain
    D. Spiking fever

Charcot's triad of jaundice, abdominal pain, and fever is present in ~70% of patients with ascending cholangitis and biliary sepsis.

284. **Which of the following statements about choledocholithiasis is false?**
    Harrison's 20th Ed. Chapter 339 Page 2431
    A. Maximum bilirubin level is 15.0 mg/dL in choledocholithiasis
    B. Rise in alkaline phosphatase often precedes clinical jaundice
    C. Pancreatitis complicates choledocholithiasis in >30% cases
    D. None of the above

285. **Which of the following statements about choledocholithiasis is false?**
    Harrison's 20th Ed. Chapter 45 Page 281
    A. Most common cause of extrahepatic cholestasis
    B. ERCP is "gold standard" for identifying choledocholithiasis
    C. Normal albumin level is suggestive of choledocholithiasis
    D. None of the above

Abdominal Swelling and Ascites

286. Which of the following is not one of the six "F" that are the causes of abdominal swelling?
Harrison's 20th Ed. Chapter 46 Page 282

- A. Flatus
- B. Fat
- C. Feces
- D. Fertile

Causes of abdominal swelling can be remembered as the six Fs: flatus, fat, fluid, fetus, feces, or a "fatal growth" (often a neoplasm).

287. The normal small intestine contains how much gas?
Harrison's 20th Ed. Chapter 46 Page 282

- A. ~ 100 mL
- B. ~ 200 mL
- C. ~ 300 mL
- D. ~ 400 mL

288. Small intestinal gas is?
Harrison's 20th Ed. Chapter 46 Page 282

- A. Oxygen
- B. Hydrogen
- C. Methane
- D. All of the above

289. Which of the following gases is produced intraluminally by bacterial fermentation?
Harrison's 20th Ed. Chapter 46 Page 282

- A. Carbon dioxide
- B. Hydrogen
- C. Methane
- D. All of the above

Normal small intestine contains ~200 mL of gas made up of nitrogen, oxygen, carbon dioxide, hydrogen & methane. Nitrogen & oxygen are swallowed from outside) whereas carbon dioxide, hydrogen & methane are produced intraluminally by bacterial fermentation.

290. Which of the following is a cause of abdominal distention?
Harrison's 20th Ed. Chapter 46 Page 282

- A. Impaired intestinal transit of gas
- B. Lack of coordination between diaphragmatic contraction & anterior abdominal wall relaxation
- C. Increased lumbar lordosis
- D. All of the above

291. Increase in abdominal size is first noted at how many weeks of gestation?
Harrison's 20th Ed. Chapter 46 Page 282

- A. 6 – 8
- B. 8 – 10
- C. 10 – 12
- D. 12 – 14

292. A minimum of how much ascitic fluid is required for detection on physical examination?
Harrison's 20th Ed. Chapter 46 Page 282

- A. 1000 mL
- B. 1500 mL
- C. 2000 mL
- D. 2500 mL

A minimum of 1500 mL of ascitic fluid is required for detection on physical examination.

293. Abdominal ultrasonography can detect how much ascitic fluid?
Harrison's 20th Ed. Chapter 46 Page 282

- A. 100 mL
- B. 200 mL
- C. 300 mL
- D. 400 mL

Abdominal ultrasonography can detect as little as 100 mL of ascitic fluid.

294. Increased hepatic resistance occurs by which of the following mechanisms?
Harrison's 20th Ed. Chapter 46 Page 283

- A. Development of hepatic fibrosis
- B. Activation of hepatic stellate cells
- C. Decrease in endothelial nitric oxide synthetase production
- D. All of the above

295. Development of cirrhosis is associated with?
Harrison's 20th Ed. Chapter 46 Page 283

- A. Increased systemic circulating levels of nitric oxide
- B. Increased levels of vascular endothelial growth factor
- C. Increased levels of tumor necrosis factor
- D. All of the above

Development of cirrhosis is associated with increased systemic circulating levels of nitric oxide (contrary to decrease seen intrahepatically), increased levels of vascular endothelial growth factor and tumor necrosis factor that result in splanchnic arterial vasodilation.

296. Vasodilation of the splanchnic circulation results in?
Harrison's 20th Ed. Chapter 46 Page 283

- A. Release of antidiuretic hormone
- B. Activation of sympathetic nervous system
- C. Activation of renin angiotensin aldosterone system
- D. All of the above

297. Cirrhosis accounts for what percentage of cases of ascites?
Harrison's 20th Ed. Chapter 46 Page 283

- A. 34%
- B. 54%
- C. 64%
- D. 84%

Cirrhosis accounts for 84% of cases of ascites.

298. Out of the following which is a less common cause of ascites?
Harrison's 20th Ed. Chapter 46 Page 283

    A. Cardiac ascites
    B. Tuberculosis
    C. Peritoneal carcinomatosis
    D. Cirrhosis + a second disease

Cardiac ascites, peritoneal carcinomatosis, and "mixed" ascites (cirrhosis and a second disease) account for 10 – 15% of cases. Less common causes of ascites include massive hepatic metastasis, tuberculosis, Chlamydia infection, pancreatitis, and nephrotic syndrome. Rare causes of ascites include hypothyroidism & familial Mediterranean fever.

299. Dark brown ascitic fluid may indicate?
Harrison's 20th Ed. Chapter 46 Page 283

    A. Familial Mediterranean fever
    B. Chlamydia infection
    C. Pancreatic necrosis
    D. Biliary tract perforation

300. Black ascitic fluid may indicate?
Harrison's 20th Ed. Chapter 46 Page 283

    A. Familial Mediterranean fever
    B. Chlamydia infection
    C. Pancreatic necrosis
    D. Biliary tract perforation

301. The serum-ascites albumin gradient (SAAG) reflects the pressure within the?
Harrison's 20th Ed. Chapter 46 Page 283

    A. Hepatic sinusoids
    B. Hepatic artery
    C. Hepatic vein
    D. Portal vein

SAAG reflects pressure within hepatic sinusoids and correlates with hepatic venous pressure gradient. According to Starling's law, high SAAG reflects oncotic pressure that counterbalances portal pressure.

302. Which of the following is false about serum-ascites albumin gradient (SAAG)?
Harrison's 20th Ed. Chapter 46 Page 284

    A. Calculated as ascitic albumin - serum albumin concentration
    B. Does not change with diuresis
    C. SAAG ≥1.1 g/dL reflects presence of portal hypertension
    D. SAAG <1.1 g/dL suggests Budd-Chiari syndrome

303. Which of the following is a cause of a high SAAG?
Harrison's 20th Ed. Chapter 46 Page 284

    A. Cardiac ascites
    B. Hepatic vein thrombosis (Budd-Chiari syndrome)
    C. Sinusoidal obstruction syndrome (veno-occlusive disease)
    D. All of the above

304. Which of the following is a cause of SAAG <1.1 g/dL?
Harrison's 20th Ed. Chapter 46 Page 284

    A. Tuberculous peritonitis
    B. Peritoneal carcinomatosis
    C. Pancreatic ascites
    D. All of the above

305. Which of the following is a cause of ascitic protein level of ≥ 2.5 g/dL?
Harrison's 20th Ed. Chapter 46 Page 284

    A. Cardiac ascites
    B. Early Budd-Chiari syndrome
    C. Sinusoidal obstruction syndrome
    D. All of the above

306. Which of the following is a cause of ascitic protein level of <2.5 g/dL?
Harrison's 20th Ed. Chapter 46 Page 284

    A. Cirrhosis
    B. Late Budd-Chiari syndrome
    C. Massive liver metastases
    D. All of the above

307. Secondary peritonitis is suggested by?
Harrison's 20th Ed. Chapter 46 Page 284

    A. Ascitic glucose level <50 mg/dL
    B. Ascitic LDH level > serum LDH level
    C. Detection of multiple pathogens on ascitic fluid culture
    D. All of the above

308. In pancreatic ascites, ascitic amylase level is typically?
Harrison's 20th Ed. Chapter 46 Page 284

    A. > 200 mg/dL
    B. > 600 mg/dL
    C. > 800 mg/dL
    D. > 1000 mg/dL

309. Estimation of ascitic adenosine deaminase level is of value in?
Harrison's 20th Ed. Chapter 46 Page 284

    A. Budd-Chiari syndrome
    B. Tuberculous peritonitis
    C. Veno-occlusive disease
    D. Peritoneal carcinomatosis

310. Maximal daily dose of furosemide in cirrhotic ascites is?
Harrison's 20th Ed. Chapter 46 Page 284

    A. 100 mg/day
    B. 200 mg/day
    C. 400 mg/day
    D. 600 mg/day

Maximal daily dose of furosemide in cirrhotic ascites is 400 mg/day.

311. Maximal daily dose of spironolactone in cirrhotic ascites is?
Harrison's 20th Ed. Chapter 46 Page 284

    A. 100 mg/day
    B. 140 mg/day
    C. 160 mg/day
    D. 180 mg/day

Maximal daily dose of spironolactone in cirrhotic ascites is 160 mg/day.

312. **In refractory ascites, which of the following is added to diuretic regimen?**

    Harrison's 20th Ed. Chapter 46 Page 284

    A. Amiloride
    B. Ethacrynic acid
    C. Clonidine
    D. Captopril

    Refractory cirrhotic ascites is defined by the persistence of ascites despite sodium restriction and maximally tolerated diuretic use. Addition of midodrine (α1-adrenergic agonist) or clonidine (α2-adrenergic agonist) to diuretic therapy is beneficial. They act as vasoconstrictors, counteracting splanchnic vasodilation.

313. **Post-paracentesis circulatory dysfunction is prevented by?**

    Harrison's 20th Ed. Chapter 46 Page 284

    A. β-adrenergic blocking agents
    B. Intravenous albumin
    C. α1-adrenergic agonist - midodrine
    D. All of the above

314. **Spontaneous bacterial peritonitis is rare in?**

    Harrison's 20th Ed. Chapter 46 Page 284

    A. Malignant ascites
    B. Nephrotic syndrome
    C. Heart failure
    D. Acute liver failure

    Spontaneous bacterial peritonitis is a common complication of cirrhotic ascites. SBP also complicates ascites caused by nephrotic syndrome, heart failure, acute hepatitis, and acute liver failure but is rare in malignant ascites.

315. **Which of the following is false about spontaneous bacterial peritonitis (SBP)?**

    Harrison's 20th Ed. Chapter 46 Page 284

    A. Abdominal tenderness is found in only 40% of patients, rebound tenderness is uncommon
    B. New onset of or exacerbation of hepatic encephalopathy
    C. Cultures of ascitic fluid typically reveal one bacterial pathogen
    D. None of the above

    SBP is the result of enteric bacteria that have translocated across an edematous bowel wall.

316. **What polymorphonuclear neutrophil count in ascitic fluid denotes spontaneous bacterial peritonitis?**

    Harrison's 20th Ed. Chapter 46 Page 284

    A. ≥ 50 / μL
    B. ≥ 150 / μL
    C. ≥ 250 / μL
    D. ≥ 350 / μL

317. **Which of the following antibiotic is recommended to prevent SBP?**

    Harrison's 20th Ed. Chapter 46 Page 284

    A. Doxycycline
    B. Norfloxacin
    C. Azithromycin
    D. Trimethoprim + sulfamethoxazole

318. **Which of the following should be avoided in hepatic hydrothorax?**

    Harrison's 20th Ed. Chapter 46 Page 284

    A. Diuretics
    B. Thoracentesis
    C. TIPS placement
    D. Chest tube placement

Diseases of the Esophagus

319. The most common esophageal symptom is?
Harrison's 20th Ed. Chapter 316 Page 2209
- A. Heartburn
- B. Regurgitation
- C. Water brash
- D. Globus sensation

Heartburn is the most common esophageal symptom. It is characterized by a discomfort or burning sensation behind sternum arising from epigastrium and radiates toward neck.

320. In which of the following situations, heartburn is most commonly experienced?
Harrison's 20th Ed. Chapter 316 Page 2209
- A. After eating
- B. During exercise
- C. While lying recumbent
- D. All of the above

Heartburn is an intermittent symptom, most commonly experienced after eating, during exercise and while lying recumbent.

321. Pyrosis is best related to?
Harrison's 20th Ed. Chapter 316 Page 2209
- A. Fever
- B. Heartburn
- C. Defervescence
- D. Pain

Heartburn, or pyrosis, is characterized by burning retrosternal discomfort.

322. Which of the following is false about esophageal chest pain?
Harrison's 20th Ed. Chapter 316 Page 2210
- A. Pressure type sensation in mid chest
- B. Radiation to mid back or arms
- C. Radiation to jaws
- D. None of the above

Similarity of esophageal chest pain to cardiac pain is because the two organs share a nerve plexus and nerve endings in esophageal wall have poor discriminative ability among stimuli.

323. Most frequent esophageal cause of chest pain is?
Harrison's 20th Ed. Chapter 316 Page 2210
- A. Gastroesophageal reflux
- B. Diffuse esophageal spasm (DES)
- C. Achalasia
- D. Esophageal hypersensitivity syndrome

Gastroesophageal reflux is the most common cause of esophageal chest pain.

324. Dysphagia for liquids as well as solid food suggests?
Harrison's 20th Ed. Chapter 316 Page 2210
- A. Esophageal stricture
- B. Esophageal ring
- C. Esophageal tumor
- D. Esophageal motility disorder

325. Solid food dysphagia is suggestive of?
Harrison's 20th Ed. Chapter 316 Page 2210
- A. Esophageal stricture
- B. Esophageal ring
- C. Esophageal tumor
- D. Any of the above

326. Which of the following is not a concomitant symptom associated with oropharyngeal dysphagia?
Harrison's 20th Ed. Chapter 316 Page 2210
- A. Odynophagia
- B. Aspiration
- C. Cough
- D. Drooling

Concomitant symptoms associated with oropharyngeal dysphagia are aspiration, nasopharyngeal regurgitation, cough, drooling.

327. Odynophagia is unusual in?
Harrison's 20th Ed. Chapter 316 Page 2210
- A. Pill-induced esophagitis
- B. Nonreflux esophagitis
- C. Esophageal perforation
- D. Uncomplicated reflux esophagitis

Odynophagia (painful swallowing) is characteristic of nonreflux esophagitis, herpes & pill-induced esophagitis. Odynophagia may occur with peptic ulcer of esophagus (Barrett's ulcer), carcinoma with periesophageal involvement, caustic damage of esophagus, and esophageal perforation. Odynophagia is unusual in uncomplicated reflux esophagitis.

328. Globus sensation or "globus hystericus" is the perception of a lump or fullness in?
Harrison's 20th Ed. Chapter 316 Page 2210
- A. Mouth
- B. Throat
- C. Chest
- D. Abdomen

Globus sensation or "globus hystericus" is the perception of a lump or fullness in the throat that is felt irrespective of swallowing, often relieved by the act of swallowing.

329. Reflex salivary hypersecretion in response to acidification of the esophageal mucosa is called?
Harrison's 20th Ed. Chapter 316 Page 2210
- A. Water brash
- B. Salivary brash
- C. Esophageal brash
- D. Barret's brash

Water brash is excessive reflex salivation resulting from a vagal reflex triggered by acidification of the esophageal mucosa. It is not regurgitation which is effortless appearance of gastric or esophageal contents in the mouth.

330. **Which of the following is an uncommon symptom of esophageal diseases?**
   Harrison's 20th Ed. Chapter 316 Page 2210
   A. Water brash
   B. Odynophagia
   C. Globus sensation
   D. Chest pain

331. **Barium radiography is better than esophagogastroduodenoscopy (EGD) in?**
   Harrison's 20th Ed. Chapter 316 Page 2210
   A. Esophageal strictures
   B. Esophageal function and morphology
   C. Disorders of the cricopharyngeus muscle
   D. All of the above

332. **Endoscopic ultrasound (EUS) is useful in which of the following esophageal condition?**
   Harrison's 20th Ed. Chapter 316 Page 2210
   A. To stage esophageal cancer
   B. To evaluate dysplasia in Barrett's esophagus
   C. To assess submucosal lesions
   D. All of the above

Endoscopic ultrasound (EUS) is useful in which of the following esophageal conditions : to stage esophageal cancer, to evaluate dysplasia in Barrett's esophagus & to assess submucosal lesions.

333. **Esophageal peristalsis is best studied in?**
   Harrison's 20th Ed. Chapter 316 Page 2210
   A. Upright position
   B. Recumbent position
   C. Lateral position
   D. Head down position

Esophageal peristalsis is best studied in the recumbent position, because in the upright position barium passage occurs largely by gravity alone.

334. **Which of the following defines gastroesophageal reflux disease (GERD)?**
   Harrison's 20th Ed. Chapter 316 Page 2210
   A. Heartburn
   B. Esophageal chest pain
   C. Esophageal dysphagia
   D. Endoscopic esophagitis

335. **Which is the most common type of hiatus hernia?**
   Harrison's 20th Ed. Chapter 316 Page 2211
   A. Type I
   B. Type II
   C. Type III
   D. Type IV

Type I or sliding hiatal hernia comprises ~95% of the overall total cases of hiatus hernia.

336. **Sliding hiatal hernias enlarge with?**
   Harrison's 20th Ed. Chapter 316 Page 2211
   A. Increased intraabdominal pressure
   B. Swallowing
   C. Respiration
   D. All of the above

337. **Sliding hiatal hernias are a result of weakening of?**
   Harrison's 20th Ed. Chapter 316 Page 2211
   A. Phrenoesophageal ligament
   B. Hepatophrenic ligament
   C. Costotransverse ligament
   D. All of the above

In sliding hiatal hernia, gastroesophageal junction & gastric cardia translocate cephalad due to weakening of phrenoesophageal ligament attaching gastroesophageal junction to diaphragm at the hiatus and dilatation of diaphragmatic hiatus.

338. **The gastroesophageal junction remains fixed at the hiatus in which type of hiatal hernia?**
   Harrison's 20th Ed. Chapter 316 Page 2211
   A. Type I
   B. Type II
   C. Type III
   D. Type IV

In type II hiatal hernia, the gastroesophageal junction remains fixed at the hiatus.

339. **When colon herniate into the mediastinum, the type of hiatus hernia is?**
   Harrison's 20th Ed. Chapter 316 Page 2211
   A. Type I
   B. Type II
   C. Type III
   D. Type IV

With type IV hiatal hernias, viscera other than stomach herniate into mediastinum, most commonly the colon.

340. **Gastric cardia does not herniate into the mediastinum in which of the following hiatal hernias?**
   Harrison's 20th Ed. Chapter 316 Page 2211
   A. Type II
   B. Type III
   C. Type IV
   D. All of the above

Type II, III, and IV hiatal hernias are subtypes of paraesophageal hernia in which herniation into mediastinum includes a visceral structure other than the gastric cardia.

341. **Intersection of squamous epithelium of tubular esophagus & columnar epithelium of stomach is termed?**
   Lancet 2009; 373:850 - 61
   A. W line
   B. X line
   C. Y line
   D. Z line

The intersection of squamous epithelium of the tubular esophagus & columnar epithelium of stomach is termed Z line, because of jagged appearance of the interface.

342. **Lower esophageal mucosal ring is also called?**
   Harrison's 20th Ed. Chapter 316 Page 2211
   A. A ring
   B. B ring
   C. C ring
   D. D ring

A lower esophageal mucosal ring, also called B ring, is a thin membranous narrowing at the squamocolumnar mucosal junction.

343. Location of 'Schatzki ring' is?
Harrison's 20th Ed. Chapter 316 Page 2211

A. Hypopharyngeal
B. Mid esophageal
C. Lower esophageal
D. Any of the above

Schatzki ring is a lower esophageal mucosal ring. It is a thin, weblike constriction located at the squamo-columnar mucosal junction at or near the border of the LES. It may result from GERD or be congenital in origin.

344. Schatzki ring invariably produces dysphagia when the lumen diameter is?
Harrison's 20th Ed. Chapter 316 Page 2211

A. < 1.3 cm
B. < 2.3 cm
C. < 3.3 cm
D. < 4.3 cm

Schatzki ring invariably produces dysphagia when the lumen diameter is <1.3 cm.

345. "Steakhouse syndrome" best relates to?
Harrison's 20th Ed. Chapter 316 Page 2211

A. Mouth
B. Esophagus
C. Stomach
D. Colon

Schatzki ring is one of the most common causes of intermittent food impaction, also called "steakhouse syndrome" as meat is a typical instigator.

346. Which of the following is false about Plummer-Vinson syndrome?
Harrison's 20th Ed. Chapter 316 Page 2211

A. Young women
B. Symptomatic proximal esophageal web
C. Iron-deficiency anemia
D. All of the above

Symptomatic hypopharyngeal webs and iron-deficiency anemia in middle-aged women constitutes Plummer-Vinson syndrome.

347. Which of the following is false about Zenker's diverticula?
Harrison's 20th Ed. Chapter 316 Page 2211

A. Hypopharyngeal
B. False diverticula
C. Associated with distal obstruction
D. None of the above

348. Which of the following is false about Zenker's diverticulum?
Harrison's 20th Ed. Chapter 316 Page 2211

A. Occurs below the Killian's triangle
B. Causes halitosis & regurgitation of saliva & food
C. Nasogastric intubation may cause perforation
D. Symptomatic pt's treated by cricopharyngeal myotomy

Zenker's diverticulum appears in natural zone of weakness in posterior hypopharyngeal wall (Killian's triangle).

349. Epiphrenic diverticula are associated with?
Harrison's 20th Ed. Chapter 316 Page 2212

A. Achalasia
B. Esophageal hypercontractile disorders
C. Distal esophageal stricture
D. All of the above

350. Esophageal cancer has poor survival because of the?
Harrison's 20th Ed. Chapter 316 Page 2212

A. Constant proximity to acidic milieu
B. Nonconvoluted pipe like structure
C. Abundant esophageal lymphatics
D. All of the above

Esophageal cancer has poor survival because of the abundant esophageal lymphatics leading to regional lymph node metastases.

351. The most common congenital esophageal anomaly is?
Harrison's 20th Ed. Chapter 316 Page 2212

A. Esophageal atresia
B. Congenital esophageal stenosis
C. Esophageal webs
D. Esophageal duplications

The most common congenital esophageal anomaly is esophageal atresia, occurring in about 1 in 5000 live births.

352. Dysphagia lusoria best relates to which of the following?
Harrison's 20th Ed. Chapter 316 Page 2213

A. Artery of Adamkiewicz
B. Aberrant right subclavian artery
C. Aberrant mast cells
D. Dieulafoy's lesion

Dysphagia lusoria is a condition wherein the esophagus is compressed by an aberrant right subclavian artery arising from the descending aorta and passing behind the esophagus.

353. Esophageal inlet patch best relates to?
Harrison's 20th Ed. Chapter 316 Page 2213

A. Esophageal atresia
B. Benign esophageal tumor
C. Heterotopic gastric mucosa
D. Zenker's diverticula

Heterotopic gastric mucosa, also known as an esophageal inlet patch, is an area of gastric type epithelium in proximal cervical esophagus. The inlet patch is due to incomplete replacement of embryonic columnar epithelium with squamous epithelium. It produces acid as most contain fundic type gastric epithelium with parietal cells.

354. Which of the following is an esophageal motility disorder?
Harrison's 20th Ed. Chapter 316 Page 2213

A. Achalasia
B. Diffuse esophageal spasm (DES)
C. Gastroesophageal reflux disease (GERD)
D. All of the above

Esophageal motility disorders are diseases attributable to esophageal neuromuscular dysfunction. The major entities are achalasia, diffuse esophageal spasm (DES) and GERD.

355. Which of the following is a secondary esophageal motility disorder?
Harrison's 20th Ed. Chapter 316 Page 2213

A. Pseudoachalasia
B. Chagas' disease
C. Scleroderma
D. Diphtheria

Motility disorders can be secondary to pseudoachalasia, Chagas' disease and scleroderma.

356. Secondary achalasia may be caused by all except?
Harrison's 20th Ed. Chapter 316 Page 2213

A. Ulcerative colitis
B. Chagas' disease
C. Eosinophilic gastroenteritis
D. Neurodegenerative disorders

Secondary achalasia may be caused by gastric carcinoma that infiltrates the esophagus, lymphoma, Chagas' disease, certain viral infections, eosinophilic gastroenteritis & neurodegenerative disorders.

357. Which of the following statements about achalasia is false?
Harrison's 20th Ed. Chapter 316 Page 2213

A. Motor disorder of esophageal smooth muscle
B. UES & LES relax normally with swallowing
C. Nonperistaltic contractions in esophageal body
D. Underlying abnormality is loss of intramural neurons

With a swallow, pressure in sphincters falls and a contraction wave starts in pharynx and progresses down the esophagus. In achalasia, esophageal body loses peristaltic contractions & are replaced by simultaneous contractions with elevated resting pressure & LES does not relax normally in response to swallowing. Prominent loss of ganglion cells within the esophageal myenteric plexus is seen in achalasia.

358. Cause of ganglion cell degeneration in achalasia is infection with?
Harrison's 20th Ed. Chapter 316 Page 2213

A. Varicella zoster virus
B. Human herpes simplex virus 1
C. Cytomegalovirus
D. Epstein-Barr virus

Cause of ganglion cell degeneration in achalasia is an autoimmune process attributable to a latent infection with human herpes simplex virus 1 combined with genetic susceptibility.

359. Sigmoid deformity of esophagus with hypertrophy of LES is suggestive of?
Harrison's 20th Ed. Chapter 316 Page 2213

A. Achalasia
B. Diffuse esophageal spasm
C. Jackhammer esophagus
D. All of the above

Long-standing achalasia is characterized by progressive dilatation and sigmoid deformity of the esophagus with hypertrophy of LES.

360. Which of the following statements about achalasia is false?
Harrison's 20th Ed. Chapter 316 Page 2213

A. Impaired LES relaxation
B. Absent peristalsis
C. Presence of GE reflux goes against achalasia
D. None of the above

Inhibitory neurons containing VIP and nitric oxide synthase are predominantly involved.

361. Which of the following is not a feature of achalasia?
Harrison's 20th Ed. Chapter 316 Page 2213

A. Dysphagia
B. Gastroesophageal reflux
C. Chest pain
D. Regurgitation

Dysphagia, chest pain, regurgitation and weight loss are the main symptoms of achalasia. Presence of gastroesophageal reflux goes against achalasia.

362. Chest X-ray in achalasia may show all except?
Harrison's 20th Ed. Chapter 316 Page 2213

A. Absence of the gastric air bubble
B. Tubular mediastinal mass beside the aorta
C. Air-fluid level in mediastinum in upright position
D. Atelectasis

A chest X-ray shows absence of the gastric air bubble and sometimes a tubular mediastinal mass beside the aorta. An air-fluid level in the mediastinum in the upright position represents retained food in the esophagus. Barium swallow shows esophageal dilation, and in advanced cases the esophagus may become sigmoid. On fluoroscopy with barium swallow, normal peristalsis is lost in the lower two-thirds of the esophagus. The terminal part of the esophagus shows a persistent beaklike narrowing representing the nonrelaxing LES.

363. Which of the following is the most sensitive diagnostic test for achalasia?
Harrison's 20th Ed. Chapter 316 Page 2213

A. Esophageal manometry
B. Barium swallow X-ray
C. Esophagogastroduodenoscopy (EGD)
D. None of the above

364. Impaired lower esophageal sphincter (LES) relaxation & absent peristalsis are seen in?
Harrison's 20th Ed. Chapter 316 Page 2213

A. Classic achalasia
B. Achalasia with esophageal compression
C. Spastic achalasia
D. All of the above

365. In CCK test, paradoxical contraction of LES is found in?
Harrison's 17th Ed. 1850

A. Achalasia
B. Gastric carcinoma
C. Scleroderma
D. Diffuse esophageal spasm

In achalasia, Cholecystokinin (CCK) paradoxically causes contraction of LES (CCK test) because neurally transmitted inhibitory effect of CCK is absent & direct excitatory effect of CCK remains unopposed.

366. Which of the following is typical of esophageal chest pain?
Harrison's 20th Ed. Chapter 316 Page 2214

A. Nonexertional
B. Prolonged
C. Interrupts sleep, meal-related
D. All of the above

Features suggesting esophageal pain include nonexertional, prolonged, interrupts sleep, meal-related, relieved with antacids, and accompanied by heartburn, dysphagia, or regurgitation.

367. **Which of the following drugs can be used in achalasia?**
Harrison's 20th Ed. Chapter 316 Page 2213
   A. Nitrates or calcium channel blockers
   B. Botulinum toxin
   C. Sildenafil
   D. All of the above

368. **In achalasia, which is the treatment of choice?**
Harrison's 20th Ed. Chapter 316 Page 2213
   A. Pneumatic dilatation
   B. Esophageal resection with gastric pull-up
   C. Laparoscopic Heller myotomy of LES
   D. Open surgical myotomy of LES

Laparoscopic Heller myotomy is currently the procedure of choice.

369. **"Corkscrew" esophagus is typical of?**
Harrison's 20th Ed. Chapter 316 Page 2215
   A. Diffuse esophageal spasm (DES)
   B. Achalasia
   C. Carcinoma esophagus
   D. GERD

Barium swallow in DES shows curling or multiple ripples in the wall, sacculations, and pseudodiverticula - termed "corkscrew" esophagus and rosary bead esophagus. Diffuse esophageal spasm is primarily defined by a short latency (premature) contraction.

370. **Which of the following about "corkscrew" esophagus is false?**
Harrison's 20th Ed. Chapter 316 Page 2214 Figure 316-7
   A. Radiographic term
   B. Spastic tertiary contraction of circular muscle in esophageal wall
   C. Normal deglutitive LES relaxation
   D. None of the above

371. **Which of the following about "Jackhammer" esophagus is false?**
Harrison's 20th Ed. Chapter 316 Page 2215 Figure 316-8
   A. Variant of esophageal spasm
   B. Vigorous & repetitive contractions with normal peristaltic onset
   C. Normal latency of the contraction
   D. None of the above

Jackhammer esophagus is defined by the extraordinarily vigorous and repetitive contractions with normal peristaltic onset and normal latency of the contraction.

372. **Which of the following is most efficacious in DES?**
Harrison's 20th Ed. Chapter 316 Page 2215
   A. Nitrates
   B. Calcium channel blockers
   C. Botulinum toxin
   D. Anxiolytics

Nitrates, calcium channel blockers, hydralazine, botulinum toxin and anxiolytics have been tried in DES with anxiolytics most efficacious.

373. **Which of the following is not a hypertensive motor disorder of esophagus?**
Harrison's 20th Ed. Chapter 316 Page 2215
   A. Diffuse esophageal spasm (DES)
   B. Nutcracker esophagus
   C. Hypercontracting LES
   D. Hypertensive LES

The hypertensive disorders of esophagus include nutcracker esophagus, hypercontracting LES and hypertensive LES. DES is characterized by nonperistaltic contractions.

374. **Motility pattern of esophagus showing reduced amplitude of contractions in lower esophagus, peristaltic or simultaneous in onset with hypotension of LES is suggestive of?**
Harrison's 20th Ed. Chapter 316 Page 2215
   A. Scleroderma
   B. Achalasia
   C. Diffuse esophageal spasm
   D. None of the above

In scleroderma, thoracic esophagus shows reduced amplitude of contractions, which may be peristaltic or simultaneous in onset & hypotension of LES.

375. **Motility pattern of esophagus showing reduced amplitude of contractions in lower esophagus, simultaneous in onset with hypertensive LES nonrelaxing on swallowing is suggestive of?**
Harrison's 20th Ed. Chapter 316 Page 2215
   A. Scleroderma
   B. Achalasia
   C. Diffuse esophageal spasm
   D. None of the above

In achalasia, lower part of esophagus shows contractions that are reduced in amplitude & simultaneous in onset. In contrast to scleroderma, LES in achalasia is hypertensive and fails to relax in response to a swallow.

376. **Motility pattern of esophagus showing large amplitude, prolonged and repetitive contractions in lower esophagus, simultaneous in onset is suggestive of?**
Harrison's 20th Ed. Chapter 316 Page 2215
   A. Scleroderma
   B. Achalasia
   C. Diffuse esophageal spasm
   D. None of the above

In diffuse esophageal spasm, lower part of esophagus shows simultaneous-onset, large-amplitude, prolonged, repetitive contractions.

377. **Esophageal motility studies are helpful in the diagnosis of all except?**
Harrison's 20th Ed. Chapter 316 Page 2215
   A. Achalasia
   B. Diffuse esophageal spasm
   C. Scleroderma
   D. Mechanical dysphagia

Esophageal motility studies are helpful in the diagnosis of esophageal motor disorders (achalasia, spasm, and scleroderma) but are of little value in the differential diagnosis of mechanical dysphagia.

378. **Esophageal contractions are normally peristaltic but hypertensive in?**
Harrison's 19th Ed. 1905
   A. Nutcracker esophagus
   B. Hypercontracting LES
   C. Hypertensive LES
   D. All of the above

In nutcracker esophagus, esophageal contractions are normally peristaltic but hypertensive. In hypercontracting LES, normal sphincter relaxation is followed by hypertensive contraction. In hypertensive LES, basal LES pressure is elevated, but sphincter relaxation and contraction are normal.

379. **Gastric distention-evoked transient lower esophageal sphincter relaxation (tLESR) is a?**
Harrison's 20th Ed. Chapter 316 Page 2215
- A. Stretch reflex
- B. Chemical reflex
- C. Vasovagal reflex
- D. All of the above

Gastric distention - evoked transient lower esophageal sphincter relaxation (tLESR) is a vagovagal reflex.

380. **Which of the following contributes to the development of gastroesophageal reflux disease (GERD)?**
Harrison's 20th Ed. Chapter 316 Page 2215
- A. Transient LES relaxations
- B. LES hypotension
- C. Anatomic distortion of esophagogastric junction
- D. All of the above

381. **Which of the following may have a protective effect in GERD patients?**
Harrison's 20th Ed. Chapter 316 Page 2216
- A. Zollinger-Ellison syndrome
- B. Chronic H. pylori gastritis
- C. Hiatus hernia
- D. Scleroderma

Chronic H. pylori gastritis may have a protective effect in GERD by inducing atrophic gastritis with concomitant hypoacidity.

382. **Which of the following acts as a cofactor in the pathogenesis of Barrett's metaplasia and esophageal adenocarcinoma?**
Harrison's 20th Ed. Chapter 316 Page 2216
- A. Pepsin
- B. Bile
- C. Pancreatic enzymes
- D. All of the above

Bile persists in refluxate despite acid-suppressing medications. Bile can transverse the cell membrane, imparting severe cellular injury in a weakly acidic environment and acts as a cofactor in the pathogenesis of Barrett's metaplasia and adenocarcinoma.

383. **Which out of the following conditions has associations with GERD?**
Harrison's 20th Ed. Chapter 316 Page 2216
- A. Pulmonary fibrosis
- B. Chronic sinusitis
- C. Cardiac arrhythmias
- D. All of the above

Extraesophageal syndromes that have established association to GERD include chronic cough, laryngitis, asthma & dental erosions. Other conditions like pharyngitis, chronic bronchitis, pulmonary fibrosis, chronic sinusitis, cardiac arrhythmias, sleep apnea, and recurrent aspiration pneumonia have proposed associations with GERD.

384. **Which of the following groups is at greatest risk of Barrett's metaplasia progressing to adenocarcinoma?**
Harrison's 20th Ed. Chapter 316 Page 2216
- A. Obese black males in fifth decade of life
- B. Obese white males in fifth decade of life
- C. Obese black males in sixth decade of life
- D. Obese white males in sixth decade of life

Barrett's metaplasia can progress to adenocarcinoma and the group at greatest risk is obese white males in their sixth decade of life.

385. **Which of the following foods is "refluxogenic"?**
Harrison's 20th Ed. Chapter 316 Page 2217
- A. Peppermint
- B. Coffee and tea
- C. Alcohol
- D. All of the above

Foods that reduce lower esophageal sphincter pressure are called "refluxogenic". These include fatty foods, alcohol, spearmint, peppermint, tomato-based foods, coffee and tea.

386. **Absorption of which of the following may be compromised on indefinite treatment with PPIs?**
Harrison's 20th Ed. Chapter 316 Page 2217
- A. Vitamin B12
- B. Calcium
- C. Iron
- D. All of the above

With indefinite treatment with PPIs, Vitamin B12, calcium, and iron absorption may be compromised and susceptibility to enteric infections, particularly Clostridium difficile colitis increased.

387. **Which of the following has been reported with indefinite treatment with PPIs?**
Harrison's 20th Ed. Chapter 316 Page 2217
- A. Interstitial nephritis
- B. Severe, reversible hypomagnesemia
- C. Clostridium difficile colitis
- D. All of the above

388. **Multiple esophageal mucosal rings are characteristic of?**
Harrison's 20th Ed. Chapter 316 Page 2217
- A. Eosinophilic esophagitis
- B. Radiation esophagitis
- C. Corrosive esophagitis
- D. Candida esophagitis

Multiple mucosal rings (feline esophagus) are characteristic of eosinophilic esophagitis.

389. **Characteristic endoscopic finding of Eosinophilic Esophagitis is?**
Harrison's 20th Ed. Chapter 316 Page 2217
- A. Multiple esophageal rings
- B. Linear furrows
- C. White punctate exudates
- D. All of the above

The characteristic endoscopic findings of Eosinophilic Esophagitis (EoE) include multiple esophageal rings, linear furrows, and white punctate exudates.

390. **For diagnosis of eosinophilic esophagitis, eosinophils in esophagal mucosa per high-power field should be?**
Harrison's 20th Ed. Chapter 316 Page 2217
- A. 5 or more
- B. 10 or more
- C. 15 or more
- D. 20 or more

The diagnosis of eosinophilic esophagitis is made histologically, with 15 or more eosinophils per high-power field in the esophagal mucosa. Normal esophagus contains almost no eosinophils.

391. Preferred treatment of eosinophilic esophagitis is?
Harrison's 20th Ed. Chapter 316 Page 2218
   A. H_2 receptor blocking agents
   B. Nifedipine
   C. Swallowed fluticasone propionate
   D. Isosorbide dinitrate

Treatment of eosinophilic esophagitis consists of a 12-week course of swallowed fluticasone propionate using a metered dose inhaler. Anti human interleukin 5, systemic steroids, montelukast or cromolyn may be useful.

392. Risk of development of esophageal adenocarcinoma in Barrett's metaplasia is increased by?
N Engl J Med. 2006;354:1403-9
   A. 5 fold
   B. 10 fold
   C. 15 fold
   D. 20 fold

Risk of development of esophageal adenocarcinoma in Barrett's metaplasia is increased by 20 fold.

393. Esophageal mucosal biopsies should be taken at least?
N Engl J Med. 2006;354:1403-9
   A. 2 cm above the LES
   B. 5 cm above the LES
   C. 7 cm above the LES
   D. 9 cm above the LES

Mucosal biopsies should be performed at least 5 cm above LES, as esophageal mucosal changes of chronic esophagitis are frequent in the most distal esophagus in otherwise normal individuals.

394. Which of the following about Bernstein test is false?
N Engl J Med. 2006;354:1403-9
   A. Infusion of 0.1 N HCl & saline in esophagus
   B. Useful in diagnosing Barrett's esophagus that is not endoscopically obvious
   C. In symptomatic esophagitis, infusion of acid, but not of saline, reproduces symptoms of heartburn
   D. Infusion of acid in normal individuals produces no symptom

Bernstein test involves infusion of solutions of 0.1 N HCl or normal saline in esophagus. In symptomatic esophagitis, infusion of acid, but not of saline, reproduces the symptoms of heartburn. Infusion of acid in normal individuals usually produces no symptoms.

395. Which of the following statements about Barrett's esophagus is false?
N Engl J Med. 2006;354:1403-9
   A. Barrett's esophagus is an acquired condition
   B. Metaplasia occurs from esophageal columnar to squamous epithelium
   C. Complication of severe reflux esophagitis
   D. Risk factor for esophageal adenocarcinoma

Metaplasia of esophageal squamous epithelium to columnar epithelium (Barrett's esophagus) is a complication of severe reflux esophagitis. Finding intestinal metaplasia with goblet cells in esophagus is diagnostic of Barrett's esophagus.

396. Methods for mucosal ablation in Barrett's esophagus include all except?
N Engl J Med. 2006;354:1403-9
   A. Electrocautery
   B. Mucosal stripping
   C. Argon-plasma-beam fulguration
   D. Chemical fulguration

397. Methods for mucosal ablation in Barrett's esophagus include all except?
N Engl J Med. 2006;354:1403-9
   A. Laser photothermal coagulation
   B. Heater-probe ablation
   C. Hyperbaric oxygen ablation
   D. Cryotherapy

398. Photosensitizing agent used in photodynamic therapy for Barrett's esophagus is?
N Engl J Med. 2006;354:1403-9
   A. Trigen sodium
   B. Porfimer sodium
   C. Sugran sodium
   D. Mofetil sodium

399. Odynophagia is a characteristic symptom of?
Harrison's 20th Ed. Chapter 316 Page 2218
   A. Pill-induced esophagitis
   B. Reflux esophagitis
   C. Esophageal perforation
   D. Infectious esophagitis

Regardless of the infectious agent, odynophagia is a characteristic symptom of infectious esophagitis. Odynophagia is uncommon with reflux esophagitis.

400. Feline esophagus best relates to which of the following?
Harrison's 20th Ed. Chapter 315 Page 2203
   A. Herpes simplex virus esophagitis
   B. Candida esophagitis
   C. Eosinophilic esophagitis
   D. Radiation esophagitis

The presence of linear furrows and multiple corrugated rings throughout a narrowed esophagus (feline esophagus) should raise suspicion for eosinophilic esophagitis.

401. Which of the following is characteristic of Candida esophagitis?
Harrison's 20th Ed. Chapter 316 Page 2218
   A. Bleeding
   B. White plaques with friability
   C. Perforation
   D. Stricture

Candida esophagitis has a characteristic appearance of white plaques with friability. Rarely, Candida esophagitis is complicated by bleeding, perforation, stricture, or systemic invasion.

402. Candida esophagitis can be treated with?
Harrison's 20th Ed. Chapter 316 Page 2218
   A. Fluconazole
   B. Echinocandin
   C. Voriconazole
   D. Any of the above

Oral fluconazole, itraconazole, voriconazole or posaconazole are effective. Poorly responsive patients or those who cannot swallow medications can be treated with an intravenous echinocandin (caspofungin).

403. "Volcano-like" esophageal ulcerations are seen in?
N Engl J Med. 2006;354:1403-9
   A. Candidiasis
   B. HSV
   C. CMV
   D. Corrosive poisoning

In HSV (1 or 2) infection of esophagus, endoscopy shows vesicles & small, discrete, punched-out ("volcano-like") superficial ulcerations with or without a fibrinous exudate.

404. Eosinophilic Cowdry's type A inclusion bodies is related to?
Harrison's 20th Ed. Chapter 316 Page 2218

A. Herpes simplex esophagitis
B. Candida esophagitis
C. Radiation esophagitis
D. Cytomegalovirus esophagitis

Herpes simplex infections are limited to squamous epithelium. Biopsies shows characteristic ground-glass nuclei, eosinophilic Cowdry's type A inclusion bodies and giant cells.

405. Herpes simplex virus (HSV) esophagitis is treated with?
Harrison's 20th Ed. Chapter 316 Page 2218

A. Acyclovir
B. Valacyclovir
C. Famciclovir
D. All of the above

406. Which of the following infections occur primarily in immunocompromised patients?
Harrison's 20th Ed. Chapter 316 Page 2218

A. Herpes simplex virus (HSV) esophagitis
B. Varicella-zoster virus (VZV) esophagitis
C. Cytomegalovirus (CMV) esophagitis
D. Candida esophagitis

Cytomegalovirus (CMV) infections occur primarily in immunocompromised patients, particularly transplant recipients.

407. Serpiginous ulcers in an otherwise normal esophageal mucosa is a feature of?
Harrison's 20th Ed. Chapter 316 Page 2218

A. Herpes simplex virus (HSV) esophagitis
B. Varicella-zoster virus (VZV) esophagitis
C. Cytomegalovirus (CMV) esophagitis
D. Candida esophagitis

Endoscopically, CMV lesions appear as serpiginous ulcers in an otherwise normal mucosa, particularly in the distal esophagus.

408. Ganciclovir is the treatment of choice for?
Harrison's 20th Ed. Chapter 316 Page 2218

A. Herpes simplex virus (HSV) esophagitis
B. Varicella-zoster virus (VZV) esophagitis
C. Cytomegalovirus (CMV) esophagitis
D. Candida esophagitis

Ganciclovir, 5 mg/kg BD IV, is the treatment of choice for Cytomegalovirus (CMV) esophagitis.

409. Boerhaave's syndrome refers to?
Harrison's 20th Ed. Chapter 316 Page 2219

A. Esophagial damage due to instrumentation
B. Esophagial damage due to vomiting or retching
C. Esophagial damage due to external trauma
D. None of the above

Boerhaave's syndrome or spontaneous rupture refers to esophageal rupture at gastroesophageal junction caused by increased intraesophageal pressure associated with forceful vomiting or retching.

410. Instrumental perforation usually occurs in?
Harrison's 20th Ed. Chapter 316 Page 2219

A. Upper esophagus
B. Mid esophagus
C. Lower esophagus
D. Any of the above

Instrumental perforation occurs in pharynx or lower esophagus, just above diaphragm in posterolateral wall.

411. Esophageal perforation may cause?
Harrison's 20th Ed. Chapter 316 Page 2219

A. Pneumomediastinum
B. Subcutaneous emphysema
C. Mediastinitis
D. All of the above

412. Mallory-Weiss syndrome can be caused by?
Harrison's 20th Ed. Chapter 316 Page 2219

A. Vomiting
B. Retching
C. Vigorous coughing
D. All of the above

Vomiting, retching, or vigorous coughing can cause a nontransmural tear at the gastroesophageal junction that is Mallory-Weiss Syndrome.

413. Which of the following is false about Mallory-Weiss syndrome?
Harrison's 20th Ed. Chapter 316 Page 2219

A. Usually involves esophageal mucosa
B. Upper gastrointestinal bleeding
C. In most patients bleeding ceases spontaneously
D. Respond to vasopressin therapy

Mallory-Weiss Syndrome refers to nontransmural tear or mucosal tear involving gastric mucosa near the squamocolumnar mucosal junction caused by vomiting, retching or vigorous coughing. Upper gastrointestinal bleeding may be severe but in mostly bleeding ceases spontaneously. Respond to vasopressin therapy or angiographic embolization.

414. Which of the following increases the risk of radiation esophagitis?
Harrison's 20th Ed. Chapter 316 Page 2219

A. Doxorubicin
B. Bleomycin
C. Cyclophosphamide
D. All of the above

Radiosensitizing drugs such as doxorubicin, bleomycin, cyclophosphamide and cisplatin increase the risk of radiation esophagitis.

415. Treatment with which of the following can reduce esophagitis during radiation treatment?
Harrison's 20th Ed. Chapter 316 Page 2219

A. Cimetidine
B. Indomethacin
C. Allopurinol
D. Sucralfate

Indomethacin treatment may reduce radiation damage of esophagus.

416. **Patients with alkaline esophagitis are treated with?**
    Harrison's 20th Ed. Chapter 316 Page 2219
    A. Cholestyramine
    B. Aluminum hydroxide
    C. Sucralfate
    D. All of the above

Treatment of alkaline esophagitis includes neutralization of bile salts with cholestyramine, aluminum hydroxide, or sucralfate.

417. **Pill-induced esophagitis can be caused by all except?**
    Harrison's 20th Ed. Chapter 316 Page 2219
    A. Alendronate
    B. Ferrous sulfate
    C. Doxycycline
    D. Medroxyprogesterone

Pill-induced esophagitis mostly occurs with ingestion of doxycycline, tetracycline, quinidine, phenytoin, potassium chloride, ferrous sulfate, nonsteroidal anti-inflammatory drugs (NSAIDs), and bisphosphonates.

418. **Most common location for the pill to lodge is in?**
    Harrison's 20th Ed. Chapter 316 Page 2219
    A. Upper esophagus
    B. Mid esophagus
    C. Lower esophagus
    D. Any of the above.

The most common location for the pill to lodge is in the mid-esophagus near the crossing of the aorta or carina.

419. **Which of the following is sometimes tried before endoscopic dislodgement of impacted food?**
    Harrison's 20th Ed. Chapter 316 Page 2219
    A. Adrenaline
    B. Isoprenaline
    C. Glucagon
    D. Atropine

420. **Esophageal lesion in systemic sclerosis consist of?**
    Harrison's 20th Ed. Chapter 316 Page 2219
    A. Atrophy of smooth muscle
    B. Weakness in lower two-thirds of esophagus
    C. Incompetence of LES
    D. All of the above

Esophageal lesions in systemic sclerosis consist of atrophy of smooth muscle, manifested by weakness in lower two-thirds of esophagus & incompetence of LES.

421. **Which of the following dermatologic disorders can cause esophagitis?**
    Harrison's 20th Ed. Chapter 316 Page 2219
    A. Pemphigus vulgaris
    B. Bullous pemphigoid
    C. Cicatricial pemphigoid
    D. All of the above

422. **What is normal integrated relaxation pressure?**
    Cleveland Clinic Journal of Medicine 2017;84(6):446
    A. < 5 mm Hg
    B. < 15 mm Hg
    C. < 25 mm Hg
    D. < 35 mm Hg

Integrated relaxation pressure is a measurement of lower esophageal relaxation. Normal is <15 mm Hg.

423. **What is normal distal latency?**
    Cleveland Clinic Journal of Medicine 2017;84(6):446
    A. > 2.5 seconds
    B. > 3.5 seconds
    C. > 4.5 seconds
    D. > 5.5 seconds

Distal latency is the time from onset to completion of the peristaltic wave during the swallow. Normal is greater than 4.5 seconds. Distal latency less than 4.5 seconds indicates a premature contraction. In distal esophageal spasm, there is normal lower esophageal sphincter relaxation (median integrated relaxation pressure < 15 mm Hg) and ≥ 20% of swallows are premature contraction in the distal esophagus (distal latency < 4.5 seconds).

424. **What is normal distal contractile integral?**
    Cleveland Clinic Journal of Medicine 2017;84(6):446
    A. 150 and 8,000 mm Hg · s · cm
    B. 250 and 8,000 mm Hg · s · cm
    C. 350 and 8,000 mm Hg · s · cm
    D. 450 and 8,000 mm Hg · s · cm

Distal contractile integral is the measure of vigor of peristaltic contraction. Normal is between 450 and 8,000 mm Hg · s · cm. Hypercontractile ('jackhammer') esophagus is characterized by distal contractile integral > 8,000 mm Hg · s · cm in at least 2 swallows.

Peptic Ulcer Disease and Related Disorders

425. Rumination is best related to?
Harrison's 20th Ed. Chapter 41 Page 253

A. Nausea
B. Vomiting
C. Regurgitation
D. All of the above

Rumination refers to repeated voluntary regurgitation of stomach contents, which may be rechewed and reswallowed.

426. Under normal conditions, frequency of slow wave cycles in the stomach is?
Harrison's 20th Ed. Chapter 41 Page 253

A. 3 cycles / minute
B. 6 cycles / minute
C. 9 cycles / minute
D. 12 cycles / minute

427. Under normal conditions, frequency of slow wave cycles in the duodenum is?
Harrison's 20th Ed. Chapter 41 Page 253

A. 4 cycles / minute
B. 8 cycles / minute
C. 11 cycles / minute
D. 15 cycles / minute

Under normal conditions, distally migrating gut contractions, the slow wave, occur at 3 cycles/minute in the stomach and 11 cycles/minute in duodenum.

428. Which of the following is termed the chemoreceptor trigger zone?
Harrison's 20th Ed. Chapter 41 Page 253

A. Area postrema
B. Nucleus tractus solitarius
C. Dorsal vagal nuclei
D. Phrenic nuclei

Area postrema, a medullary nucleus, responds to bloodborne emetic stimuli and is termed the chemoreceptor trigger zone.

429. Which of the following act on the area postrema?
Harrison's 20th Ed. Chapter 41 Page 253

A. Uremia
B. Hypoxia
C. Ketoacidosis
D. All of the above

Uremia, hypoxia, and ketoacidosis act on the area postrema and are emetogenic.

430. Which of the following stimulate induction of vomiting in labyrinthine disorders is?
Harrison's 20th Ed. Chapter 41 Page 253

A. Muscarinic M_1 receptors
B. Histaminergic H_2 receptors
C. Serotonin 5-HT_3 receptors
D. Dopamine D_2 receptors

Neurotransmitters that mediate induction of vomiting in labyrinthine disorders is vestibular muscarinic M_1 and histaminergic H_1 receptors, whereas vagal afferent stimuli activate serotonin 5-HT_3 receptors. Area postrema is richly served by nerves acting on 5-HT_3, M_1, H_1, and dopamine D_2 subtypes.

431. Gastroparesis occurs after which of the following?
Harrison's 20th Ed. Chapter 41 Page 254

A. Pancreatic adenocarcinoma
B. Mesenteric vascular insufficiency
C. Scleroderma
D. All of the above

Gastroparesis or a delay in gastric emptying of food occurs after vagotomy, with pancreatic adenocarcinoma, with mesenteric vascular insufficiency, or in systemic diseases such as diabetes, scleroderma, and amyloidosis. Anorexia nervosa, bulimia nervosa, anxiety, and depression may cause significant nausea that may be associated with delayed gastric emptying.

432. Gastroparesis does not occur with which of the following?
Harrison's 20th Ed. Chapter 41 Page 254

A. Diabetes
B. Amyloidosis
C. Scleroderma
D. Cyclic vomiting syndrome

Cyclic vomiting syndrome produces periodic discrete episodes of relentless nausea & vomiting and has a strong association with migraine headaches. Cyclic vomiting is most common in children, although adult cases occur in association with rapid gastric emptying & with chronic cannabis use.

433. Which of the following drugs is a highly emetogenic agent?
Harrison's 20th Ed. Chapter 41 Page 254

A. Digoxin
B. Oral contraceptives
C. Cisplatin
D. Erythromycin

Acute emesis from intensely emetogenic cisplatin is mediated by 5-HT_3 pathways.

434. What proportion of pregnant women experience nausea in the first trimester?
Harrison's 20th Ed. Chapter 41 Page 254

A. 25%
B. 50%
C. 70%
D. 90%

Nausea affects 70% of pregnant women in first trimester.

435. Relief of abdominal pain by emesis is characteristic of?
Harrison's 20th Ed. Chapter 41 Page 255

A. Pancreatitis
B. Zenker's diverticulum
C. Gastric obstruction
D. Intestinal obstruction

Relief of abdominal pain by emesis characterizes intestinal obstruction, whereas vomiting has no effect on pancreatitis or cholecystitis pain.

436. Which of the following antiemetic agent is a Serotonin5-HT$_3$ antagonist?
Harrison's 20th Ed. Chapter 41 Page 256

   A. Meclizine
   B. Granisetron
   C. Mirtazapine
   D. Dimenhydrinate

Antiemetic agent ondansetron and granisetron are Serotonin5-HT$_3$ antagonists. Meclizine & dimenhydrinate are antihistamines. Scopolamine is an anticholinergic drug.

437. Which of the following is a combined 5-HT$_4$ agonist and D$_2$ antagonist?
Harrison's 20th Ed. Chapter 41 Page 256

   A. Metoclopramide
   B. Domperidone
   C. Erythromycin
   D. Octreotide

Metoclopramide is a combined 5-HT$_4$ agonist & D$_2$ antagonist. Domperidone is a D$_2$ antagonist. Erythromycin increases gastroduodenal motility by action on receptors for motilin. Somatostatin analogue octreotide induces propagative small intestinal motor complexes.

438. Which of the following is a Neurokinin NK$_1$ antagonist?
Harrison's 20th Ed. Chapter 41 Page 255 Table 41-2

   A. Aprepitant
   B. Kevetiracetam
   C. Cyproheptadine
   D. Sumatriptan

Aprepitant is a neurokinin NK$_1$ antagonist that has antiemetic & antinausea effects during acute and delayed periods after chemotherapy.

439. Gastric pits of stomach branch into?
Harrison's 20th Ed. Chapter 317 Page 2220

   A. 1 or 2 gastric glands
   B. 3 or 4 gastric glands
   C. 4 or 5 gastric glands
   D. 6 or 7 gastric glands

Microscopic gastric pits (foveolus) of gastric epithelial lining branch into four or five gastric glands made up of highly specialized epithelial cells.

440. Which of the following cells is found deepest in the oxyntic gastric gland?
Harrison's 20th Ed. Chapter 317 Page 2220 Figure 317-1

   A. Mucous neck cells
   B. Parietal cells
   C. Endocrine cells
   D. Chief cells

441. Parietal cell is also known as?
Harrison's 20th Ed. Chapter 317 Page 2220

   A. Mucous cell
   B. Oxyntic cell
   C. Endocrine cell
   D. Enterochromaffin-like (ECL) cell

Parietal cell is also known as oxyntic cell and is found in neck, or isthmus, or in oxyntic gland.

442. Peptic ulcer disease (PUD) occurs due to constant attack on gastroduodenal mucosa by all noxious agents except?
Harrison's 20th Ed. Chapter 317 Page 2220

   A. Hydrochloric acid (HCl)
   B. Pepsinogen/pepsin
   C. Bile acids
   D. Salivary amylase

443. PUD occurs due to constant attack on gastroduodenal mucosa by all noxious agents except?
Harrison's 20th Ed. Chapter 317 Page 2220

   A. Pancreatic enzymes
   B. Alcohol
   C. Virus
   D. Bacteria

PUD occurs due to constant attack on gastroduodenal mucosa by endogenous noxious agents like acid, pepsin, bile acids, pancreatic enzymes or exogenous substances like medications, alcohol & bacteria.

444. Which of the following is an element of gastric mucosal defense system?
Harrison's 20th Ed. Chapter 317 Page 2221

   A. Preepithelial
   B. Epithelial
   C. Subepithelial
   D. All of the above

Gastric mucosal defense is a 3-level barrier composed of preepithelial, epithelial & subepithelial elements.

445. First line of defense of gastric epithelium is?
Harrison's 20th Ed. Chapter 317 Page 2221

   A. Mucus layer
   B. Bicarbonate-phospholipid layer
   C. Phospholipid layer
   D. Mucus-bicarbonate-phospholipid layer

The first line of defense of gastric epithelium is a mucus-bicarbonate-phospholipid layer that serves as a physicochemical barrier. Surface epithelial cells provide the next line of defense.

446. Surface epithelial cells generate which of the following?
Harrison's 20th Ed. Chapter 317 Page 2221 Figure 317-3

   A. Heat shock proteins
   B. Trefoil peptides
   C. Antimicrobial cathelicidins
   D. All of the above

Surface epithelial cells generate heat shock proteins that prevent protein denaturation, trefoil factor family peptides and antimicrobial cathelicidins, which play a role in surface cell protection and regeneration.

447. Trefoil factor family (TFF) peptides were formerly known as?
Cellular and Molecular Life Sciences. 2009; 66(8):1350-1369

   A. C-domain peptides
   B. D-domain peptides
   C. G-domain peptides
   D. P-domain peptides

Trefoil factor family peptides (TFF1, TFF2, TFF3) were formerly called P-domain peptides promote wound healing in the gut through epithelial restitution. TFF peptides are found in mucous membranes of stomach, conjunctiva, Brunner's glands, intestine, salivary glands, uterus and respiratory tract.

448. Cathelicidin is best related to?
Mol Biol Rep. 2012; 39(12):10957-10970
- A. P-domain peptides
- B. Antimicrobial peptides (AMPs)
- C. Angiogenesis
- D. All of the above

Antimicrobial peptides (AMPs) have the capacity to rapidly inactivate infectious agents. The two major AMP families in mammals are the defensins and cathelicidin peptides.

449. Continuous cell renewal accomplished by proliferation of progenitor cells is regulated by?
Gastroenterology. 2008;135:41-60
- A. Growth factors
- B. PGE2
- C. Survivin
- D. All of the above

Survivin is a member of the inhibitor of apoptosis (IAP) protein family that inhibits caspases & blocks cell death. It is highly expressed in most cancers and is associated with a poor clinical outcome.

450. In seriously ill patients, which of the following cause reperfusion injury?
N Engl J Med. 2018;378:2506-16
- A. Proinflammatory state
- B. Splanchnic hypoperfusion
- C. Impaired microcirculation
- D. All of the above

In seriously ill patients, proinflammatory states, splanchnic hypoperfusion, and impaired microcirculation induce ischemia, reperfusion injury, and low gastric intramucosal pH.

451. Surface epithelial cells secrete which of the following?
N Engl J Med. 2018;378:2506-16
- A. Mucus
- B. Bicarbonate
- C. Prostaglandins
- D. All of the above

Beneath the layer of alkaline mucus gel lining are surface epithelial cells that secrete mucus, bicarbonate, prostaglandins. Surface epithelial cells are regenerated by mucosal progenitor cells.

452. Which of the following is a predictor of clinically important upper gastrointestinal bleeding in patients in ICU?
N Engl J Med. 2018;378:2506-16
- A. Coagulopathy
- B. Renal-replacement therapy
- C. Use of acid suppressants
- D. All of the above

Predictors of clinically important upper gastrointestinal bleeding in patients in the ICU include invasive mechanical ventilation for 48 hours or longer, coagulopathy, three or more coexisting diseases, liver disease, renal-replacement therapy, a high organ-failure score, & use of acid suppressants.

453. Which of the following define clinically important upper GI bleeding?
N Engl J Med. 2018;378:2506-16
- A. Orthostatic increase in pulse of ≥20 beats/minute and decrease in systolic BP of 10 mm Hg
- B. Decrease in hemoglobin of ≥2 g/dL over a 24-hour period
- C. Transfusion of ≥2 units of PRBCs within 24 hour after start of bleeding
- D. All of the above

454. With acid suppression, there is evidence of an increased risk of?
N Engl J Med. 2018;378:2506-16
- A. Gastric perforation
- B. Pancreatitis
- C. Pneumonia
- D. All of the above

Pharmacoepidemiologic studies provide support for an increased risk of pneumonia with acid suppression.

455. With acid suppression, there is evidence of an increased risk of?
N Engl J Med. 2018;378:2506-16
- A. Achalasia
- B. Duodenitis
- C. C. difficile infection
- D. Ileus

Hospital-acquired C. difficile infection showed an association with proton-pump inhibitors among patients in medical & surgical units.

456. Restitution of gastric mucosa means?
Harrison's 20th Ed. Chapter 317 Page 2221
- A. Proliferation of damaged gastric mucosa
- B. Regeneration of damaged gastric mucosa
- C. Migration of normal gastric epithelium to damaged areas
- D. All of the above

Restitution is migration of gastric epithelial cells bordering site of injury when preepithelial barrier is breached.

457. Which of the following statements about restitution is false?
Harrison's 20th Ed. Chapter 317 Page 2222
- A. Occurs independent of cell division
- B. Requires uninterrupted blood flow
- C. Requires an alkaline pH in surroundings
- D. None of the above

Restitution occurs independent of cell division and requires uninterrupted blood flow and an alkaline pH in the surrounding environment.

458. Restitution of gastric mucosa is modulated by?
Harrison's 20th Ed. Chapter 317 Page 2222
- A. Epidermal growth factor (EGF)
- B. Transforming growth factor alpha (TGF-α)
- C. Fibroblast growth factor (FGF)
- D. All of the above

Growth factors like epidermal growth factor (EGF), transforming growth factor (TGF) alpha and basic fibroblast growth factor (FGF) modulate restitution.

459. Gastric epithelial cell regeneration is regulated by?
Harrison's 20th Ed. Chapter 317 Page 2222
- A. Prostaglandins
- B. Epidermal growth factor (EGF)
- C. Transforming growth factor-alpha (TGF-α)
- D. All of the above

Larger defects not effectively repaired by restitution require cell proliferation. Epithelial cell regeneration is regulated by prostaglandins, EGF & TGF-alpha.

460. **Angiogenesis in the gastric mucosa is regulated by?**
    Harrison's 20th Ed. Chapter 317 Page 2222
    A. Fibroblast growth factor (FGF)
    B. Vascular endothelial growth factor (VEGF)
    C. Gastric peptide gastrin
    D. All of the above

461. **Bicarbonate secretion in stomach is stimulated by all except?**
    Harrison's 20th Ed. Chapter 317 Page 2222
    A. Calcium
    B. Prostaglandins
    C. VIP
    D. Luminal acidification

462. **Which of the following plays a central role in gastric epithelial defense / repair?**
    Harrison's 20th Ed. Chapter 317 Page 2222
    A. Mucosal bicarbonate
    B. Mucus
    C. Prostaglandins
    D. Growth factor

463. **Prostaglandins are important in gastric epithelial defense / repair due to all except?**
    Harrison's 20th Ed. Chapter 317 Page 2222
    A. Release of mucosal bicarbonate and mucus
    B. Inhibition of parietal cell secretion
    C. Maintaining mucosal lymphatic flow
    D. Epithelial cell restitution

Pg's in gastric mucosa play a central role in gastric epithelial defense/repair. Pg regulate release of mucosal bicarbonate & mucus, inhibit parietal cell secretion & maintain mucosal blood flow & epithelial cell restitution.

464. **Key enzyme that controls the rate-limiting step in prostaglandin synthesis is?**
    Harrison's 20th Ed. Chapter 317 Page 2222
    A. Thromboxane A_2 (TXA_2)
    B. Phospholipase A_2
    C. Cyclooxygenase (COX)
    D. Prostacyclin (PGI_2)

Prostaglandins are derived from esterified arachidonic acid which is formed from phospholipids (cell membrane) by the action of phospholipase A2. Key enzyme that controls the rate-limiting step in prostaglandin synthesis is cyclooxygenase (COX) which is present in two isoforms - COX-1 & COX-2.

465. **COX-1 is expressed in all except?**
    Harrison's 20th Ed. Chapter 317 Page 2222
    A. Stomach
    B. Platelets
    C. Kidneys
    D. Liver

COX-1 is expressed in stomach, platelets, kidneys, and endothelial cells. Gastro-intestinal mucosal ulceration & renal dysfunction is due to inhibition of COX-1.

466. **COX-2 is expressed in all except?**
    Harrison's 20th Ed. Chapter 317 Page 2222
    A. Macrophages
    B. Leukocytes
    C. Platelets
    D. Synovial cells

COX-2, induced by inflammatory stimuli is expressed in macrophages, leukocytes, fibroblasts & synovial cells.

467. **Selective COX-2 inhibitors increase the risk of?**
    Harrison's 20th Ed. Chapter 317 Page 2222
    A. Myocardial infarction
    B. Blindness
    C. Acute renal failure
    D. Fulminant hepatitis

Selective COX-2 inhibitors has adverse effects on the cardiovascular system, leading to increased risk of myocardial infarction. Valdecoxib and rofecoxib are banned by USFDA.

468. **Which of the following is a function of Nitric oxide (NO)?**
    Harrison's 20th Ed. Chapter 317 Page 2222
    A. Stimulates gastric mucus
    B. Increases mucosal blood flow
    C. Maintains epithelial cell barrier function
    D. All of the above

Nitric oxide (NO) is important in the maintenance of gastric mucosal integrity. The key enzyme NO synthase is constitutively expressed in the mucosa and contributes to cytoprotection by stimulating gastric mucus, increasing mucosal blood flow and maintaining epithelial cell barrier function.

469. **Gastric acid & pepsinogen play a physiologic role in?**
    Harrison's 20th Ed. Chapter 317 Page 2222
    A. Protein digestion
    B. Absorption of iron, calcium, magnesium & vitamin B_{12}
    C. Killing ingested bacteria
    D. All of the above

Gastric acid and pepsinogen play a physiologic role in protein digestion, absorption of iron, calcium, magnesium and vitamin B12 and killing ingested bacteria.

470. **Which of the following is capable of inducing mucosal injury?**
    Harrison's 20th Ed. Chapter 317 Page 2222
    A. Amylin
    B. Phospholipase A_2
    C. Pepsinogen
    D. Ghrelin

Hydrochloric acid and pepsinogen are the two principal gastric secretory products capable of inducing mucosal injury.

471. **Which of the following about acid production in stomach is false?**
    Harrison's 20th Ed. Chapter 317 Page 2222
    A. Basal acid production occurs in a circadian pattern
    B. Cholinergic & histaminergic input are the principal contributors to basal acid secretion
    C. Stimulated gastric acid secretion occurs in cephalic, gastric & intestinal phases
    D. Cephalic phase stimulates gastric secretion via hormones

Cephalic phase stimulates gastric secretion via vagus nerve.

472. Which of the following about acid production in stomach is false?
Harrison's 20th Ed. Chapter 317 Page 2222

A. Cephalic phase stimulates gastric secretion via vagus
B. Gastric phase is activated when food enters stomach
C. Amino acids stimulate vagus to release gastrin
D. Intestinal phase is mediated by luminal distention

Gastric phase is activated once food enters stomach. Amino acids and amines directly stimulate G cell to release gastrin, which in turn activate parietal cell.

473. Gastric acid production is inhibited by?
Harrison's 20th Ed. Chapter 317 Page 2222

A. Prostaglandins
B. Somatostatin
C. EGF
D. All of the above

Gastric acid production is inhibited by prostaglandins, somatostatin & epidermal growth factor (EGF).

474. Which of the following is a part of innate immune system?
Harrison's 20th Ed. Chapter 317 Page 2222

A. Dendritic cell
B. Epithelial cells
C. Macrophages
D. All of the above

475. Which of the following about basal acid secretion is false?
Harrison's 20th Ed. Chapter 317 Page 2222

A. Highest levels during night & lowest during morning hours
B. Cholinergic input via the vagus nerve play a role
C. Histaminergic input from local gastric sources play a role
D. None of the above

476. Histamine is released in stomach from?
Harrison's 20th Ed. Chapter 317 Page 2222

A. D cells
B. ECL cells
C. Gr cells
D. G cells

477. Somatostatin is released from D cells in response to?
Harrison's 20th Ed. Chapter 317 Page 2222

A. Pepsinogen
B. HCl
C. Secretin
D. All of the above

GI hormone somatostatin is released from endocrine cells in gastric mucosa (D cells) in response to HCl.

478. Somatostatin inhibits acid production by?
Harrison's 20th Ed. Chapter 317 Page 2222

A. Decreasing histamine release from ECL cells
B. Decreasing ghrelin release from Gr cells
C. Decreasing gastrin release from G cells
D. All of the above

479. Somatostatin acts by?
Harrison's 20th Ed. Chapter 317 Page 2222

A. Direct inhibition of parietal cells
B. Decreased histamine release from ECL cells
C. Decreased gastrin release from G cells
D. All of the above

Somatostatin is released from endocrine cells in gastric mucosa (D cells) in response to HCl. Somatostatin inhibits acid production by direct action on parietal cell, decreased histamine release from enterochromaffin-like (ECL) cells and gastrin release from G cells.

480. Which of the following hormone play a role in counterbalancing acid secretion?
Harrison's 20th Ed. Chapter 317 Page 2222

A. Atrial natriuretic peptide (ANP)
B. Cholecystokinin
C. Obestatin
D. All of the above

Amylin, atrial natriuretic peptide (ANP), cholecystokinin, ghrelin, interleukin 11 (IL-11), obestatin, secretin, and serotonin play a role in counterbalancing acid secretion.

481. Which of the following is the appetite-regulating hormone?
Harrison's 20th Ed. Chapter 317 Page 2222

A. Amylin
B. Obestatin
C. Secretin
D. Ghrelin

Ghrelin is the appetite-regulating hormone expressed in Gr cells in the stomach, may increase gastric acid secretion through stimulation of histamine release from ECL cells.

482. Which of the following about Ghrelin is false?
Journal of Clinical Endocrinology and Metabolism, 2005;90(4):2205-2211

A. Only peptide hormone modified by a fatty acid
B. Natural ligand for growth hormone secretagogue receptor (GHS-R)
C. Influences secretion of growth hormone
D. None of the above

Orexigenic Ghrelin is the only known peptide hormone modified by a fatty acid. Ghrelin is the natural ligand for the growth hormone secretagogue (GHS) receptor (GHS-R). Major biological functions of ghrelin include secretion of growth hormone, stimulation of appetite & food intake, modulation of gastric acid secretion & motility, and modulation of endocrine and exocrine pancreatic secretions.

483. Ghrelin is expressed in?
Journal of Clinical Endocrinology and Metabolism, 2005;90(4):2205-2211

A. Stomach
B. Lung
C. Testis
D. All of the above

Suffix "Ghre" means "to grow". It was discovered in 1999 as a peptide hormone. In addition to stomach, ghrelin is expressed in duodenum, jejunum, ileum, colon, lung, heart, pancreas, kidney, testis, pituitary, and hypothalamus.

484. Which of the following is called ghrelin's antagonistic hormone?
Journal of Clinical Endocrinology and Metabolism, 2005;90(4):2205-2211

A. Nucleobindin2 / Nesfatin-1
B. Leptin
C. Neuropeptide Y
D. All of the above

Orexigenic and anorexigenic peptides control appetite. Orexigenic peptides include neuropeptides Y (NPY), agouti-related peptide (AGRP), orexins, melanin-concentrating hormone (MCH), galanin, & ghrelin. Ghrelin is the only one acting peripherally to stimulate appetite, while all other orexigenic peptides act centrally. Anorexigenic peptides include melanocortin (a-MSH), cocaine- and amphetamine- regulated transcript (CART), corticotrophin-releasing hormone (CRH), cholecystokinin (CCK), gastrin-related peptide (GRP), glucagon like peptides 1 and 2 (GLP1, GLP2), pancreatic polypeptide (PP), peptide YY (PYY)), and leptin.

485. Which of the following is a cell type in gastric mucosa?
Journal of Clinical Endocrinology and Metabolism, 2005;90(4):2205-2211

A. Enterochromaffin-like cells (ECL)
B. D cells
C. P/D1 cell
D. All of the above

Gastric mucosa is composed of five endocrine cell types: enterochromaffin cells (EC), enterochromaffin-like cells (ECL), D cells, G cells, and X/A like cells or P/D1 cell which, respectively, secrete serotonin, histamine, somatostatin, gastrin, and ghrelin.

486. X/A-like cells or P/D1 cells release which of the following?
J Neurogastroenterol Motil. 2012;18(2):138-149

A. Desacyl ghrelin
B. Obestatin
C. Nesfatin-1
D. All of the above

X/A-like cells produce desacyl ghrelin, obestatin and nesfatin-1.

487. Which of the following about parietal cells is false?
Harrison's 20th Ed. Chapter 317 Page 2222

A. Located in oxyntic gland
B. Does not secrete intrinsic factor
C. Express receptors for histamine, gastrin & acetylcholine
D. Express receptors for ligands that inhibit acid production

Acid-secreting parietal cell secretes intrinsic factor (IF) and IL-11.

488. Activation of which of the following receptor on D-cells inhibits somatostatin release?
Harrison's 20th Ed. Chapter 317 Page 2223

A. H2 receptor
B. H3 receptor
C. M3 receptor
D. All of the above

489. Which of the following statements about enzyme H^+, K^+-ATPase is false?
Harrison's 20th Ed. Chapter 317 Page 2223

A. Responsible for generating large concentration of H^+
B. Membrane-bound protein consisting of α & β subunits
C. Active catalytic site is found within α subunit
D. Active catalytic site is found within β subunit

Active catalytic site is found within α subunit.

490. Which of the following statements about enzyme H^+, K^+-ATPase is false?
Harrison's 20th Ed. Chapter 317 Page 2223

A. Transfers H^+ ions from parietal cell cytoplasm to secretory canaliculi in exchange for K^+
B. Located within secretory canaliculus & in nonsecretory cytoplasmic tubulovesicles
C. Tubulovesicles are impermeable to K^+
D. At rest, 50% of pumps are within secretory canaliculus

Distribution of proton pumps between nonsecretory vesicles & secretory canaliculus varies according to parietal cell activity. They are recycled back to inactive state in cytoplasmic vesicles once parietal cell activation ceases.

491. Which of the following is an actin binding protein?
Harrison's 20th Ed. Chapter 317 Page 2223

A. Carin
B. Hamartin
C. Ezrin
D. Tuberin

492. Which of the following about chief cell is false?
Harrison's 20th Ed. Chapter 317 Page 2223

A. Found primarily in gastric fundus
B. Synthesize & secrete pepsinogen
C. Acid environment converts pepsinogen to pepsin
D. Pepsin activity is irreversibly inactivated & denatured at a pH of ≥4

Pepsin activity is significantly diminished at a pH of 4 and irreversibly inactivated and denatured at a pH of ≥7.

493. Which out of the following is the strongest risk factor for PUD?
Harrison's 20th Ed. Chapter 317 Page 2223

A. Chronic obstructive lung disease
B. Chronic renal insufficiency
C. Current tobacco use
D. Older age

Risk factors (odds ratio) for PUD are chronic obstructive lung disease (2.34), chronic renal insufficiency (2.29), current tobacco use (1.99), former tobacco use (1.55), older age (1.67), three or more doctor visits in a year (1.49), coronary heart disease (1.46), former alcohol use (1.29), African-American race (1.20), obesity (1.18) & diabetes (1.13).

494. All of the following about gastric ulcer are true except?
Harrison's 20th Ed. Chapter 317 Page 2223

A. A break in mucosal surface >5 mm in size
B. Depth to submucosa
C. More than half of gastric ulcers occur in males
D. Peak incidence is in the 4th decade of life

Gastric & duodenal ulcers are defined as breaks in mucosal surface >5 mm in size with depth to submucosa. Peak incidence of gastric ulcers is in the sixth decade & more than half of GUs occur in males.

495. ~90% of DU's occur within what distance from pylorus?
Harrison's 20th Ed. Chapter 317 Page 2223

A. 3 cm
B. 5 cm
C. 7 cm
D. 9 cm

~90% of DU's are located within 3 cm of the pylorus.

496. Which of the following statements about DU is false?
Harrison's 20th Ed. Chapter 317 Page 2223

A. Most often occur in first part of duodenum
B. Usually <=1 cm in diameter
C. Malignant DUs are extremely rare
D. Base of ulcer consists of neutrophilic necrosis with surrounding fibrosis

Base of DU consists of a zone of eosinophilic necrosis with surrounding fibrosis. Malignant DUs are rare.

497. Which of the following statements about GU is false?
Harrison's 20th Ed. Chapter 317 Page 2223

A. Can represent malignancy
B. Benign GUs are found distal to junction between antrum & acid secretory mucosa
C. Benign GUs are common in gastric fundus
D. Gastric acid output is normal or decreased in GU

Benign GUs are rare in the gastric fundus.

498. A chemical gastropathy is typified by?
Harrison's 20th Ed. Chapter 317 Page 2223

A. Foveolar hyperplasia
B. Edema of lamina propria
C. Epithelial regeneration in the absence of H. pylori
D. All of the above

499. Type IV Gastric Ulcers are found in?
Harrison's 20th Ed. Chapter 317 Page 2224

A. Cardia
B. Gastric body
C. Gastric antrum
D. Pylorus

Gastric ulcers are classified based on their location. Type I occur in gastric body, type II occur in antrum, type III occur within 3 cm of pylorus and type IV are found in the cardia.

500. Which of the following Gastric Ulcers has high gastric acid production?
Harrison's 20th Ed. Chapter 317 Page 2224

A. Type I
B. Type II
C. Type III
D. Type IV

Type III GU's occur within 3 cm of the pylorus and are commonly accompanied by duodenal ulcers and normal or high gastric acid production.

501. Helicobacter pylori was discovered by?
N Engl J Med. 2010;362:1597-604

A. Marshall B & Warren R
B. Julie Parsonnet & Jennings R
C. Banatvala N & Mayo K
D. Deeks JJ & Feldman RA

Helicobacter pylori is a gram-negative helical rod shaped bacterium found on the luminal surface of gastric epithelium. It was first isolated by Warren and Marshall in 1983.

502. Gastric infection with H. pylori can lead to?
Harrison's 20th Ed. Chapter 317 Page 2224

A. Peptic ulcer disease (PUD)
B. Gastric mucosal-associated lymphoid tissue lymphoma
C. Gastric adenocarcinoma
D. All of the above

H. pylori plays a role in the development of majority of PUD, gastric mucosal-associated lymphoid tissue (MALT) lymphoma and gastric adenocarcinoma.

503. Which of the following statements about H. pylori is false?
Harrison's 20th Ed. Chapter 317 Page 2224

A. It is a gram-positive microaerophilic rod
B. Found between mucous layer & gastric epithelium
C. Normally, it does not invade gastric epithelial cells
D. S-shaped & contains multiple sheathed flagella

H. pylori is a gram-negative microaerophilic rod found most commonly between the mucous layer and the gastric epithelium.

504. pH-gated urea channel in H. pylori bacterium is called?
N Engl J Med. 2002:347,1175

A. UreI
B. UreJ
C. UreK
D. UreL

505. Which of the following statements about H. pylori is false?
Harrison's 20th Ed. Chapter 317 Page 2224

A. Its genome contains 1.65 million base pairs
B. May transform into coccoid dormant form
C. Produces urease to convert urea to NH_3 and water
D. Single strain of H. pylori exist

Multiple strains of H. pylori exist. Different diseases related to H. pylori infection can be attributed to different strains with distinct pathogenic features.

506. Which of the following statements about H. pylori is false?
N Engl J Med. 2002:347,1175

A. 80% population by age 20 years is infected in developing countries
B. Transmission occurs through faeco-oral route
C. Infection is associated with chronic active gastritis
D. BabA is vital for entry into gastric epithelial cell

507. Which of the following statements about H. pylori is false?
Harrison's 20th Ed. Chapter 317 Page 2224

A. Express vacuolating cytotoxin VacA
B. Cag A and pic B are virulence factors
C. Its LPS has high immunologic activity
D. Neutrophil response is strong in acute & chronic H. pylori infection

508. Which out of the following factors has a central role in H. pylori infection?
N Engl J Med. 2002:347,1175

A. Interleukin-1β
B. Interleukin-2
C. Interleukin-6
D. Interleukin-8

509. Which of the following statements about H. pylori is false?
N Engl J Med. 2002:347, 1175

A. Most pathogenic strains contain VacA pathogenicity island
B. 5 of its genes are similar to Agrobacterium tumefaciens
C. Pathogenicity island proteins are involved in interleukin-8 production by gastric epithelial cells
D. Pathogenicity island proteins are involved in translocation of CagA from bacterium into host cell

510. **Adhesins for *H. pylori* include all except?**
    N Engl J Med. 2002:347,1175
    A. BabA
    B. AlpA
    C. AlpB
    D. HopY

    H. pylori expresses adhesins which facilitate attachment of the bacteria to gastric epithelial cells.

511. **Which of the following statements about *H. pylori* is false?**
    N Engl J Med. 2002:347,1175
    A. *H. pylori* is usually acquired in childhood
    B. Acute infection causes transient hypochlorhydria
    C. 80-90% with chronic gastritis will never have symptoms
    D. After eradication, reinfection rates are high

    Reinfection after successful eradication of H. pylori is rare in US. If recurrent infection occurs within first 6 months after completing therapy, most likely explanation is recrudescence and not reinfection.

512. **Which of the following enzymes is not related to *H. pylori*-induced gastrointestinal disease?**
    Harrison's 20th Ed. Chapter 317 Page 2224 Table 317-6
    A. Urease
    B. Vac A
    C. GAD
    D. Cag A

    Bacterial enzymes that cause H. pylori-induced gastrointestinal disease are Urease, Vac A & Cag A.

513. **"cag" stands for?**
    Harrison's 20th Ed. Chapter 317 Page 2224
    A. Cytotoxin-associated gene
    B. Cytotoxin-assembly gene
    C. Cytotoxin-augmented gene
    D. Cytotoxin-apoptotic gene

514. **Which of the following secretion system is associated with *H. pylori* infection?**
    N Engl J Med. 2002:347,1175
    A. Type I
    B. Type II
    C. Type III
    D. Type IV

515. **Which of the following about Cag A is false?**
    Harrison's 20th Ed. Chapter 317 Page 2224
    A. Virulence factor in pathogenicity island (cag-PAI)
    B. Cytotoxin-associated gene A
    C. Oncoprotein
    D. None of the above

516. **Chronic *H. pylori* infection may lead to?**
    Harrison's 20th Ed. Chapter 317 Page 2224 Figure 317-8
    A. Antral predominant gastritis
    B. Nonatrophic pangastritis
    C. Corpus predominant atrophic gastritis
    D. All of the above

517. **Asymptomatic *H. pylori* infection may be a consequence of?**
    Harrison's 20th Ed. Chapter 317 Page 2224 Figure 317-8
    A. Antral predominant gastritis
    B. Nonatrophic pangastritis
    C. Corpus predominant atrophic gastritis
    D. All of the above

518. **Which of the following consequences of chronic *H. pylori* infection leads to gastric cancer?**
    Harrison's 20th Ed. Chapter 317 Page 2224 Figure 317-8
    A. Antral predominant gastritis
    B. Nonatrophic pangastritis
    C. Corpus predominant atrophic gastritis
    D. All of the above

    Chronic H. pylori infection leading to corpus predominant atrophic gastritis going on to intestinal metaplasia is an important predisposing factor for gastric cancer.

519. **Which of the following consequences of chronic *H. pylori* infection leads to DU?**
    Harrison's 20th Ed. Chapter 317 Page 2224 Figure 317-8
    A. Antral predominant gastritis
    B. Nonatrophic pangastritis
    C. Corpus predominant atrophic gastritis
    D. All of the above

    Presence of antral-predominant gastritis is associated with DU formation.

520. **Which of the following consequences of chronic H. pylori infection leads to MALT lymphoma?**
    Harrison's 20th Ed. Chapter 317 Page 2224 Figure 317-8
    A. Antral predominant gastritis
    B. Nonatrophic pangastritis
    C. Corpus predominant atrophic gastritis
    D. All of the above

    Chronic infection with H. pylori is associated with development of a low-grade B cell lymphoma, gastric MALT lymphoma. (MALT refers to mucosal-associated lymphoid tissue).

521. **Which of the following in *H. pylori* may be associated with development of DUs?**
    Harrison's 20th Ed. Chapter 317 Page 2225
    A. Cag A
    B. dupA
    C. pic B
    D. Vac A

    In H. pylori, bacterial factor DU-promoting gene A (dupA) may be associated with development of DUs.

522. **Antral-predominant gastritis is associated with the development of?**
    Harrison's 20th Ed. Chapter 317 Page 2225
    A. DU
    B. GU
    C. Gastric atrophy
    D. Gastric carcinoma

523. Gastritis involving primarily corpus predisposes to development of?
Harrison's 20th Ed. Chapter 317 Page 2225

A. GU
B. Gastric atrophy
C. Gastric carcinoma
D. All of the above

524. Risk factors that increase morbidity and mortality related to NSAID usage are all except?
Harrison's 20th Ed. Chapter 317 Page 2226

A. Advanced age
B. History of PUD
C. Concomitant use of iron
D. Multisystem disease

525. Risk factors that increase morbidity and mortality related to NSAID usage are all except?
Harrison's 20th Ed. Chapter 317 Page 2226

A. High dose NSAIDs
B. Multiple NSAIDs
C. Concomitant use of anticoagulants
D. Spicy food

Established risk factors for serious gastrointestinal complications from NSAIDs include advanced age, history of ulcer, concomitant use of glucocorticoids, high-dose NSAIDs, multiple NSAIDs, concomitant use of anticoagulants, and serious or multisystem disease. Possible risk factors include concomitant infection with H. pylori, cigarette smoking, and alcohol consumption.

526. Disorders that are associated with PUD include all except?
Harrison's 20th Ed. Chapter 317 Page 2226

A. Systemic mastocytosis
B. Chronic pulmonary disease
C. Chronic renal failure
D. Acute pancreatitis

527. Disorders that are associated with PUD include all except?
Harrison's 20th Ed. Chapter 317 Page 2226

A. Cirrhosis
B. Nephrolithiasis
C. Hyperthyroidism
D. α1 antitrypsin deficiency

Chronic disorders that have a strong association with PUD are systemic mastocytosis, chronic pulmonary disease, chronic renal failure, cirrhosis, nephrolithiasis, and alpha$_1$-antitrypsin deficiency. Those with a possible association are hyperparathyroidism, coronary artery disease, polycythemia vera, and chronic pancreatitis.

528. Which of the following blood group has been implicated in the pathogenesis of PUD?
Harrison's 20th Ed. Chapter 317 Page 2226

A. Blood group A
B. Blood group B
C. Blood group AB
D. Blood group O

Increased frequency of blood group O has been implicated as genetic risk factors for peptic diathesis.

529. The typical pain pattern in DU occurs?
Harrison's 20th Ed. Chapter 317 Page 2227

A. 15 minutes to 1 hour after a meal
B. 30 minutes to 2 hour after a meal
C. 60 minutes to 3 hour after a meal
D. 90 minutes to 3 hour after a meal

Typical pain pattern in DU occurs 90 minutes to 3 hours after a meal and is frequently relieved by antacids or food.

530. Which of the following is a feature of pain pattern in GU?
Harrison's 20th Ed. Chapter 317 Page 2227

A. Awakes patient from sleep between midnight and 3 AM
B. Discomfort may be precipitated by food
C. Nausea & weight loss occur more commonly
D. All of the above

Pain that awakes the patient from sleep (between midnight and 3 AM) is the most discriminating symptom. In GU, nausea & weight loss occur more commonly & discomfort may be precipitated by food.

531. Which of the following infectious agents can cause PUD?
Harrison's 20th Ed. Chapter 317 Page 2227 Table 317-1

A. Cytomegalovirus
B. Herpes simplex virus
C. Helicobacter heilmannii
D. All of the above

532. Which of the following is the most frequent finding in patients with GU or DU?
Harrison's 20th Ed. Chapter 317 Page 2227

A. Succussion splash
B. Epigastric tenderness
C. Dehydration secondary to vomiting
D. Abdominal distension

533. Most common complication observed in PUD is?
Harrison's 20th Ed. Chapter 317 Page 2227

A. Gastrointestinal bleeding
B. Perforation
C. Gastric Outlet Obstruction
D. Malignancy

Gastrointestinal bleeding is the most common complication observed in PUD followed by perforation and gastric outlet obstruction. >50% of patients with ulcer-related hemorrhage bleed without any preceding warning signs or symptoms.

534. Which of the following is the least common cause of mortality in PUD-related bleeding?
Harrison's 20th Ed. Chapter 317 Page 2227

A. Exsanguination
B. Multiorgan failure
C. Pulmonary complications
D. Malignancy

Most of the mortality in PUD-related bleeding is due to nonbleeding causes like multiorgan failure (24%), pulmonary complications (24%), and malignancy (34%).

535. Out of the following, which is the least common ulcer-related complication?
Harrison's 20th Ed. Chapter 317 Page 2227

A. Gastric outlet obstruction
B. Gastrointestinal bleeding
C. Perforation
D. Malignancy

Gastric outlet obstruction is the least common ulcer-related complication.

536. GUs tend to perforate into?
Harrison's 20th Ed. Chapter 317 Page 2227

A. Spleen
B. Pancreas
C. Left hepatic lobe
D. Left kidney

537. DUs tend to perforate into?
Harrison's 20th Ed. Chapter 317 Page 2227

A. Spleen
B. Pancreas
C. Right hepatic lobe
D. Left kidney

GUs tend to penetrate into the left hepatic lobe while DUs tend to penetrate posteriorly into pancreas.

538. Functional dyspepsia or essential dyspepsia is typified by?
Harrison's 20th Ed. Chapter 317 Page 2227

A. Heartburn
B. Upper abdominal pain
C. Water brash
D. Loss of appetite

NUD (functional dyspepsia / essential dyspepsia) is typified by upper abdominal pain without presence of ulcer.

539. Postprandial distress syndrome & epigastric pain syndrome are a type of?
Harrison's 20th Ed. Chapter 317 Page 2227

A. Functional dyspepsia
B. Gastric outlet obstruction
C. Coronary artery disease
D. Neuroticism

Postprandial distress syndrome (PDS) and epigastric pain syndrome (EPS) are subcategories of functional dyspepsia (FD).

540. Ulcers are more often malignant when their size is?
Harrison's 20th Ed. Chapter 317 Page 2228

A. > 1 cm
B. > 2 cm
C. > 3 cm
D. > 4 cm

Ulcers are more often malignant when their size is > 3 cm or those associated with a mass.

541. Tests for diagnosing H. pylori include?
Harrison's 20th Ed. Chapter 317 Page 2229 Table 317-2

A. Biopsy urease test
B. Fecal H. pylori antigen test
C. ^{13}C- or ^{14}C-urea breath test
D. All of the above

Tests for diagnosing H. pylori include serologic testing, ^{13}C- or ^{14}C-urea breath test & fecal H. pylori (Hp) antigen test (monoclonal antibody test). Urinary Hp antigen test appear promising.

542. Rapid urease invasive test for detection of H. pylori is false negative with recent use of?
Harrison's 20th Ed. Chapter 317 Page 2229 Table 317-2

A. PPIs
B. Antibiotics
C. Bismuth compounds
D. All of the above

543. Milk-alkali syndrome includes all except?
Harrison's 20th Ed. Chapter 317 Page 2229

A. Hypercalcemia
B. Hypophosphatemia
C. Renal calcinosis
D. Progression to renal insufficiency

Milk-alkali syndrome comprises of hypercalcemia, hyperphosphatemia, renal calcinosis & progression to renal insufficiency.

544. Initial mild hypercalcemia in Milk-alkali syndrome first leads to?
Harrison's 20th Ed. Chapter 403 Page 2933

A. Alkalosis
B. Bicarbonate retention
C. Renal calcium retention
D. Severe hypercalcemia

545. Burnett's syndrome is best related to?
Harrison's 20th Ed. Chapter 403 Page 2933

A. Aluminum intoxication
B. Vitamin A intoxication
C. Milk-alkali syndrome
D. Hypethyroidism

The chronic form of Milk-alkali syndrome is termed as Burnett's syndrome. It is associated with irreversible renal damage.

546. Phrase "no acid, no ulcer" is best related to?
N Engl J Med. 1971; 285:620

A. Palmer
B. Piper
C. Schwarz
D. Bralow

"No acid - no ulcer" statement has been referred to as Schwarz's dictum. Dragutin (Carl) Schwarz (1868-1917) is primarily remembered for his dictum 'No acid, no ulcer' (1910).

547. Structure of H_2 receptor antagonists share structural homology with?
Harrison's 20th Ed. Chapter 317 Page 2229

A. Pepsin
B. Secretin
C. Gastrin
D. Histamine

H_2 receptor antagonists (cimetidine, ranitidine, famotidine & nizatidine) have structural homology with histamine.

548. Which of the following about cimetidine is false?
Harrison's 20th Ed. Chapter 317 Page 2229

A. First H₂ receptor antagonist used in acid peptic disorders
B. Antiandrogenic side effects
C. Inhibit cytochrome P450
D. None of the above

549. Monitoring of which of the following drugs is needed when used with cimetidine?
Harrison's 20th Ed. Chapter 317 Page 2229

A. Warfarin
B. Phenytoin
C. Theophylline
D. All of the above

Caution is needed when using theophylline, warfarin, diazepam, atazanavir & phenytoin with PPIs.

550. Which of the following H₂ receptor antagonist does not bind to hepatic cytochrome P450?
Harrison's 20th Ed. Chapter 317 Page 2229

A. Cimetidine
B. Ranitidine
C. Famotidine
D. All of the above

Famotidine and nizatidine do not bind to hepatic cytochrome P450.

551. Which of the following is the most recent PPI approved for clinical use?
Harrison's 20th Ed. Chapter 317 Page 2229

A. Esomeprazole
B. Dexlansoprazole
C. Tenatoprazole
D. Rabeprazole

Dexlansoprazole is an R-isomer of lansoprazole, and is the most recent PPI approved for clinical use.

552. The half-life of PPIs is?
Harrison's 20th Ed. Chapter 317 Page 2229

A. ~ 8 hours
B. ~ 12 hours
C. ~ 14 hours
D. ~ 18 hours

The half-life of PPIs is ~18 hours.

553. Which of the following occurs with the use of PPIs?
Harrison's 20th Ed. Chapter 317 Page 2229

A. Hypergastrinemia
B. IF production is inhibited
C. Hypomagnesemia
D. All of the above

Long-term use of PPIs may lead to development of iron, vitamin B12, and magnesium deficiency.

554. Proton pump inhibitors may interfere with absorption of?
Harrison's 20th Ed. Chapter 317 Page 2230

A. Ketoconazole
B. Iron
C. Digoxin
D. All of the above

PPIs may interfere with absorption of ketoconazole, ampicillin, iron & digoxin.

555. Hepatic cytochrome P450 can be inhibited by?
Harrison's 20th Ed. Chapter 317 Page 2230

A. Lansoprazole
B. Rabeprazole
C. Pantoprazole
D. Esomeprazole

Hepatic cytochrome P450 can be inhibited by omeprazole & lansoprazole and not by rabeprazole, pantoprazole and esomeprazole.

556. Long-term acid suppression with PPIs has been associated with a higher incidence of?
Harrison's 20th Ed. Chapter 317 Page 2230

A. Bacterial meningitis
B. Community-acquired pneumonia
C. Urinary tract infection
D. Gall stones

557. Long-term acid suppression with PPIs has been associated with a higher incidence of?
Harrison's 20th Ed. Chapter 317 Page 2230

A. Nail dystrophy
B. Clostridium difficile - associated disease
C. Gingivitis
D. Cataract

Long-term acid suppression with PPIs is associated with higher incidence of community-acquired pneumonia and community and hospital acquired Clostridium difficile-associated disease.

558. Which of the following cytochrome P450 is involved in the competition of PPI & clopidogrel?
Harrison's 20th Ed. Chapter 317 Page 2230

A. CYP2B6
B. CYP2D6
C. CYP2C19
D. CYP3A

PPIs may exert a negative effect on the antiplatelet effect of clopidogrel. If PPIs are to be given, there should be a 12 hour separation between administration of PPI & clopidogrel.

559. PPI containing an imidazopyridine ring instead of a benzimidazole ring is?
Harrison's 20th Ed. Chapter 317 Page 2230

A. Rabeprazole
B. Pantoprazole
C. Tenatoprazole
D. Esomeprazole

Tenatoprazole is a PPI containing an imidazopyridine ring instead of a benzimidazole ring.

560. Which of the following is a potassium-competitive acid pump antagonists (P-CABs)?
Harrison's 20th Ed. Chapter 317 Page 2230

A. Vilazodone
B. Revaprazan
C. Gadoteridol
D. All of the above

Revaprazan & venoprazan are potassium-competitive acid pump antagonists (P-CABs).

561. **Sucralfate is a complex sucrose salt in which hydroxyl groups are substituted by?**
Harrison's 20th Ed. Chapter 317 Page 2231
   A. Aluminum acetate
   B. Aluminum chloride
   C. Aluminum hydroxide
   D. Aluminum phosphate

Sucralfate is a complex sucrose salt in which the hydroxyl groups are substituted by aluminum hydroxide & sulfate.

562. **Which of the following is false about Sucralfate?**
Harrison's 20th Ed. Chapter 317 Page 2231
   A. Complex sucrose salt
   B. Insoluble in water
   C. To be avoided in chronic renal insufficiency
   D. None of the above

563. **Sir William Osler considered which of the following the drug of choice for treating PUD?**
Harrison's 20th Ed. Chapter 317 Page 2231
   A. Antacids
   B. Bismuth-containing compounds
   C. Sucralfate
   D. H_2 receptor antagonists

Sir William Osler considered bismuth-containing compounds the drug of choice for treating PUD.

564. **Black stools & darkening of tongue are adverse effects of?**
Harrison's 20th Ed. Chapter 317 Page 2231
   A. Misoprostol
   B. Sucralfate
   C. Colloidal bismuth subcitrate (CBS)
   D. Proton Pump Inhibitors (PPI)

Adverse effects with short-term usage of Colloidal bismuth subcitrate (CBS) and bismuth subsalicylate (BSS) include black stools, constipation and darkening of tongue.

565. **Maastricht IV/Florence Consensus Report recommends a test-and-treat approach for patients with uninvestigated dyspepsia if the local incidence of H. pylori is?**
Harrison's 20th Ed. Chapter 317 Page 2231
   A. > 10%
   B. > 20%
   C. > 30%
   D. > 40%

566. **ACG clinical guidelines recommend testing & offering H. pylori eradication to patients with?**
Harrison's 20th Ed. Chapter 317 Page 2231
   A. Enteric fever
   B. Idiopathic thrombocytopenic purpura
   C. Nephrolithiasis
   D. Asthma

ACG clinical guidelines recommend testing & offering H. pylori eradication to patients with unexplained iron deficiency anemia & idiopathic thrombocytopenic purpura.

567. **Which of the following about therapy of H. pylori is false?**
Harrison's 20th Ed. Chapter 317 Page 2231
   A. No single agent is effective in eradicating the organism
   B. Combination therapy for 14 days provides greatest efficacy
   C. Aim for initial eradication rates should be 85 – 90%
   D. None of the above

568. **Combination therapy for H. pylori infection should be given for a period of?**
Harrison's 20th Ed. Chapter 317 Page 2231
   A. 7 days
   B. 14 days
   C. 21 days
   D. 28 days

Combination therapy for H. pylori infection for 14 days provides the greatest efficacy.

569. **First triple regimen therapy against H. pylori was?**
Harrison's 20th Ed. Chapter 317 Page 2231
   A. Amoxicillin + omeprazole + metronidazole
   B. Bismuth + metronidazole + tetracycline
   C. Clarithromycin + omeprazole + metronidazole
   D. Lansoprazole + clarithromycin + amoxicillin

First triple regimen therapy against H. pylori was bismuth, metronidazole & tetracycline.

570. **Most feared complication with amoxicillin is?**
Harrison's 20th Ed. Chapter 317 Page 2232
   A. Antibiotic-associated diarrhea
   B. Pseudomembranous colitis
   C. Hepatotoxicity
   D. Anaphylaxis

571. **Which of the following statements about H. pylori is false?**
Harrison's 20th Ed. Chapter 317 Page 2232
   A. H. pylori should be eradicated in documented PUD
   B. No single agent is effective in eradicating H. pylori
   C. Rifabutin used to treat resistant strains of H. pylori
   D. H. pylori is implicated in pathogenesis of acute pancreatitis

572. **Which of the following is a treatment regimen for eradication of H. pylori infection?**
Harrison's 20th Ed. Chapter 317 Page 2232
   A. Triple therapy
   B. Quadruple therapy
   C. Sequential therapy
   D. All of the above

573. **Which of the following drugs can be used for eradication of H. pylori?**
Harrison's 20th Ed. Chapter 317 Page 2232
   A. Tinidazole
   B. Levofloxacin
   C. Furazolidone
   D. All of the above

574. Which of the following drugs can be used for eradication of H. pylori?
Harrison's 20th Ed. Chapter 317 Page 2234

   A. N-acetylcysteine
   B. Lactobacillus spp.
   C. Saccharomyces spp.
   D. All of the above

575. Which of the following can heal GUs or DUs, independent of whether NSAIDs are discontinued?
Harrison's 20th Ed. Chapter 317 Page 2234

   A. H_2 receptor antagonist
   B. PPIs
   C. Misoprostol
   D. Sucralfate

Only PPIs can heal GUs or DUs, independent of whether NSAIDs are discontinued.

576. H. pylori eradication should be documented how many weeks after completing antibiotics?
Harrison's 20th Ed. Chapter 317 Page 2235

   A. 1
   B. 2
   C. 3
   D. 4

H. pylori eradication should be documented 4 weeks after completing antibiotics.

577. Test of choice for documenting eradication of H. pylori is?
Harrison's 20th Ed. Chapter 317 Page 2235

   A. Biopsy urease test
   B. Fecal H. pylori antigen test
   C. ^{13}C- or ^{14}C-urea breath test
   D. Urinary Hp antigen test

The test of choice for documenting eradication is the urea breath test (UBT).

578. A GU is considered refractory if it fails to heal after how many weeks of therapy?
Harrison's 20th Ed. Chapter 317 Page 2235

   A. 4 weeks
   B. 8 weeks
   C. 12 weeks
   D. 16 weeks

579. A DU is considered refractory if it fails to heal after how many weeks of therapy?
Harrison's 20th Ed. Chapter 317 Page 2235

   A. 4 weeks
   B. 8 weeks
   C. 12 weeks
   D. 16 weeks

GU that fails to heal >12 weeks & a DU that does not heal >8 weeks of therapy is considered refractory.

580. Etiologies of refractory ulcers (GU / DU) include all except?
Harrison's 20th Ed. Chapter 317 Page 2235

   A. Ischemia
   B. Crohn's disease
   C. Ulcerative colitis
   D. Amyloidosis

581. Etiologies of refractory ulcers (GU / DU) include all except?
Harrison's 20th Ed. Chapter 317 Page 2235

   A. Sarcoidosis
   B. Lymphoma
   C. Eosinophilic gastroenteritis
   D. HIV

582. Etiologies of refractory ulcers (GU / DU) include all except?
Harrison's 20th Ed. Chapter 317 Page 2235

   A. Leprosy
   B. Cytomegalovirus (CMV)
   C. Tuberculosis
   D. Syphilis

Rare etiologies of refractory GU/DU's include ischemia, Crohn's disease, amyloidosis, sarcoidosis, lymphoma, eosinophilic gastroenteritis, cytomegalovirus (CMV), tuberculosis or syphilis.

583. Posterior DU can penetrate into?
Harrison's 20th Ed. Chapter 317 Page 2236

   A. Pancreas
   B. Colon
   C. Liver
   D. All of the above

Posterior DU can penetrate into pancreas, colon, liver or biliary tree.

584. Which of the following is a component of Zollinger-Ellison Syndrome (ZES)?
Harrison's 20th Ed. Chapter 317 Page 2238

   A. Severe peptic ulcer diathesis
   B. Gastric acid hypersecretion
   C. Unregulated gastrin from a non-β cell neuroendocrine tumor
   D. None of the above

ZES is typified by severe peptic ulcer diathesis secondary to gastric acid hypersecretion due to unregulated gastrin release from gastrinoma - a non-β cell well-differentiated neuroendocrine tumor.

585. Which of the following is not a typical feature of Zollinger-Ellison Syndrome (ZES)?
Harrison's 20th Ed. Chapter 317 Page 2238

   A. Gastrin release from beta cell endocrine tumor
   B. Hypergastrinemia
   C. Erosive esophagitis
   D. Diarrhea

The increased gastric acid output leads to peptic ulcer diathesis, erosive esophagitis, and diarrhea.

586. In ZES, majority of patients are diagnosed between ages of?
Harrison's 20th Ed. Chapter 317 Page 2238

   A. 01 and 10 years
   B. 10 and 30 years
   C. 30 and 50 years
   D. 50 and 70 years

In ZES, males are more commonly affected than females, and majority of patients are diagnosed between the ages of 30 and 50 years.

587. Average time from symptom onset to diagnosis of Zollinger–Ellison syndrome is?
N Engl J Med. 2018;378:73-9

A. > 3 years
B. > 5 years
C. > 7 years
D. > 10 years

Average time from symptom onset to diagnosis of Zollinger–Ellison syndrome is more than 5 years.

588. Multiple endocrine neoplasia (MEN) type 1 is characterized by all except?
Harrison's 20th Ed. Chapter 369 Page 2649

A. Parathyroid tumor
B. Pancreatic islet tumor
C. Pheochromocytoma
D. Pituitary tumor

Gastrinomas are classified into sporadic tumors (80%) and those associated with multiple endocrine neoplasia (MEN) type 1.

589. Which of the following is the action of gastrin?
Harrison's 20th Ed. Chapter 317 Page 2238

A. Stimulates acid secretion through gastrin receptors on parietal cells
B. Stimulates acid secretion by inducing histamine release from ECL cells
C. Has a trophic action on gastric epithelial cells
D. All of the above

Gastrin stimulates acid secretion through gastrin receptors on parietal cells and by inducing histamine release from ECL cells. Gastrin also has a trophic action on gastric epithelial cells.

590. 'Gastrinoma triangle' is formed by all except?
Harrison's 20th Ed. Chapter 317 Page 2238

A. Cystic and common bile ducts
B. Junction of II and III portions of duodenum
C. Inferior surface of liver
D. Junction of neck & body of pancreas

Hypothetical gastrinoma triangle is formed by confluence of cystic & common bile ducts superiorly, junction of second & third portions of duodenum inferiorly, and junction of neck & body of pancreas medially.

591. What proportion of gastrinoma are found within the hypothetical gastrinoma triangle?
Harrison's 20th Ed. Chapter 317 Page 2238

A. 20%
B. 40%
C. 60%
D. 80%

Gastrinomas occur within pancreas or may be extrapancreatic. Over 80% of gastrinoma are found within the hypothetical gastrinoma triangle.

592. Which of the following is the most common extrapancreatic site of gastrinoma?
Harrison's 20th Ed. Chapter 317 Page 2238

A. Stomach
B. Duodenum
C. Liver
D. Lymph nodes

Duodenal gastrinoma tumors constitute the most common nonpancreatic lesion (50 to 75%). Less-common extrapancreatic sites include stomach, bones, ovaries, heart, liver, and lymph nodes.

593. What proportion of gastrinoma are malignant?
Harrison's 20th Ed. Chapter 317 Page 2238

A. 20%
B. 40%
C. 60%
D. 80%

More than 60% of gastrinoma tumors are considered malignant, with up to 30–50% of patients having multiple lesions or metastatic disease at presentation.

594. Marker typically found in endocrine neoplasms is?
Harrison's 20th Ed. Chapter 74 Page 538

A. Chromogranin
B. Neuron-specific enolase
C. Synaptophysin
D. All of the above

Markers for neuroendocrine differentiation within a tumor are neuron-specific enolase (NSE), CD56 or NCAM, synaptophysin, chromogranin, and Leu7.

595. Which of the following suggest the diagnosis of ZES?
Harrison's 20th Ed. Chapter 317 Page 2238

A. Ulcer in second part of duodenum & beyond
B. Ulcers refractory to standard medical therapy
C. Ulcer presenting with frank complication
D. All of the above

Gastrinoma should be suspected when ulcers occur unusual locations like II part of duodenum & beyond, ulcers refractory to standard medical therapy, ulcer recurrence after acid-reducing surgery, ulcers presenting with frank complications (bleeding, obstruction, and perforation), or ulcers in the absence of H. pylori or NSAID ingestion.

596. What proportion of ZES patients have diarrhea?
Harrison's 20th Ed. Chapter 317 Page 2238

A. 25%
B. 50%
C. 75%
D. 100%

After peptic ulcer (90%), diarrhea is the next most common clinical manifestation after peptic ulcer and is found in up to 50% of patients of ZES.

597. Etiology of the diarrhea in ZES is?
Harrison's 20th Ed. Chapter 317 Page 2238

A. Volume overload to the small bowel
B. Pancreatic enzyme inactivation by acid
C. Damage of the intestinal epithelial surface by acid
D. All of the above

In ZES, etiology of diarrhea is multifactorial, resulting from marked volume overload to small bowel, pancreatic enzyme inactivation by acid & damage of intestinal epithelial surface by acid.

598. Gastrinomas develop in the presence of MEN 1 syndrome in what percentage of patients?
Harrison's 20th Ed. Chapter 317 Page 2238

A. ~ 10%
B. ~ 25%
C. ~ 50%
D. ~ 75%

Gastrinomas can develop in the presence of MEN 1 syndrome in ~25% of patients.

599. Organs involved in MEN 1 syndrome are all except?
Harrison's 20th Ed. Chapter 317 Page 2238

A. Parathyroid
B. Thyroid
C. Pancreas
D. Pituitary

MEN I syndrome (autosomal dominant) involves parathyroid glands (80–90%), pancreas (40–80%), pituitary gland (30–60%) and gastrinomas (~25%).

600. Genetic defect in MEN 1 is in?
Harrison's 20th Ed. Chapter 317 Page 2238

A. Short arm of chromosome 11
B. Long arm of chromosome 11
C. Short arm of chromosome 12
D. Long arm of chromosome 12

The genetic defect in MEN I is in the long arm of chromosome 11 (11q11-q13).

601. MEN1 tumor suppressor gene encodes for?
Harrison's 20th Ed. Chapter 317 Page 2238

A. β-catenin
B. Parafibromin
C. Menin
D. Neurokinin B

MEN1 tumor suppressor gene encodes for Menin, 610-amino-acid protein. Pathophysiology of MEN 1 follows the Knudson two-hit hypothesis.

602. Distinguishing feature between MEN I associated ZES & sprodic ZES is?
Harrison's 20th Ed. Chapter 317 Page 2239

A. Incidence of gastric carcinoid tumor
B. Size, number & location of gastrinoma
C. Disease free period after surgery
D. All of the above

Gastrinomas tend to be smaller, multiple, and located in the duodenal wall more often than is seen in patients with sporadic ZES. An additional distinguishing feature in ZES patients with MEN I is the higher incidence of gastric carcinoid tumor development (as compared to patients with sporadic gastrinomas). Gastrinomas tend to be smaller, multiple, and located in the duodenal wall more often than is seen in patients with sporadic ZES.

603. First step in the evaluation of a patient suspected of ZES is?
Harrison's 20th Ed. Chapter 317 Page 2239

A. Assess acid secretion
B. Obtain a fasting gastrin level
C. Secretin stimulation test
D. Calcium infusion study

The first step in evaluation of a patient suspected of ZES is to obtain a fasting gastrin level.

604. Patients with gastrinoma have gastrin level more than?
Harrison's 20th Ed. Chapter 317 Page 2239

A. 25 pg/mL
B. 50 pg/mL
C. 100 pg/mL
D. 150 pg/mL

Fasting gastrin levels are <150 pg/mL. All gastrinoma patients have a gastrin level >150 – 200 pg/mL.

605. The most frequent condition that leads to an elevated fasting gastrin level is?
Harrison's 20th Ed. Chapter 317 Page 2239

A. Nonsteroidal antiinflammatory drug ingestion
B. *H. pylori* infection
C. Gastric hypochlorhydria and achlorhydria
D. Hypercalcemia

Most frequent condition that leads to an elevated fasting gastrin level is gastric hypochlorhydria / achlorhydria, with or without pernicious anemia.

606. PPI should be stopped for a minimum of how many days before estimation of fasting gastrin level?
Harrison's 20th Ed. Chapter 317 Page 2239

A. 3
B. 7
C. 10
D. 14

PPI should be stopped for a minimum of 7 days before fasting gastrin level testing.

607. Elevated fasting gastrin level are due to all except?
Harrison's 20th Ed. Chapter 317 Page 2239

A. Hypochlorhydria
B. Renal insufficiency
C. Diabetes mellitus
D. Hypertension

608. Elevated fasting gastrin level are due to all except?
Harrison's 20th Ed. Chapter 317 Page 2239

A. Rheumatoid arthritis
B. Ankylosing arthritis
C. Pheochromocytoma
D. Vitiligo

Elevated fasting gastrin level are due to gastric hypochlorhydria or achlorhydria, renal insufficiency, massive small-bowel obstruction, rheumatoid arthritis, vitiligo, diabetes mellitus & pheochromocytoma.

609. Patients with gastrinoma have a BAO level more than?
Harrison's 20th Ed. Chapter 317 Page 2239

A. 4 meq/hour
B. 8 meq/hour
C. 12 meq/hour
D. 15 meq/hour

Normal BAO in nongastric surgery patients is typically <5 meq/hour.

610. What value of BAO / MAO is highly suggestive of ZES?
Harrison's 20th Ed. Chapter 317 Page 2239

A. < 0.3
B. < 0.6
C. > 0.3
D. > 0.6

BAO/MAO ratio using pentagastrin infusion of >0.6 is highly suggestive of ZES.

611. What level of basal gastric pH excludes gastrinoma?
Harrison's 20th Ed. Chapter 317 Page 2239

A. ≥ 1
B. ≥ 1.5
C. ≥ 2
D. ≥ 3

A basal gastric pH ≥ 3 virtually excludes a gastrinoma.

612. Which of the following is the most sensitive & specific gastrin provocative test?

Harrison's 20th Ed. Chapter 317 Page 2239

A. Secretin stimulation test
B. Calcium infusion study
C. Standard meal test
D. None of the above

Most sensitive & specific gastrin provocative test for diagnosis of gastrinoma is secretin study. Increase in gastrin of ≥120 pg within 15 minutes of secretin injection has a sensitivity & specificity of >90% for ZES. Calcium infusion study is less sensitive & specific with greater potential for adverse effects.

613. Which of the following tests has maximum sensitivity in detecting primary gastrinoma?

Harrison's 20th Ed. Chapter 317 Page 2240 Table 317-10

A. Selective arterial secretin injection (SASI)
B. Octreoscan imaging with ^{111}In-pentreotide
C. Endoscopic ultrasonography (EUS)
D. Magnetic resonance imaging

Sensitivity of EUS in Zollinger-Ellison Syndrome is 80 – 100%.

614. In surgery-naive ZES patients, PPI dosing should be adjusted to achieve a BAO of?

Harrison's 20th Ed. Chapter 317 Page 2240

A. <1 meq/hour
B. <3 meq/hour
C. <7 meq/hour
D. <10 meq/hour

615. Which of the following is a favorable prognostic indicator in ZES?

Harrison's 20th Ed. Chapter 317 Page 2240

A. Primary duodenal wall tumor
B. Isolated lymph node tumor
C. Undetectable tumor upon surgical exploration
D. All of the above

In ZES, favorable prognostic indicators include primary duodenal wall tumors, isolated lymph node tumor, and undetectable tumor upon surgical exploration. Poor outcome indicators are shorter disease duration; higher gastrin levels (>10,000 pg/mL); large pancreatic primary tumors (>3 cm); metastatic disease to lymph nodes, liver, and bone and Cushing's syndrome. Rapid growth of hepatic metastases is also predictive of poor outcome.

616. Procedure that provides the lowest rates of peptic ulcer recurrence but has highest complication rate is?

Harrison's 20th Ed. Chapter 317 Page 2236

A. Vagotomy
B. Billroth I
C. Vagotomy in combination with antrectomy
D. Billroth II

617. Cushing's ulcer refers to?

Harrison's 20th Ed. Chapter 317 Page 2241

A. Stress ulceration after head trauma
B. Stress ulceration after severe burns
C. Stress ulceration after mechanical ventilation
D. Stress ulceration after sepsis

Elevated gastric acid secretion may be noted in patients with stress ulceration after head trauma (Cushing's ulcer).

618. Curling's ulcer refers to?

Harrison's 20th Ed. Chapter 317 Page 2241

A. Stress ulceration after head trauma
B. Stress ulceration after severe burns
C. Stress ulceration after mechanical ventilation
D. Stress ulceration after sepsis

Elevated gastric acid secretion may be noted in patients with stress ulceration after severe burns (Curling's ulcer).

619. To avoid stress ulceration, gastric pH should be maintained at?

Harrison's 20th Ed. Chapter 317 Page 2241

A. > 1.5
B. > 2.0
C. > 2.5
D. > 3.5

Maintenance of gastric pH >3.5 with continuous infusion of H_2 blockers or liquid antacids administered every 2–3 hours are viable options to avoid stress ulceration.

620. Treatment of choice for stress ulcer prophylaxis is?

Harrison's 20th Ed. Chapter 317 Page 2241

A. H_2 blocker
B. PPI
C. Sucralfate
D. All of the above

PPIs are the treatment of choice for stress ulcer prophylaxis.

621. 'Phlegmonous gastritis' refers to?

Harrison's 20th Ed. Chapter 317 Page 2241

A. Viral infection of stomach
B. Bacterial infection of stomach
C. Vascular congestion of stomach
D. All of the above

Bacterial infection of the stomach or phlegmonous gastritis although rare is a potentially life-threatening disorder characterized by marked & diffuse acute inflammatory infiltrates of entire gastric wall, at times accompanied by necrosis.

622. Which of the following are affected by phlegmonous gastritis?

Harrison's 20th Ed. Chapter 317 Page 2241

A. Elderly individuals
B. Alcoholics
C. AIDS patients
D. All of the above

Elderly individuals, alcoholics, and AIDS patients may be affected by Phlegmonous gastritis.

623. Organism associated with phlegmonous gastritis is?

Harrison's 20th Ed. Chapter 317 Page 2241

A. Staphylococci
B. Escherichia coli
C. Haemophilus
D. All of the above

Organisms associated with Phlegmonous gastritis include streptococci, staphylococci, Escherichia coli, Proteus, and Haemophilus species.

624. Bouveret's Syndrome best relates to?
N Engl J Med. 2018:378,1335

- A. Pneumoperitoneum
- B. Retroperitoneal fibrosis
- C. Situs inversus
- D. Gallstone ileus

625. Rigler's triad includes all except?
N Engl J Med. 2018:378,1335

- A. Pneumobilia
- B. Small-bowel obstruction
- C. Large-bowel obstruction
- D. Ectopic gallstone

Bouveret's syndrome is a form of gallstone ileus that is characterized by gastric outlet obstruction caused by impaction of a gallstone in pylorus or proximal duodenum after its passage through a cholecystoduodenal fistula. Patients with gallstone ileus may present with radiographic findings of Rigler's triad i.e., pneumobilia, small-bowel obstruction, and ectopic gallstone.

626. The final stage of chronic gastritis is?
Harrison's 20th Ed. Chapter 317 Page 2241

- A. Superficial gastritis
- B. Atrophic gastritis
- C. Gastric atrophy
- D. Intestinal metaplasia

Early phase of chronic gastritis is superficial gastritis in which inflammatory changes are limited to lamina propria and intact gastric glands. Next stage is atrophic gastritis in which inflammatory infiltrate extends deeper into mucosa, with destruction of gastric glands. Final stage of chronic gastritis is gastric atrophy in which glandular structures are lost, and there is a paucity of inflammatory infiltrates. Endoscopically, mucosa is thin and underlying blood vessels can be visualized. Intestinal metaplasia refers to the conversion of gastric glands to small-bowel mucosal glands containing goblet cells. Intestinal metaplasia is an important predisposing factor for gastric cancer.

627. Antral-predominant form of chronic gastritis is called?
Harrison's 20th Ed. Chapter 317 Page 2241

- A. Type A gastritis
- B. Type B gastritis
- C. Type AB gastritis
- D. Type O gastritis

Chronic gastritis is also classified according to the predominant site of involvement. Type A refers to fundus and body predominant form, with antral sparing (autoimmune) and type B is the antral-predominant form (H. pylori–related). AB gastritis refers to a mixed antral/body picture.

628. Which of the following types of chronic gastritis is associated with pernicious anemia?
Harrison's 20th Ed. Chapter 317 Page 2241

- A. Type A gastritis
- B. Type B gastritis
- C. Type AB gastritis
- D. Type O gastritis

Type A gastritis, also called autoimmune gastritis is associated with pernicious anemia with circulating antibodies against parietal cells and IF.

629. Parietal cell antibodies are directed against which of the following?
Harrison's 20th Ed. Chapter 317 Page 2242

- A. Gastrin receptors
- B. Acetylcholine receptors
- C. Histamine receptors
- D. H^+,K^+-ATPase

Antibodies to parietal cells are detected in >90% of patients with pernicious anemia and in up to 50% of patients with type A gastritis. The parietal cell antibody is directed against H^+,K^+-ATPase.

630. Varioliform gastritis best relates to?
Harrison's 20th Ed. Chapter 317 Page 2242

- A. Lymphocytic gastritis
- B. Eosinophilic gastritis
- C. Granulomatous gastritis
- D. Sarcoidosis

A subgroup of patients with lymphocytic gastritis have thickened folds noted on endoscopy. These folds are often capped by small nodules that contain a central depression or erosion; this form of the disease is called varioliform gastritis.

631. Which of the following is false about Ménétrier's disease?
Harrison's 20th Ed. Chapter 317 Page 2243

- A. Protein-losing gastropathy
- B. Large gastric mucosal folds in body and fundus
- C. Hyperplasia of surface & glandular mucous cells
- D. None of the above

Ménétrier's disease is not considered a form of gastritis. It is characterized by large, tortuous gastric mucosal folds.

632. Large gastric folds can be seen in?
Harrison's 20th Ed. Chapter 317 Page 2243

- A. ZES
- B. Gastric malignancy
- C. Sarcoidosis
- D. All of the above

Large gastric folds are due to ZES, malignancy (lymphoma, infiltrating carcinoma), infectious etiologies (CMV, histoplasmosis, syphilis, tuberculosis), gastritis polyposa profunda & infiltrative disorders like sarcoidosis.

633. Which of the following is most useful in the treatment of Ménétrier's disease?
Harrison's 20th Ed. Chapter 317 Page 2243

- A. Octreotide
- B. Prednisone
- C. Cetuximab
- D. PPIs

Medical therapy with EGF inhibitory antibody cetuximab, anticholinergic agents, prostaglandins, octreotide, PPIs, prednisone, and H_2 receptor antagonists yields varying results. Anticholinergics decrease protein loss.

Disorders of Absorption

634. In malabsorption syndrome, intestinal absorption is increased in?
Harrison's 20th Ed. Chapter 318 Page 2244

A. Cirrhosis
B. Jejunal diverticulosis
C. Hemochromatosis
D. Crohn's disease

635. In malabsorption syndrome, intestinal absorption is increased in?
Harrison's 20th Ed. Chapter 318 Page 2244

A. Cirrhosis
B. Jejunal diverticulosis
C. Wilson's disease
D. Crohn's disease

Only clinical malabsorption situations in which absorption is increased are hemochromatosis & Wilson's disease, where absorption of iron and copper is increased respectively.

636. Steatorrhea is defined as an increase in stool fat excretion of how much of dietary fat intake?
Harrison's 20th Ed. Chapter 318 Page 2244

A. > 2%
B. > 4%
C. > 5%
D. > 7%

Most malabsorption syndrome disorders are associated with an increase in stool fat excretion of >7% of dietary fat intake (steatorrhea).

637. Malabsorption disorder that is not associated with steatorrhea is?
Harrison's 20th Ed. Chapter 318 Page 2244

A. Primary lactase deficiency
B. Celiac sprue
C. Abetalipoproteinemia
D. Intestinal lymphangiectasia

638. Malabsorption disorder that is not associated with steatorrhea is?
Harrison's 20th Ed. Chapter 318 Page 2244

A. Tropical sprue
B. Celiac sprue
C. Pernicious anemia
D. Bacterial overgrowth syndrome

Most, but not all, malabsorption syndromes are associated with steatorrhea. Primary lactase deficiency and pernicious anemia are not associated with steatorrhea.

639. In a western-type diet, diarrhea as a sign is a quantitative increase in stool water or weight of?
Harrison's 20th Ed. Chapter 318 Page 2244

A. > 100 – 200 gram/day
B. > 200 – 225 gram/day
C. > 300 – 425 gram/day
D. > 400 – 500 gram/day

Diarrhea as a sign quantitative increase in stool weight of >200–225 mL or gram per day, when a western-type diet is consumed.

640. Which of the following diarrhea would undoubtedly cease during a prolonged fast?
Harrison's 20th Ed. Chapter 318 Page 2244

A. Enterotoxin-induced traveler's diarrhea
B. Primary lactase deficiency
C. VIPoma
D. All of the above

Diarrhea secondary to lactose malabsorption in primary lactase deficiency ceases during a prolonged fast.

641. Stool osmolality is?
Harrison's 20th Ed. Chapter 318 Page 2244

A. 250 mosmol/kg H_2O
B. 275 mosmol/kg H_2O
C. 300 mosmol/kg H_2O
D. 325 mosmol/kg H_2O

Stool osmotic gap = 2 x (stool Na + stool K). Stool osmolality is assumed to be 300 mosmol/kg H_2O.

642. Fecal osmotic gap is calculated as?
Gastroenterology. 1999;116:1461-1463

A. 90 - 2([Na^+] + [K^+])
B. 190 - 2([Na^+] + [K^+])
C. 290 - 2([Na^+] + [K^+])
D. 390 - 2([Na^+] + [K^+])

Osmotic diarrheas are characterized by osmotic gaps >125 mOsm/kg (nonelectrolytes account for most of the osmolality of stool water), whereas secretory diarrheas typically have osmotic gaps <50 mOsm/kg (electrolytes account for most of stool osmolality).

643. The lengths of the small intestine and colon are?
Harrison's 20th Ed. Chapter 318 Page 2244

A. ~200 cm and ~50 cm, respectively
B. ~250 cm and ~70 cm, respectively
C. ~300 cm and ~80 cm, respectively
D. ~400 cm and ~100 cm, respectively

Lengths of small intestine and colon are ~300 cm and ~80 cm respectively.

644. Effective functional surface area of intestines is about how many times greater than that of a hollow tube?
Harrison's 20th Ed. Chapter 318 Page 2244

A. 200 times
B. 400 times
C. 600 times
D. 800 times

Effective functional surface area is about 600-fold greater than that of a hollow tube due to the presence of folds, villi (in small intestine), and microvilli.

645. Intestinal mucosa synthesizes & secretes which of the following immunoglobulin?
Harrison's 20th Ed. Chapter 318 Page 2244
- A. Secretory IgA
- B. Secretory IgG
- C. Secretory IgM
- D. Secretory IgE

Intestinal mucosa synthesizes and secretes secretory IgA.

646. Daily salivary, gastric, pancreatic, biliary, and intestinal fluid amounts to?
Harrison's 20th Ed. Chapter 318 Page 2244
- A. 3 to 4 L/day
- B. 5 to 6 L/day
- C. 6 to 7 L/day
- D. 7 to 8 L/day

The intestine absorbs ~7 to 8 liters of fluid daily, comprising dietary fluid intake (1 to 2 L/day) and salivary, gastric, pancreatic, biliary, and intestinal fluid (6 to 7 L/day).

647. The intestine produces which of the following?
Harrison's 20th Ed. Chapter 318 Page 2245
- A. IgA
- B. Apolipoproteins
- C. 5-hydroxytryptophan
- D. All of the above

648. Which of the following statements is false?
Harrison's 20th Ed. Chapter 318 Page 2245
- A. Villi are present in small intestine & colon
- B. Nutrient digestion & absorption occurs in small intestine but not in colon
- C. Digestive hydrolytic enzymes are present in brush border of villus epithelial cells
- D. Secretory function is present in crypts of both small & large intestine

Villi are present in small intestine but are absent in colon.

649. Na^+, K^+ - ATPase in the Na^+ pump is located on?
Harrison's 20th Ed. Chapter 318 Page 2245
- A. Apical membrane
- B. Basolateral membrane
- C. Basomedial membrane
- D. All of the above

Na^+ pump is located on the basolateral membrane, which expels Na^+ and maintains a low intracellular Na^+ through Na^+, K^+ - ATPase.

650. Transport protein SGLT is located on?
Harrison's 20th Ed. Chapter 318 Page 2245
- A. Apical membrane
- B. Basolateral membrane
- C. Basomedial membrane
- D. All of the above

Active glucose (monosaccharide) absorption & glucose-stimulated Na^+ absorption require both apical membrane transport protein SGLT (sodium/glucose cotransporter) & basolateral Na^+, K^+ - ATPase. A competitive inhibitor of SGLT, phlorizin exerts a hypoglycemic effect in diabetics. Gene for SGLT is SLC5A.

651. Which of the following about bile acids is false?
Harrison's 20th Ed. Chapter 318 Page 2245
- A. Primary bile acids are synthesized in liver from cholesterol
- B. Secondary bile acids are synthesized from primary in intestine
- C. Cholic & deoxycholic acids are primary bile acids
- D. Lithocholic acid is a secondary bile acid

Bile acids are not present in the diet but are synthesized in liver. Primary bile acids are synthesized in liver from cholesterol and secondary bile acids are synthesized from primary bile acids in intestine by colonic bacterial enzymes. Primary bile acids are cholic acid & chenodeoxycholic acid. Secondary bile acids are deoxycholic acid and lithocholic acid.

652. What quantity of bile acids are synthesized in liver every day?
Harrison's 20th Ed. Chapter 318 Page 2245
- A. 200 mg
- B. 300 mg
- C. 400 mg
- D. 500 mg

About 500 mg bile acids are synthesized in liver daily, conjugated to either taurine or glycine to form tauro-conjugated or glyco-conjugated bile acids, respectively, and then secreted into duodenum as bile.

653. Primary functions of bile acids is?
Harrison's 20th Ed. Chapter 318 Page 2245
- A. To promote bile flow
- B. To solubilize cholesterol & phospholipid in gallbladder
- C. To enhance dietary lipid digestion & absorption
- D. All of the above

Primary functions of bile acids are to promote bile flow, to solubilize cholesterol and phospholipid in gallbladder and to enhance dietary lipid digestion and absorption by forming mixed micelles in proximal small intestine.

654. Bile acids are primarily absorbed "actively" in?
Harrison's 20th Ed. Chapter 318 Page 2245
- A. Duodenum
- B. Jejunum
- C. Ileum
- D. Colon

Bile acids are primarily absorbed by an active, Na^+-dependent process exclusively in ileum. To a lesser extent, they are absorbed by non-carrier-mediated transport processes in the jejunum, ileum and colon.

655. The bile acid pool size is approximately?
Harrison's 20th Ed. Chapter 318 Page 2245
- A. 4 grams
- B. 8 grams
- C. 12 grams
- D. 16 grams

656. How many times bile acid pool is circulated via enterohepatic circulation?
Harrison's 20th Ed. Chapter 318 Page 2245
- A. 2 to 4 times / day
- B. 4 to 6 times / day
- C. 6 to 8 times / day
- D. 8 to 12 times / day

Bile acid pool size is ~4 grams and is circulated via the enterohepatic circulation about twice during each meal, or six to eight times daily.

657. Daily bile acids excretion in stool (fecal loss) equals?
Harrison's 20th Ed. Chapter 318 Page 2245

A. Half of total fat intake
B. Half of enterohepatic circulation
C. Hepatic bile acid synthesis
D. None of the above

A relatively small quantity of bile acids (~500 mg) is not absorbed and is excreted in stool daily; this fecal loss is matched by hepatic bile acid synthesis.

658. Secondary bile acids are formed in?
Harrison's 20th Ed. Chapter 318 Page 2245

A. Duodenum
B. Jejunum
C. Ileum
D. Colon

Colonic bacterial enzymes dehydroxylate bile acids to secondary bile acids.

659. Bile acid synthesis is autoregulated by?
Harrison's 20th Ed. Chapter 318 Page 2245

A. 7 α-hydroxylase
B. 7 β-hydroxylase
C. 7 δ-hydroxylase
D. 7 γ-hydroxylase

Bile acid synthesis is autoregulated by 7 alpha-hydroxylase, an initial enzyme in cholesterol degradation.

660. Steatorrhea can be caused by abnormalities in?
Harrison's 20th Ed. Chapter 318 Page 2245

A. Bile-acid synthesis & excretion
B. Physical state of bile-acids in the intestinal lumen
C. Bile-acid reabsorption
D. All of the above

661. Small ileal dysfunction leads to?
Harrison's 20th Ed. Chapter 318 Page 2246

A. Bile acid diarrhea
B. Fatty acid diarrhea
C. Chloride diarrhea
D. Protein diarrhea

Due to limited ileal disease or resection increased amount of bile acids are delivered into colon that stimulate active Cl− secretion producing diarrhea but not steatorrhea because hepatic synthesis of bile acids increases to compensate for the rate of fecal bile acid losses up to a limit. It is called bile acid diarrhea, or cholorrheic enteropathy. It responds promptly to cholestyramine until ileal size is severely reduced.

662. Large ileal dysfunction leads to?
Harrison's 20th Ed. Chapter 318 Page 2246

A. Bile acid diarrhea
B. Fatty acid diarrhea
C. Carbohydrate diarrhea
D. Protein diarrhea

Patients with greater degrees of ileal disease and/or resection have diarrhea & steatorrhea that do not respond to cholestyramine. Increased quantities of bile acids enter colon. Hepatic synthesis proves insufficient resulting in impaired micelle formation and steatorrhea. This is called fatty acid diarrhea. Low-fat diet can be effective.

663. Reabsorption defect in enterohepatic circulation of bile acids is due to?
Harrison's 20th Ed. Chapter 318 Page 2246

A. Cirrhosis
B. Primary biliary cirrhosis
C. Jejunal diverticulosis
D. Crohn's disease

Ileal dysfunction caused by Crohn's disease results in a decrease in bile acid reabsorption in ileum and an increase in the delivery of bile acids to large intestine leading to diarrhea with or without steatorrhea.

664. Which of the following is not a feature of bile acid diarrhea?
Harrison's 20th Ed. Chapter 318 Page 2246 Table 318-2

A. Normal bile acid pool size
B. None or mild steatorrhea
C. Responds to cholestyramine
D. Responds to low-fat diet

Features of bile acid diarrhea are—extent of ileal disease is limited, ileal bile acid absorption is reduced, fecal bile acid excretion is increased, fecal bile acid loss is compensated by hepatic synthesis, bile acid pool size is normal, steatorrhea is absent or mild, response obtained with cholestyramine & no response to low-fat diet.

665. Which of the following is not a feature of fatty acid diarrhea?
Harrison's 20th Ed. Chapter 318 Page 2246 Table 318-2

A. Reduced bile acid pool size
B. Steatorrhea
C. Responds to cholestyramine
D. Responds to low-fat diet

Features of fatty acid diarrhea are extensive ileal disease, ileal bile acid absorption reduced, fecal bile acid excretion increased, fecal bile acid loss is not compensated by hepatic synthesis, bile acid pool size is reduced, steatorrhea (>20 grams) that does not respond to cholestyramine but responds to a low-fat diet.

666. Which of the following is a negative regulator of bile acid synthesis?
Harrison's 20th Ed. Chapter 318 Page 2246

A. FGF17
B. FGF18
C. FGF19
D. FGF20

FGF19 is a negative regulator of bile acid synthesis. Bile acids in intestine release fibroblast growth factor 19 (FGF19) into circulation, which is transported to liver where it suppresses synthesis of bile acids from cholesterol by inhibiting the rate-limiting enzyme cytochrome P450 7A1 (CYP7A1) and also promotes gallbladder relaxation.

667. Which of the following type of fatty acids compose fats?
Harrison's 20th Ed. Chapter 318 Page 2246

A. Long-chain fatty acids (LCFAs)
B. Medium-chain fatty acids (MCFAs)
C. Short-chain fatty acids (SCFAs)
D. All of the above

Three types of fatty acids compose fats: long-chain fatty acids (LCFAs), medium-chain fatty acids (MCFAs), and short-chain fatty acids (SCFAs).

668. Dietary fat is in the form of?
Harrison's 20th Ed. Chapter 318 Page 2246

A. Long-chain triglycerides (LCTs)
B. Medium-chain fatty acids (MCFAs)
C. Short-chain fatty acids (SCFAs)
D. All of the above

Dietary fat is exclusively composed of long-chain triglycerides (LCTs), i.e., glycerol that is bound via ester-linkages to three LCFAs.

669. Majority of dietary long chain fatty acids (LCFAs) have carbon chain lengths of?
Harrison's 20th Ed. Chapter 318 Page 2246 Table 318-3

A. 6 - 8
B. 8 - 10
C. 10 - 12
D. > 12

3 types of fatty acids compose fats—long chain fatty acids (LCFAs), medium-chain fatty acids (MCFAs) & short-chain fatty acids (SCFAs). Majority of dietary LCFAs have carbon chain lengths of 16 or 18.

670. Dietary MCFAs have carbon chain lengths of?
Harrison's 20th Ed. Chapter 318 Page 2246 Table 318-3

A. 6 - 8
B. 8 - 12
C. 12 - 16
D. 16 - 20

Medium-chain triglycerides (MCTs) or medium-chain fatty acids, composed of fatty acids with carbon chain lengths of 8 to 10, are present in large amounts in coconut oil.

671. Which of the following fatty acids requires pancreatic lipolysis?
Harrison's 20th Ed. Chapter 318 Page 2246 Table 318-3

A. Long-chain fatty acids (LCFAs)
B. Medium-chain fatty acids (MCFAs)
C. Short-chain fatty acids (SCFAs)
D. All of the above

672. Which of the following fatty acids requires micelle formation?
Harrison's 20th Ed. Chapter 318 Page 2246 Table 318-3

A. Long-chain fatty acids (LCFAs)
B. Medium-chain fatty acids (MCFAs)
C. Short-chain fatty acids (SCFAs)
D. All of the above

673. Which of the following fatty acids is not present in diet?
Harrison's 20th Ed. Chapter 318 Page 2246 Table 318-3

A. Long-chain fatty acids (LCFAs)
B. Medium-chain fatty acids (MCFAs)
C. Short-chain fatty acids (SCFAs)
D. All of the above

674. Colon is the primary site of absorption of which of the following fatty acids?
Harrison's 20th Ed. Chapter 318 Page 2246 Table 318-3

A. Long-chain fatty acids (LCFAs)
B. Medium-chain fatty acids (MCFAs)
C. Short-chain fatty acids (SCFAs)
D. All of the above

675. Substantial amounts of which of the fatty acids is present in stool?
Harrison's 20th Ed. Chapter 318 Page 2246 Table 318-3

A. Long-chain fatty acids (LCFAs)
B. Medium-chain fatty acids (MCFAs)
C. Short-chain fatty acids (SCFAs)
D. All of the above

676. Steatorrhea results due to defect in which phase of dietary lipid assimilation?
Harrison's 20th Ed. Chapter 318 Page 2246

A. Intraluminal or digestive phase
B. Mucosal or absorptive phase
C. Delivery or postabsorptive phase
D. Any of the above

Assimilation of dietary lipid occurs in intraluminal or digestive phase, mucosal or absorptive phase and delivery or postabsorptive phase. An abnormality at any site of this process can cause steatorrhea.

677. "Micellar formation" belongs to which phase of dietary lipid assimilation?
Harrison's 20th Ed. Chapter 318 Page 2246

A. Intraluminal or digestive phase
B. Mucosal or absorptive phase
C. Delivery or postabsorptive phase
D. Any of the above

The digestive phase has two components, lipolysis and micellar formation.

678. Which of the following statements is false?
Harrison's 20th Ed. Chapter 318 Page 2247

A. Dietary lipid is in the form of long-chain triglycerides (LCTs)
B. Intestinal mucosa does not absorb triglycerides
C. All fatty acids of carbon chain length >12 are metabolized in the same manner
D. None of the above

679. Lipolysis is initiated in?
Harrison's 20th Ed. Chapter 318 Page 2247

A. Stomach
B. Duodenum
C. Jejunum
D. Iliem

680. In lipolysis, hydrolysis of triglycerides by lipase leads to the formation of?
Harrison's 20th Ed. Chapter 318 Page 2247

A. Free fatty acids
B. Monoglycerides
C. Glycerol
D. All of the above

Lipolysis i.e. hydrolysis of Tg to free fatty acids, β-monoglycerides & glycerol by lipase is "initiated" in stomach by gastric lipase. ~20 – 30% of total lipolysis occurs in stomach.

681. Pancreatic lipolysis is greatly enhanced by?
Harrison's 20th Ed. Chapter 318 Page 2247

A. Gastric lipase
B. Pancreatic lipase
C. Colipase
D. All of the above

Pancreatic lipolysis is greatly enhanced by the presence of pancreatic enzyme, colipase, which facilitates the movement of lipase to triglyceride.

682. Normal lipolysis can be maintained by what percentage of maximal pancreatic lipase secretion?
Harrison's 20th Ed. Chapter 318 Page 2247

A. 5%
B. 15%
C. 25%
D. 35%

Normal lipolysis can be maintained by ~5% of maximal pancreatic lipase secretion.

683. Pancreatic lipase is inactivated at?
Harrison's 20th Ed. Chapter 318 Page 2247

A. pH < 7
B. pH < 7.5
C. pH < 8
D. pH < 8.5

Lipolysis is completed in the duodenum and jejunum by pancreatic lipase, which is inactivated by pH <7.0 leading to altered lipolysis.

684. Mixed micelles are molecular aggregates composed of all except?
Harrison's 20th Ed. Chapter 318 Page 2247

A. Fatty acids
B. Triglycerides
C. Cholesterol
D. Conjugated bile acids

Mixed micelles are molecular aggregates composed of fatty acids, monoglycerides, phospholipids, cholesterol, and conjugated bile acids. Mixed micelles are formed when concentration of conjugated bile acids is greater than its CMC.

685. Which of the following relates best with absorptive phase of lipid digestion-absorption?
Harrison's 20th Ed. Chapter 318 Page 2247

A. Micellar formation
B. Uptake and reesterification
C. Formation of chylomicrons
D. Colonic bacterial enzymes

Uptake and reesterification constitute the absorptive phase of lipid digestion-absorption.

686. In which form lipids exit from intestinal epithelial cell?
Harrison's 20th Ed. Chapter 318 Page 2247

A. Free fatty acids
B. Reesterified triglyceride
C. Cholesterol
D. Monoglyceride

Fatty acids and monoglycerides are reesterified by a series of enzymatic steps in the endoplasmic reticulum to form triglycerides, the form in which lipid exits from the intestinal epithelial cell. Reesterified triglycerides require formation of chylomicrons for their exit from small-intestinal epithelial cell & their delivery to liver via lymphatics.

687. Chylomicrons are composed of?
Harrison's 20th Ed. Chapter 318 Page 2247

A. α-lipoprotein
B. β-lipoprotein
C. δ-lipoprotein
D. γ-lipoprotein

688. Chylomicrons contain?
Harrison's 20th Ed. Chapter 318 Page 2247

A. Triglyceride
B. Cholesterol and Cholesterol ester
C. Phospholipid
D. All of the above

689. Reesterified triglyceride exit from intestinal epithelial cell into?
Harrison's 20th Ed. Chapter 318 Page 2247

A. Lymphatics
B. Portal vein
C. Systemic vein
D. All of the above

Chylomicrons are composed of beta-lipoprotein and contain triglycerides, cholesterol, cholesterol esters, and phospholipids and enter the lymphatics, not the portal vein.

690. In abetalipoproteinemia, the defect is in?
Harrison's 20th Ed. Chapter 318 Page 2247

A. Lipolysis
B. Micelle formation
C. Lipid uptake
D. Reesterified triglyceride exit from epithelial cell

691. Which of the following is normal in patients with abetalipoproteinemia?
Harrison's 20th Ed. Chapter 318 Page 2247

A. Lipolysis
B. Micelle formation
C. Lipid uptake
D. All of the above

Abetalipoproteinemia, or acanthocytosis is a disorder of impaired synthesis of beta-lipoprotein. In abetalipoproteinemia, lipolysis, micelle formation & lipid uptake are all normal, but reesterified triglyceride cannot exit from intestinal epithelial cell because of the failure to produce chylomicrons.

692. Coconut oil contains mainly?
Harrison's 20th Ed. Chapter 318 Page 2247

A. Long-chain triglycerides (LCTs)
B. Medium-chain triglycerides (MCT)
C. Short-chain fatty acids (SCFA)
D. All of the above

Medium-chain triglycerides (MCTs), composed of fatty acids with carbon chain lengths of 8 to 10, are present in large amounts in coconut oil and are used as a nutritional supplement.

693. Which of the following statements about Medium-chain triglycerides (MCTs) is false?
Harrison's 20th Ed. Chapter 318 Page 2248

A. Do not require pancreatic lipolysis
B. Micelle formation is not necessary for absorption
C. Following absorption, not reesterified
D. Route of exit is via lymphatics

Unlike LCTs, MCTs do not require pancreatic lipolysis as Tg can be absorbed intact by intestinal epithelial cell & micelle formation is not necessary for absorption of MCTs, following absorption are not reesterified, do not require chylomicron formation for their exit from intestinal epithelial cells, & their route of exit is via portal vein & not via lymphatics.

694. The SCFA present in stool is?
Harrison's 20th Ed. Chapter 318 Page 2248

A. Acetate
B. Propionate
C. Butyrate
D. All of the above

The SCFAs present in stool are primarily acetate, propionate, and butyrate, whose carbon chain lengths are 2, 3, and 4, respectively.

695. The primary nutrient for colonic epithelial cells is?
Harrison's 20th Ed. Chapter 318 Page 2248

A. Acetate
B. Propionate
C. Butyrate
D. All of the above

Butyrate is the primary nutrient for colonic epithelial cells & its deficiency may be associated with colitis.

696. Which of the following statements about SCFAs is false?
Harrison's 20th Ed. Chapter 318 Page 2248

A. SCFAs are dietary lipids
B. Synthesized by colonic bacterial enzymes from nonabsorbed carbohydrate
C. SCFAs in stool are acetate, propionate, & butyrate
D. SCFAs are rapidly absorbed & stimulate colonic Na-Cl & fluid absorption

SCFAs are not dietary lipids but are synthesized by colonic bacterial enzymes from nonabsorbed carbohydrate. SCFAs present in stool are primarily acetate, propionate, and butyrate. SCFAs are rapidly absorbed and stimulate colonic Na-Cl and fluid absorption.

697. C. difficile accounts for what percentage of all antibiotic-associated diarrhea?
Harrison's 20th Ed. Chapter 318 Page 2248

A. ~ 10 - 15%
B. ~ 25 - 40%
C. ~ 40 - 75%
D. ~ 75 - 95%

C. difficile accounts for ~10 - 15% of all antibiotic-associated diarrhea.

698. Carbohydrates in the diet are present in the form of?
Harrison's 20th Ed. Chapter 318 Page 2248

A. Starch
B. Disaccharides (sucrose & lactose)
C. Glucose
D. All of the above

Carbohydrates in the diet are present in the form of starch, disaccharides (sucrose and lactose), and glucose.

699. Which of the following statements about carbohydrates is false?
Harrison's 20th Ed. Chapter 318 Page 2248

A. Absorbed only in the small intestine
B. Absorbed only in the form of monosaccharides
C. Absorption occurs by a Na-dependent process
D. None of the above

700. Brush border transport protein that mediates monosaccharide absorption is?
Harrison's 20th Ed. Chapter 318 Page 2248

A. AGLT1
B. MGLT1
C. SGLT1
D. TGLT1

Carbohydrates are absorbed only in the small intestine and only in the form of monosaccharides whose absorption occurs by a Na-dependent process mediated by the brush border transport protein SGLT1.

701. Which of the following about lactose malabsorption is false?
Harrison's 20th Ed. Chapter 318 Page 2248

A. Glucose and galactose are constituents of lactose
B. Primary lactase deficiency patients have severe symptoms
C. Secondary lactase deficiency is seen in celiac sprue
D. Symptoms may be similar to IBS

Most individuals with primary lactase deficiency do not have symptoms.

702. Congenital absence of SGLT leads to?
Harrison's 20th Ed. Chapter 318 Page 2248

A. Glucose, galactose malabsorption
B. Lactose malabsorption
C. Maltose malabsorption
D. Sucrose malabsorption

Congenital absence of SGLT leads to glucose-galactose or monosaccharide malabsorption diarrhea.

703. Which of the following carbohydrate is absorbed by brush border transport protein - GLUT 5?
Harrison's 20th Ed. Chapter 318 Page 2248

A. Glucose
B. Galactose
C. Fructose
D. Sorbitol

Fructose is absorbed by the brush border transport protein GLUT 5, a facilitated diffusion process that is not Na-dependent and is distinct from SGLT.

704. Actively transported monosaccharides are all except?
Harrison's 20th Ed. Chapter 318 Page 2248

A. Glucose
B. Galactose
C. Fructose
D. All of the above

Actively transported monosaccharides are glucose and galactose.

705. Sugar used in diabetic candy is?
Harrison's 20th Ed. Chapter 318 Page 2248

A. Sorbitol
B. Galactose
C. Fructose
D. None of the above

Sugar used in diabetic candy is sorbitol which is only minimally absorbed due to absence of an intestinal absorptive transport mechanism for sorbitol.

706. What value of stool pH is consistent with carbohydrate malabsorption?
Gastroenterology 1999;116:1461-1463

A. < 5.6
B. < 6.6
C. < 7.6
D. < 8.6

Stool pH <5.6 is consistent with carbohydrate malabsorption.

707. Protein is present in food almost exclusively as?
Harrison's 20th Ed. Chapter 318 Page 2248

A. Polypeptides
B. Dipeptides
C. Tripeptides
D. Amino acids

Protein is present in food almost exclusively as polypeptides and requires extensive hydrolysis to di- and tripeptides and amino acids before absorption.

708. Brush border enzyme that converts the proenzyme trypsinogen to trypsin is?
Harrison's 20th Ed. Chapter 318 Page 2249

A. Enterokinase
B. Colipase
C. Pepsinogen
D. Amylase

Proenzyme trypsinogen is activated to trypsin by the intestinal brush border enzyme enterokinase, and subsequently by trypsin.

709. Alterations in protein or amino acid digestion and absorption is seen in which of the following?
Harrison's 20th Ed. Chapter 318 Page 2249

A. Enterokinase deficiency
B. Hartnup syndrome
C. Cystinuria
D. All of the above

Enterokinase deficiency leads to failure to convert proenzyme trypsinogen to trypsin and is manifested as diarrhea, growth retardation and hypoproteinemia. Hartnup syndrome, a defect in neutral amino acid transport, is characterized by a pellagra-like rash and neuropsychiatric symptoms. Cystinuria, a defect in dibasic amino acid transport, is associated with renal calculi and chronic pancreatitis.

710. The proximal small intestine is the site for the absorption of all of the following except?
Harrison's 20th Ed. Chapter 318 Page 2249

A. Calcium
B. Iron
C. Folic acid
D. Bile acids

Calcium, iron and folic acid are exclusively absorbed by active transport processes in proximal small intestine especially the duodenum.

711. Ileum is the absorption site of all of the following except?
Harrison's 20th Ed. Chapter 318 Page 2249

A. Cobalamin
B. Bile acids
C. Calcium
D. None of the above

Active transport mechanisms for cobalamin & bile acids are present only in ileum.

712. Glucose, amino acids and lipids are absorbed in?
Harrison's 20th Ed. Chapter 318 Page 2249

A. Duodenum
B. Jejunum
C. Ileum
D. Throughout the small intestine

Glucose, amino acids & lipids are absorbed throughout the small intestine, although their rate of absorption is greater in the proximal than in the distal segments.

713. Which of the following is critical for survival of individuals with massive resection of small intestine and/or colon?
Harrison's 20th Ed. Chapter 318 Page 2249

A. Adaptation
B. Acclimation
C. Adaption
D. Accommodation

After segmental resection of small intestine/colon, remaining segments undergo morphologic & functional "adaptation" to enhance absorption.

714. Estimation of which of the following in stool helps distinguish pancreatic from nonpancreatic etiologies of steatorrhea?
Harrison's 20th Ed. Chapter 318 Page 2249

A. Stool trypsin
B. Stool chymotrypsin
C. Stool lipase
D. All of the above

Assays for stool chymotrypsin & elastase can distinguish pancreatic from nonpancreatic etiologies of steatorrhea. Indirect tests like assay of fecal elastase or chymotrypsin activity or a bentiromide test have fallen out of favor because of low sensitivity & specificity.

715. Which of the following is false about urinary D-xylose test?
Harrison's 20th Ed. Chapter 318 Page 2249

A. Assesses proximal small-intestinal mucosal function
B. D-Xylose is a pentose carbohydrate
C. 25 g of D-xylose & collecting urine for 5 hours
D. < 12 g excretion means an abnormal test

D-Xylose is a pentose absorbed almost exclusively in proximal small intestine. Urinary D-xylose test (<4.5 gram excretion) reflects presence of duodenal / jejunal mucosal disease.

716. Samples of which of the following are collected in the D-xylose test?
Harrison's 20th Ed. Chapter 318 Page 2249

A. Urine
B. Stool
C. Blood
D. All of the above

D-xylose test is performed by administering 25 grams of D-xylose and collecting urine for 5 hours.

717. Urinary D-xylose test can be false-positive in?
Harrison's 20th Ed. Chapter 318 Page 2249

A. Head injury
B. Myocardial infarction
C. Ascitis
D. Pneumonia

Urinary D-xylose test is false-positive in large fluid collections in third space (ascites, pleural fluid).

718. D-Xylose Test is normal in which of the following?
Harrison's 20th Ed. Chapter 318 Page 2252 Table 318-7
- A. Chronic pancreatitis
- B. Ileal disease
- C. Intestinal lymphangiectasia
- D. All of the above

719. Which of the following is suspected when macrophages in lamina propria contain material positive on PAS staining?
Harrison's 20th Ed. Chapter 318 Page 2251 Table 318-6
- A. Amyloidosis
- B. Celiac disease
- C. Whipple's disease
- D. Crohn's disease

720. Short villi, decreased mitosis in crypts and megalocytosis is a feature of all except?
Harrison's 20th Ed. Chapter 318 Page 2251 Table 318-6
- A. Folate deficiency
- B. Vitamin B12 deficiency
- C. Radiation enteritis
- D. Drug-induced enteritis

721. Noncaseating granulomas in small-intestinal mucosal biopsies is a feature of?
Harrison's 20th Ed. Chapter 318 Page 2251 Table 318-6
- A. Tropical sprue
- B. Crohn's disease
- C. Intestinal lymphangiectasia
- D. Amyloidosis

722. Normal villi with epithelial cells vacuolated with fat postprandially in small-intestinal mucosal biopsies is a feature of?
Harrison's 20th Ed. Chapter 318 Page 2251 Table 318-6
- A. Whipple's disease
- B. Agammaglobulinemia
- C. Abetalipoproteinemia
- D. Protein-calorie malnutrition

723. Clubbed villi in small-intestinal mucosal biopsies is a feature of?
Harrison's 20th Ed. Chapter 318 Page 2251 Table 318-6
- A. Tropical sprue
- B. Crohn's disease
- C. Intestinal lymphangiectasia
- D. Amyloidosis

724. Schilling test is performed to determine the cause for?
Harrison's 20th Ed. Chapter 327 Page 2323 Table 327-2
- A. Cobalamin malabsorption
- B. Folic acid malabsorption
- C. Iron malabsorption
- D. All of the above

Schilling test is performed to determine the cause for cobalamin malabsorption.

725. Cobalamin is present primarily in?
Harrison's 20th Ed. Chapter 95 Page 699
- A. Fruits
- B. Green vegetables
- C. Meat
- D. Egg

Cobalamin is present primarily in meat.

726. Cyanide toxicity is a possibility with which of the following forms of vitamin B12?
N Engl J Med. 2013;368:2041
- A. Cyanocobalamin
- B. Hydroxocobalamin
- C. Methylcobalamin
- D. All of the above

A 1000-μg dose of cyanocobalamin contains 20 μg (0.78 μmol) of cyanide. Oral vitamin B12 at a daily dose of 2000 μg (20 μg absorbed on average) is equivalent to weekly injections of cyanocobalamin at a dose of 1000 μg (150 μg retained).

727. Haptocorrin was previously named as?
BMC Res Notes. 2011; 4: 208
- A. Transcobalamin I
- B. Transcobalamin III
- C. R-binder
- D. All of the above

Haptocorrin (previously named transcobalamin I and III, and R-binder) is a glycoprotein, which is present in human milk in relatively large amounts. It is characterized by its ability to bind vitamin B12 and other corrinoids, and exists in two forms in human milk - apo-haptocorrin, which is unsaturated with vitamin B12, and holo-haptocorrin, which is saturated with vitamin B12.

728. Intrinsic factor is synthesized and released by?
Harrison's 20th Ed. Chapter 317 Page 2222
- A. Gastric parietal cells
- B. Gastric oxyntic cells
- C. Gastric chief cells
- D. Gastric G cells

Intrinsic factor (IF) is absolutely required for the absorption of cobalamin. IF is a glycoprotein synthesized & released by gastric parietal cells, to promote its uptake by specific cobalamin receptors on the brush border of ileal enterocytes. Pancreatic protease enzymes split the cobalamin–R binder complex to release cobalamin in proximal small intestine, where cobalamin is then bound by intrinsic factor (IF).

729. Cobalamin absorption may be abnormal in which of the following?
Harrison's 20th Ed. Chapter 95 Page 707
- A. Pernicious anemia
- B. Chronic pancreatitis
- C. Bacterial overgrowth syndromes
- D. All of the above

Cobalamin absorption may be abnormal in pernicious anemia, chronic pancreatitis, achlorhydria, bacterial overgrowth syndromes, and Ileal dysfunction.

730. Which isotope is used in Schilling test?
Harrison's 20th Ed. Chapter 95 Page 703
- A. ^{58}Co-labeled cobalamin
- B. ^{68}Co-labeled cobalamin
- C. ^{78}Co-labeled cobalamin
- D. ^{88}Co-labeled cobalamin

Schilling test is performed by administering ^{58}Co-labeled cobalamin orally and collecting urine for 24 hours. It is dependent on normal renal and bladder function. Radioactive B_{12} is no longer available, and Schilling tests are no longer performed.

731. **Synonym of Celiac sprue is?**
   Harrison's 20th Ed. Chapter 318 Page 2251
   A. Nontropical sprue
   B. Celiac disease
   C. Gluten sensitive enteropathy
   D. All of the above

   Celiac sprue has also been known as nontropical sprue, celiac disease (in children), adult celiac disease, and gluten sensitive enteropathy.

732. **Which of the following about Celiac disease is false?**
   N Engl J Med. 2012;367:2419-26
   A. Systemic disorder
   B. Immune-mediated disorder
   C. Triggered by dietary gluten
   D. None of the above

   Celiac disease is a systemic immune-mediated disorder triggered by dietary gluten in genetically susceptible persons.

733. **The word "sprue" comes from which language?**
   N Engl J Med. 2007;357:1731-43
   A. Dutch
   B. Latin
   C. Greek
   D. English

734. **Which of the following respond to elimination of gluten from the diet in celiac sprue?**
   Harrison's 20th Ed. Chapter 318 Page 2251
   A. Symptoms
   B. Evidence of malabsorption
   C. Histopathologic changes in small-intestinal biopsy
   D. All of the above

   In celiac sprue, symptoms, evidence of malabsorption and histopathologic changes on small-intestinal biopsy respond to elimination of gluten from diet.

735. **Gliadin (a component of gluten) is present in all except?**
   Harrison's 20th Ed. Chapter 318 Page 2252
   A. Wheat
   B. Barley
   C. Rice
   D. Rye

   Gluten is a protein complex. Gliadin is a component of gluten present in wheat, barley, rye & in smaller amounts in oats. Antiendomysial antibody tTG deaminates gliadin.

736. **Which of the following is considered as "safe grains" (gluten-free)?**
   N Engl J Med. 2007;357:1731-43
   A. Rice
   B. Corn
   C. Millet
   D. All of the above

   Safe grains (gluten-free) include rice, amaranth, buckwheat, corn, millet, quinoa, sorghum, teff (an Ethiopian cereal grain), & oats.

737. **Gliadin is which component of gluten?**
   N Engl J Med. 2007;357:1731-43
   A. Heat resistant fraction
   B. Alcohol-soluble fraction
   C. Water soluble fraction
   D. Contaminated fraction

   "Gluten" refers to the entire protein component of wheat. Gliadin is the alcohol-soluble fraction of gluten that contains bulk of toxic components.

738. **Which of the following enzyme in intestine deamidates gliadin peptides?**
   N Engl J Med. 2007;357:1731-43
   A. Tissue transaminase
   B. Tissue transmurase
   C. Tissue transglutaminase
   D. Tissue transpeptidase

   Enzyme tissue transglutaminase in intestine deamidates gliadin peptides increasing their immunogenicity.

739. **The most sensitive antibody tests for the diagnosis of celiac disease are of which class?**
   N Engl J Med. 2007;357:1731-43
   A. IgA
   B. IgG
   C. IgM
   D. IgE

   Most sensitive antibody tests for diagnosis of celiac disease are of IgA class.

740. **Serum antibodies found in celiac sprue include all except?**
   Harrison's 20th Ed. Chapter 318 Page 2252
   A. IgA antigliadin
   B. IgA antiendomysial antibodies
   C. IgA anti-tissue transglutaminase
   D. IgA anti-tissue transpeptidase

   "Celiac serologies" in celiac sprue include serum antibodies like IgA antigliadin, IgA antiendomysial and IgA anti-tTG antibodies are present suggesting an immunologic component to etiology.

741. **Antiendomysial antibodies are directed against?**
   N Engl J Med. 2007;357:1731-43
   A. Epithelial tissue
   B. Enzyme
   C. Connective-tissue
   D. All of the above

   Serological tests in celiac disease include antigliadin antibodies, connective-tissue antibodies (antireticulin & antiendomysial antibodies), & antibodies against tissue transglutaminase, enzyme responsible for deamidation of gliadin in lamina propria.

742. **Antigen recognized by the antiendomysial antibody test is?**
   Harrison's 20th Ed. Chapter 318 Page 2252
   A. Tissue transaminase
   B. Tissue transmurase
   C. Tissue transglutaminase
   D. Tissue transpeptidase

   In celiac sprue, antigen recognized by antiendomysial antibody test is tissue transglutaminase (tTG).

743. **Negative predictive value of which of the following HLA allele is almost 100% in celiac sprue?**
   N Engl J Med. 2007;357:1731-43

   A. HLA-DQ2
   B. HLA-DQ3
   C. HLA-DQ4
   D. HLA-DQ5

   In patients with doubtful celiac sprue, HLA-DQ2 or HLA-DQ8 typing is useful, since negative predictive value of this test is almost 100%. Almost all patients with celiac sprue express HLA-DQ2 allele. Absence of DQ2 excludes the diagnosis of celiac sprue. All patients with celiac disease express the HLA-DQ2 or HLA-DQ8 allele.

744. **The HLA-DQ2 haplotype (DQA1*0501/DQB1*0201) is expressed in what proportion of the general population?**
   N Engl J Med. 2012;367:2419-26

   A. One third
   B. One half
   C. Three fourth
   D. None

   *The HLA-DQ2 haplotype (DQA1*0501/DQB1*0201) is expressed in the majority of patients with celiac disease (90%), whereas it is expressed in one third of the general population. In another 5% of patients with celiac disease, the HLA-DQ8 haplotype (DQA1*0301/DQB1*0302) is expressed, whereas almost all the remaining 5% of patients have at least one of the two genes encoding DQ2 (DQB1*0201 or DQA1*0501). DQ2 & DQ8 haplotypes are necessary but not sufficient for the development of celiac disease. At least 39 non-HLA genes that predispose to celiac disease have been identified, mostly involved in inflammatory and immune responses.*

745. **Which of the following tests have a high negative predictive value in the diagnosis of celiac disease?**
   N Engl J Med. 2012;367:2419-26

   A. IgA anti-tTG antibodies
   B. IgG anti-tTG antibodies
   C. IgA antiendomysial antibodies
   D. HLA-DQ2 or HLA-DQ8

   Testing for HLA-DQ2 and HLA-DQ8 may be useful in at-risk persons (e.g., family members of patients with celiac disease). Such testing has a high negative predictive value, which means that the disease is very unlikely to develop in persons who are negative for both HLA-DQ2 and HLA-DQ8. Absence of HLA DQ2/DQ8 excludes the diagnosis of celiac disease.

746. **Which of the following tests have usefulness in patients with IgA deficiency?**
   N Engl J Med. 2012;367:2419-26

   A. IgA anti-tTG antibodies
   B. IgG anti-tTG antibodies
   C. IgA antiendomysial antibodies
   D. HLA-DQ2 or HLA-DQ8

747. **Which of the following tests have usefulness in patients with an uncertain diagnosis?**
   N Engl J Med. 2012;367:2419-26

   A. IgA anti-tTG antibodies
   B. IgG anti-tTG antibodies
   C. IgA antiendomysial antibodies
   D. HLA-DQ2 or HLA-DQ8

748. **Absence of DQ2/DQ8 which of the following excludes the diagnosis of celiac disease?**
   Harrison's 20th Ed. Chapter 318 Page 2253

   A. DQ1 / DQ8
   B. DQ2 / DQ8
   C. DQ3 / DQ8
   D. DQ4 / DQ8

   All patients with celiac disease express HLA-DQ2 or HLA-DQ8 allele. Absence of DQ2/DQ8 excludes the diagnosis of celiac disease.

749. **Which of the following is false about duodenal/jejunal biopsy histopathology in celiac sprue?**
   Harrison's 20th Ed. Chapter 318 Page 2253

   A. Reduced height of villi
   B. Crypt hyperplasia
   C. Increased lymphocytes & plasma cells in lamina propria
   D. None of the above

   A small-intestinal biopsy is required to establish a diagnosis of celiac disease. In celiac sprue, changes seen on duodenal/jejunal biopsy are restricted to mucosa and include absence or reduced height of villi (flat appearance), crypt hyperplasia and villus atrophy and increased lymphocytes and plasma cells in the lamina propria.

750. **Histopathologic features characteristic of celiac sprue can also be seen in all except?**
   Harrison's 20th Ed. Chapter 318 Page 2253

   A. Tropical sprue
   B. Ulcerative colitis
   C. Milk-protein intolerance in children
   D. Eosinophilic enteritis

751. **Histopathologic features characteristic of celiac sprue can also be seen in all except?**
   Harrison's 20th Ed. Chapter 318 Page 2253

   A. Lymphoma
   B. Intestinal lymphangiectasis
   C. Crohn's disease
   D. Gastrinoma with acid hypersecretion

   Histopathologic features of celiac sprue is seen in tropical sprue, eosinophilic enteritis & milk-protein intolerance in children, lymphoma, bacterial overgrowth, Crohn's disease & gastrinoma with acid hypersecretion.

752. **Which of the following about "Celiac crisis" is false?**
   N Engl J Med. 2012;367:2419-26

   A. Mostly observed in adults
   B. Severe diarrhea
   C. Hypoproteinemia
   D. Metabolic and electrolyte imbalances

   Celiac crisis is a rare life-threatening syndrome, mostly observed in children, characterized by severe diarrhea, hypoproteinemia, and metabolic and electrolyte imbalances.

753. **After how many months of a strict gluten free diet, celiac disease is termed refractory?**
   N Engl J Med. 2012;367:2419-26

   A. 3 months
   B. 6 months
   C. 9 months
   D. 12 months

   Refractory celiac disease is diagnosed when there are persistent or recurrent malabsorptive symptoms and signs with villous atrophy detected on biopsy despite maintenance of a strict gluten free diet for more than 12 months.

754. Which of the following is true for refractory celiac disease type 2?

   N Engl J Med. 2012;367:2419-26

   A. Abnormal intraepithelial lymphocytes
   B. Clonal intraepithelial lymphocytes without CD3
   C. Clonal intraepithelial lymphocytes without CD8
   D. All of the above

Refractory celiac disease can be classified as type 1 (normal intraepithelial lymphocytes) or type 2 (abnormal intraepithelial lymphocytes; clonal intraepithelial lymphocytes lacking surface markers CD3, CD8, and T-cell receptors; or both). Type 2 is associated with a higher risk of ulcerative jejunoileitis and lymphoma than type 1.

755. In celiac disease, the lowest amount of daily gluten that causes damage to celiac intestinal mucosa over time (gluten threshold) is?

   N Engl J Med. 2012;367:2419-26

   A. 1 to 5 mg per day
   B. 10 to 50 mg per day
   C. 100 to 500 mg per day
   D. 1000 to 2500 mg per day

In celiac disease, the lowest amount of daily gluten that causes damage to celiac intestinal mucosa over time (gluten threshold) is 10 to 50 mg per day (a 25 gram slice of bread contains ~1.6 grams of gluten). New Codex Alimentarius regulation permits a maximum gluten contamination of 20 ppm in gluten-free products.

756. Interval between exposure to gluten and onset of symptoms in Celiac disease is?

   N Engl J Med. 2012;367:2419-26

   A. Minutes to hours
   B. Hours to days
   C. Weeks to years
   D. Any of the above

757. Interval between exposure to gluten and onset of symptoms in wheat allergy is?

   N Engl J Med. 2012;367:2419-26

   A. Minutes to hours
   B. Hours to days
   C. Weeks to years
   D. Any of the above

758. Interval between exposure to gluten and onset of symptoms in gluten sensitivity is?

   N Engl J Med. 2012;367:2419-26

   A. Minutes to hours
   B. Hours to days
   C. Weeks to years
   D. Any of the above

759. Mechanism of diarrhea in celiac disease is?

   Harrison's 20th Ed. Chapter 318 Page 2253

   A. Steatorrhea
   B. Secondary lactase deficiency
   C. Bile acid malabsorption
   D. All of the above

The diarrhea in celiac disease may be secondary to steatorrhea (due to changes in jejunal mucosal function), secondary lactase deficiency (due to changes in jejunal brush border enzymatic function), bile acid malabsorption (due to bile acid–induced fluid secretion in the colon) and endogenous fluid secretion resulting from crypt hyperplasia.

760. The diarrhea in celiac sprue is due to all except?

   Harrison's 20th Ed. Chapter 318 Page 2253

   A. Steatorrhea
   B. Lipase deficiency
   C. Bile acid malabsorption
   D. Endogenous fluid secretion

Diarrhea in celiac sprue may be secondary to steatorrhea, secondary lactase deficiency, bile acid malabsorption and endogenous fluid secretion.

761. Celiac disease patients may improve temporarily with restriction of?

   Harrison's 20th Ed. Chapter 318 Page 2253

   A. Soy
   B. Dietary lactose
   C. Fat
   D. All of the above

762. Celiac sprue may be associated with following diseases except?

   Harrison's 20th Ed. Chapter 318 Page 2253, N Engl J Med. 2002;346:181

   A. Dermatitis herpetiformis (DH)
   B. Type 1 diabetes mellitus
   C. IgA deficiency
   D. Chronic pancreatitis

Celiac disease is associated with dermatitis herpetiformis (DH), diabetes mellitus type 1, IgA deficiency, Down syndrome, Turner's syndrome, Autoimmune thyroid disease, Sjögren's syndrome, Microscopic colitis, Rheumatoid arthritis.

763. Patients with DH have characteristic papulovesicular lesions that respond to?

   Harrison's 20th Ed. Chapter 318 Page 2253

   A. Azathioprine
   B. Dapsone
   C. Thalidomide
   D. All of the above

764. Prevalence of celiac disease is increased in which of the following conditions?

   N Engl J Med. 2012;367:2419-26

   A. Hashimoto's thyroiditis
   B. Turner's syndrome
   C. IgA deficiency
   D. All of the above

Prevalence of celiac disease is 1.5 to 2 times as high among women as among men and is increased among persons who have an affected first-degree relative (10 to 15%), type 1 diabetes (3 to 16%), Hashimoto's thyroiditis (5%) or other autoimmune diseases (including autoimmune liver diseases, Sjögren's syndrome, and IgA nephropathy), Down's syndrome (5%), Turner's syndrome (3%), and IgA deficiency (9%).

765. Complications of Celiac sprue include all except?

   Harrison's 20th Ed. Chapter 318 Page 2253

   A. Malignancy
   B. Intestinal ulceration
   C. Collagenous sprue
   D. Fistulas

Complications of celiac sprue include gastrointestinal and nongastrointestinal neoplasms, intestinal ulceration and collagenous sprue.

766. **Complications associated with untreated celiac disease include?**
Harrison's 20th Ed. Chapter 318 Page 2253, N Engl J Med. 2012;367:2419-26
   A. Infertility or recurrent abortion
   B. Impaired splenic function
   C. Neurologic disorders
   D. All of the above

Complications associated with untreated celiac disease include osteoporosis, impaired splenic function, neurologic disorders, infertility or recurrent abortion, ulcerative jejunoileitis, and cancer. Enteropathy-associated T-cell lymphoma and adenocarcinoma of the jejunum are rare complications of celiac disease.

767. **Endocrine and metabolic disorders that can cause malabsorption syndrome include?**
Harrison's 20th Ed. Chapter 318 Page 2257, Table 318-8
   A. Hypoparathyroidism
   B. Hyperthyroidism
   C. Carcinoid syndrome
   D. All of the above

Endocrine & metabolic disorders that can cause malabsorption syndrome include diabetes, hypoparathyroidism, adrenal insufficiency, hyperthyroidism & carcinoid syndrome.

768. **Circulatory disorders that can cause malabsorption syndrome include?**
Harrison's 20th Ed. Chapter 318 Page 2257, Table 318-8
   A. Congestive heart failure
   B. Constrictive pericarditis
   C. Mesenteric artery atherosclerosis
   D. All of the above

769. **Dermatitis in malabsorption syndrome is due to deficiency of?**
Harrison's 20th Ed. Chapter 318 Page 2257, Table 318-9
   A. Vitamin A
   B. Zinc
   C. Essential fatty acid
   D. All of the above

770. **Glossitis, cheilosis, stomatitis in malabsorption syndrome is due to deficiency of?**
Harrison's 20th Ed. Chapter 318 Page 2257, Table 318-9
   A. Iron
   B. Vitamin B12, folate
   C. Vitamin A
   D. All of the above

771. **Tropical sprue is manifested by all except?**
Harrison's 20th Ed. Chapter 318 Page 2253
   A. Acute diarrhea
   B. Steatorrhea
   C. Weight loss
   D. Nutritional deficiencies

Tropical sprue is manifested by chronic diarrhea, steatorrhea, weight loss, and nutritional deficiencies.

772. **Chronic diarrhea in a tropical environment is most often caused by all except?**
Harrison's 20th Ed. Chapter 318 Page 2253
   A. Yersinia enterocolitica
   B. Cryptosporidium parvum
   C. Giardia lamblia
   D. Entamoeba histolytica

Chronic diarrhea in a tropical environment is most often caused by G. lamblia, Yersinia enterocolitica, C. difficile, Cryptosporidium parvum and Cyclospora cayetanensis.

773. **Which of the following is similar to Tropical sprue?**
Harrison's 20th Ed. Chapter 318 Page 2254
   A. Sprue-like enteropathy
   B. Environmental enteropathy
   C. Protein-wasting enteropathy
   D. Autoimmune enteropathy

Environmental enteropathy ("impoverished gut"; blunted small-intestinal villi with lamina propria inflammation) is observed in tropical developing areas with endemic enteric infections like amebiasis.

774. **Patients of Tropical sprue are rarely found in?**
Harrison's 20th Ed. Chapter 318 Page 2254
   A. South India
   B. Philippines
   C. Caribbean islands
   D. Africa

Tropical sprue is found in South India, Philippines and Caribbean islands, but is rarely observed in Africa, Jamaica, or Southeast Asia.

775. **Which of the following in tropical sprue differentiate it from celiac disease?**
Harrison's 20th Ed. Chapter 318 Page 2254
   A. More mononuclear cell infiltrate in the lamina propria
   B. Less villous architectural alteration
   C. Similar degree of severity throughout small intestine
   D. All of the above

Further, gluten-free diet does not result in either clinical or histologic improvement in tropical sprue.

776. **Treatment of tropical sprue includes?**
Harrison's 20th Ed. Chapter 318 Page 2254
   A. Vitamin B12
   B. Folic acid
   C. Iron
   D. Calcium

777. **Treatment of tropical sprue includes?**
Harrison's 20th Ed. Chapter 318 Page 2254
   A. Gluten-free diet
   B. Broad-spectrum antibiotics
   C. Glucocorticoids
   D. All of the above

Broad-spectrum antibiotics and folic acid are curative in tropical sprue.

778. **In tropical sprue, tetracycline should be used for up to?**
Harrison's 20th Ed. Chapter 318 Page 2254
   A. 4 weeks
   B. 12 weeks
   C. 24 weeks
   D. 48 weeks

In tropical sprue, tetracycline should be used for up to 6 months.

779. Diseases that may arise following small-intestinal resection include all except?
Harrison's 20th Ed. Chapter 318 Page 2254

A. Colonic diverticulosis
B. Cholesterol gallstones
C. Gastric hypersecretion of acid
D. Hyperoxaluria

Following large resections of small intestine, enteric hyperoxaluria, cholesterol gallstones and gastric hypersecretion of acid occurs.

780. "Intestinal failure" best relates to?
Harrison's 20th Ed. Chapter 318 Page 2255

A. Inability to maintain nutrition with parenteral support
B. Inability to maintain nutrition without parenteral support
C. Inability to maintain nutrition by all means
D. All of the above

Intestinal failure refers to an inability to maintain nutrition without parenteral support.

781. Enteric hyperoxaluria is best treated with?
Harrison's 20th Ed. Chapter 318 Page 2255

A. Allopurinol
B. Aspirin
C. Codeine
D. Cholestyramine

Cholestyramine, an anion-binding resin & calcium are useful in reducing hyperoxaluria.

782. Which of the following hormones has a role in the treatment of short bowel syndrome?
Harrison's 20th Ed. Chapter 318 Page 2255

A. Glucagon-like peptide 2 (GLP-2)
B. VIP
C. Cholecystokinin
D. TSH

A recombinant analogue of glucagon-like peptide 2 (teduglutide) is approved for short bowel syndrome.

783. Which of the following is not a presentation of bacterial overgrowth syndrome?
Harrison's 20th Ed. Chapter 318 Page 2255

A. Diarrhea
B. Steatorrhea
C. Macrocytic anemia
D. Microcytic anemia

Bacterial overgrowth syndromes comprise a group of disorders with diarrhea, steatorrhea & macrocytic anemia. The common feature is proliferation of colonic-type bacteria within small intestine like E. coli or Bacteroides.

784. Stagnant bowel or blind loop syndrome refers to?
Harrison's 20th Ed. Chapter 318 Page 2255

A. Stasis due to impaired peristalsis
B. Changes in intestinal anatomy
C. Direct communication between small & large intestine
D. All of the above

Bacterial proliferation in bacterial overgrowth syndrome or stagnant bowel syndrome or blind loop syndrome is due to stasis caused by impaired peristalsis (functional stasis), changes in intestinal anatomy (anatomic stasis) or direct communication between small and large intestine.

785. In bacterial overgrowth syndromes, macrocytic anemia is due to deficiency of?
Harrison's 20th Ed. Chapter 318 Page 2255

A. Cobalamin
B. Folate
C. Cobalamin + Folate
D. Any of the above

In bacterial overgrowth syndromes, macrocytic anemia is due to cobalamin, not folate deficiency.

786. Diagnosis of the bacterial overgrowth syndrome is done by all except?
Harrison's 20th Ed. Chapter 318 Page 2255

A. Low serum cobalamin level
B. Low serum folate level
C. Increased aerobic &/or anaerobic colonic-type bacteria in jejunal aspirate
D. Schilling test

Diagnosis of the bacterial overgrowth syndrome is done by a low serum cobalamin level, elevated serum folate level, increased levels of aerobic and/or anaerobic colonic-type bacteria in a jejunal aspirate, Schilling test. Following tetracycline for 5 days, Schilling test will become normal.

787. For frequent recurrences of bacterial overgrowth syndrome, which of the following treatment strategies is most effective?
Harrison's 20th Ed. Chapter 318 Page 2255

A. Antibiotics for 1 week per month
B. Antibiotics for ~3 weeks
C. Antibiotics until symptoms remit
D. Antibiotics continuously

In the presence of frequent recurrences, use of antibiotics for 1 week per month whether or not symptoms are present is most effective.

788. Bacterial overgrowth may occur in?
Harrison's 20th Ed. Chapter 318 Page 2256

A. Scleroderma
B. Crohn's disease
C. Radiation enteritis
D. All of the above

789. Whipple's disease is caused by the bacteria named?
Harrison's 20th Ed. Chapter 318 Page 2256

A. Tropheryma whippeli
B. Treponema whippeli
C. Toxoplasma whippeli
D. Trenoderma whippeli

Whipple's disease is a chronic multisystem disease that presents as diarrhea, steatorrhea, weight loss, arthralgia & CNS and cardiac problems. It is caused by bacteria Tropheryma whipplei.

790. Which of the following statements about Tropheryma whippeli is false?
Harrison's 20th Ed. Chapter 318 Page 2256

A. Gram-positive
B. Actinobacterium
C. Low virulence, low infectivity
D. PAS+ macrophages in small intestine

Hallmark of Whipple's disease is the presence of PAS-positive macrophages in small intestine. T. whipplei is a small gram-positive, actinobacterium bacillus, with low virulence but high infectivity.

791. Which of the following about Whipple's disease is false?
Harrison's 20th Ed. Chapter 318 Page 2256

A. Multisystem disease
B. T. whippelii outside macrophages indicates active disease
C. T. whipplei cannot be grown on culture
D. Drug of first choice is TMP/SMX for 1 year

Presence of T. whipplei bacillus outside of macrophages is a more important indicator of active disease than within macrophages. T. whipplei has been grown in culture. The current drug of choice is double-strength trimethoprim/sulfamethoxazole for ~1 year.

792. Which of the following about Whipple's disease is false?
Harrison's 20th Ed. Chapter 318 Page 2256

A. Drug of second choice is Chloramphenicol
B. Antibiotic therapy has to be prolonged
C. Disease recurrence with dementia is a poor prognostic sign
D. None of the above

If TMP/SMX is not tolerated, chloramphenicol is an appropriate second choice. Recurrence of disease activity, especially with dementia, is an extremely poor prognostic sign.

793. Which of the following is the most common neurologic manifestations of classic Whipple's disease?
N Engl J Med. 2007;356:55-66

A. Cognitive change
B. Supranuclear ophthalmoplegia
C. Oculomasticatory or oculofacioskeletal myorhythmia
D. Ataxia

Cognitive changes and later dementia are commonest neurologic signs. Movement disorders of eye muscles (oculomasticatory or oculofacioskeletal myorhythmia) are considered pathognomonic for Whipple's disease.

794. Which of the following about protein-losing enteropathy is false?
Harrison's 20th Ed. Chapter 318 Page 2256

A. Hypoproteinemia
B. Edema
C. Proteinuria
D. No defects in protein synthesis

Protein-losing enteropathy is not a specific disease but rather a group of gastrointestinal & nongastrointestinal disorders with hypoproteinemia & edema in absence of either proteinuria or defects in protein synthesis.

795. Normally, what percentage of total protein catabolism occurs via gastrointestinal tract?
Harrison's 20th Ed. Chapter 318 Page 2256

A. ~ 5%
B. ~ 10%
C. ~ 15%
D. ~ 20%

Normally, ~10% of total protein catabolism occurs via the gastrointestinal tract.

796. Which of the following about protein-losing enteropathy is false?
Harrison's 20th Ed. Chapter 318 Page 2256

A. Excess protein loss into gastrointestinal tract
B. Low serum albumin & globulin both in absence of renal & hepatic disease
C. α_1-antitrypsin clearance can be useful in diagnosis
D. Lymphocytosis supports diagnosis

Protein-losing enteropathy is characterized by excess protein loss into gastrointestinal tract. With loss of protein, peripheral lymphocytes are also lost via lymphatics, resulting in a relative lymphopenia. Thus, presence of lymphopenia in a patient with hypoproteinemia supports the presence of increased loss of protein into gastrointestinal tract.

797. Which of the following can cause protein-losing enteropathy?
Harrison's 20th Ed. Chapter 318 Page 2256

A. Peripheral vascular disease
B. Chronic pericarditis
C. Hemolytic uremic syndrome
D. Hypothyroidism

798. Hypoproteinemia in intestinal lymphangiectasia should be treated with?
Harrison's 20th Ed. Chapter 318 Page 2256

A. SCFA
B. MCT
C. LCFA
D. All of the above

Treatment of hypoproteinemia in intestinal lymphangiectasia is done by low-fat diet and administration of MCTs, which do not exit from intestinal epithelial cells via lymphatics but are delivered to the body via portal vein.

799. Which of the following disorders is associated with lymphedema?
Harrison's 20th Ed. Chapter 276 Page 1934

A. Meige's disease
B. Milroy's disease
C. Yellow nail syndrome
D. All of the above

800. Mutations in which of the following genes causes Milroy's disease?
Harrison's 20th Ed. Chapter 276 Page 1933

A. LSC1
B. FOXC2
C. VEGFR3
D. CCBE1

Mutations in genes expressing vascular endothelial growth factor receptor 3 (VEGFR3), which is a determinant of lymphangiogenesis, cause Milroy's disease.

801. Adherence to colonic mucin by E. histolytica trophozoites is mediated by?
N Engl J Med. 2003;348:16

A. Gal/GalNAc–specific lectin
B. Gal/GalNAc–specific pepsin
C. Gal/GalNAc–specific trypsin
D. Gal/GalNAc–specific capsin

Inflammatory Bowel Disease

802. Which of the following about IBD is false?
Harrison's 20th Ed. Chapter 319 Page 2258

A. Immune-mediated
B. Chronic intestinal condition
C. Dysregulated tridirectional relationship between commensal (microbiota), intestinal epithelial cells (IEC) and mucosal immune system
D. None of the above

803. Which out of the following countries has the highest incidence of IBD?
Harrison's 20th Ed. Chapter 319 Page 2258

A. Canada
B. Israel
C. Greece
D. China

The highest reported incidence rates are in Canada (19.2 per 100,000 for UC and 20.2 per 1 00,000 for CD. ~0.6% of the Canadian population has IBD.

804. Out of the following, which ethnic group has the highest prevalence of IBD?
Harrison's 20th Ed. Chapter 319 Page 2258 Table 319-1

A. Jewish
B. African American
C. Hispanic
D. Asian

Prevalence of IBD in Ashkenazi Jews is ~twice that of Israeli-born, Sephardic, or Oriental Jews. Prevalence decreases progressively in non-Jewish Caucasian, African-American, Hispanic, and Asian populations.

805. All of the following are predisposing factors for UC except?
Harrison's 20th Ed. Chapter 319 Page 2258

A. Jewish ethnicity
B. High socio-economic status
C. Smoking
D. Hermansky-Pudlak syndrome

806. Which of the following statements about ulcerative colitis (UC) and Crohn's disease (CD) is false?
Harrison's 20th Ed. Chapter 319 Page 2258

A. Peak age of onset of UC & CD is second to fourth decades
B. Second peak occurs in seventh and ninth decades
C. Appendectomy aggravates UC
D. IBD is not gender specific

Appendectomy is protective against UC but increases the risk of CD.

807. Very early onset IBD (VEOIBD) is defined as IBD that occurs in children below the age of?
Harrison's 20th Ed. Chapter 319 Page 2258

A. 4 years
B. 6 years
C. 8 years
D. 10 years

Very early onset IBD (VEOIBD) is defined as IBD that occurs in children below the age of <6 years.

808. Infantile IBD is defined as IBD that occurs in children below the age of?
Harrison's 20th Ed. Chapter 319 Page 2258

A. 3 months
B. 12 months
C. 18 months
D. 24 months

Infantile IBD is defined as IBD that occurs in children below the age of <2 years.

809. Which of the following is false about VEOIBD and infantile IBD?
Harrison's 20th Ed. Chapter 319 Page 2258

A. Mainly affect the colon
B. Resistant to standard medications
C. Patients have a strong family history of IBD
D. None of the above

810. What percentage of patients with VEOIBD and infantile IBD have underlying immunodeficiency?
Harrison's 20th Ed. Chapter 319 Page 2258

A. 10%
B. 15%
C. 25%
D. 40%

Twenty-five percent of patients with VEOIBD and infantile IBD have an underlying immunodeficiency. In some cases, infantile IBD or VEOIBD can be caused by rare, single genetic mutations.

811. Which of the following is not associated with increased risk of UC?
Harrison's 20th Ed. Chapter 319 Page 2258

A. Urban domicile
B. High socio-economic status
C. Former smoker
D. Appendectomy

Urban areas, high socioeconomic classes have a higher prevalence of IBD. Former smokers have a 1.7-fold increased risk for UC than people who have never smoked. Appendectomy is protective against UC.

812. If a patient has IBD, the lifetime risk that a first degree relative will be similarly affected is?
Harrison's 20th Ed. Chapter 319 Page 2258

A. 10%
B. 20%
C. 30%
D. 40%

Lifetime risk of a first-degree relative of IBD patient is ~10%. If two parents have IBD, each child has a 36% chance of being affected. In twin studies, 58% of monozygotic twins are concordant for CD and 6% are concordant for UC, whereas 4% of dizygotic twins are concordant for CD and none are concordant for UC.

813. If two parents have IBD, what chance does each child has of being affected?
Harrison's 20th Ed. Chapter 319 Page 2258

A. 36%
B. 45%
C. 66%
D. 72%

If two parents have IBD, each child has a 36% chance of being affected.

814. Term "supraorganism" in IBD is best related to?
Harrison's 20th Ed. Chapter 319 Page 2259

A. Microbiota
B. IECs
C. Immune cells
D. All of the above

Under normal physiologic conditions, homeostasis exists between commensal microbiota, intestinal epithelial cells and immune cells within tissues. They function together as an integrated "supraorganism". They are affected by specific environmental (smoking, antibiotics, enteropathogens) and genetic factors in a susceptible host, cumulatively & interactively disrupting homeostasis. This leads to a chronic state of dysregulated inflammation, i.e. IBD.

815. Nonmalignant mortality in IBD cases is maximum during?
Harrison's 18th Ed. 2477

A. First year of disease
B. After five years of disease
C. After ten years of disease
D. After fifteen years of disease

Highest mortality is during first year of IBD & in long-duration disease due to risk of colon cancer.

816. Which genetic disorder is a predisposing factor for IBD?
Harrison's 20th Ed. Chapter 319 Page 2260 Table 319-2

A. Turner's syndrome
B. Down syndrome
C. Patau syndrome
D. Edward syndrome

817. IBD is associated with all of the following except?
Harrison's 20th Ed. Chapter 319 Page 2260 Table 319-2

A. Turner's syndrome
B. Down syndrome
C. Hermansky-Pudlak syndrome
D. Wiskott-Aldrich syndrome

UC and CD are associated with Turner's syndrome and Hermansky-Pudlak syndrome, Wiskott-Aldrich syndrome and chronic granulomatous disease. Immunodeficiency disorders like hypogammaglobulinemia, selective IgA deficiency and hereditary angioedema also have increased association with IBD.

818. Disease that are shares genetic risk factors with IBD is?
Harrison's 20th Ed. Chapter 319 Page 2261

A. Rheumatoid arthritis
B. Psoriasis
C. Systemic lupus erythematosus
D. All of the above

Diseases and genetic risk factors that are shared with IBD include rheumatoid arthritis (TNFAIP3), psoriasis (IL23R,IL12B), ankylosing spondylitis (IL23R), type 1 diabetes mellitus (IL10,PTPN2), asthma (ORMDL3), and systemic lupus erythematosus (TNFAIP3, IL10).

819. Which of the following single gene defects can cause IBD?
Harrison's 20th Ed. Chapter 319 Page 2260

A. IL10
B. CTLA4
C. NCF2
D. All of the above

IBD occurs with genetic syndromes and development of severe, refractory IBD in early life in single gene defects that affect the immune system. These include mutations in genes encoding interleukin-10 (IL-10), IL-10 receptor (IL-10R), cytotoxic T-lymphocyte associated protein-4 (CTLA4), neutrophil cytosolic factor 2 protein (NCF2), X linked inhibitor of apoptosis protein (XIAP), lipopolysaccharide responsive and beige-like anchor protein (LRBA), or tetratricopeptide repeat domain 7A protein (TTC7).

820. Which of the following genes is associated with innate immunity and autophagy?
Harrison's 20th Ed. Chapter 319 Page 2260 Table 319-3

A. NOD2
B. ATG16L1
C. IRGM
D. All of the above

Genes that are associated with innate immunity and autophagy are NOD2, ATG16L1, IRGM, JAK2, STAT3 that function in innate immune cells (both parenchymal and hematopoietic) to respond to and clear bacteria, mycobacteria and viruses.

821. Which of the following genes is associated with endoplasmic reticulum (ER) and metabolic stress?
Harrison's 20th Ed. Chapter 319 Page 2261

A. XBP1
B. ORMDL3
C. OCTN
D. All of the above

Genes that are associated with endoplasmic reticulum (ER) and metabolic stress are XBP1, ORMDL3, OCTN, which serve to regulate the secretory activity of cells involved in responses to the commensal microbiota such as Paneth and goblet cells and the manner in which intestinal cells respond to the metabolic products of bacteria.

822. Which of the following genes is associated with regulation of adaptive immunity?
Harrison's 20th Ed. Chapter 319 Page 2260 Table 319-3

A. IL23R
B. IL12B
C. IL10
D. All of the above

Genes that are associated with regulation of adaptive immunity are IL23R, IL12B, IL10, PTPN2, which regulate the balance between inflammatory and regulatory cytokines.

823. Which of the following genes is involved in the development and resolution of inflammation?
Harrison's 20th Ed. Chapter 319 Page 2260 Table 319-3

A. MST1
B. CCR6
C. TNFAIP3
D. All of the above

Genes that are involved in the development and resolution of inflammation are MST1, CCR6, TNFAIP3, PTGER4 and ultimately leukocyte recruitment and inflammatory mediator production.

824. NOD1 gene is now known as?
   A. CARD1
   B. CARD2
   C. CARD3
   D. CARD4

825. NOD2 gene is now known as?
   Harrison's 20th Ed. Chapter 355 Page 2573
   A. CARD1
   B. CARD5
   C. CARD15
   D. CARD18

Gene CARD4 was formerly called NOD1, and CARD15 was formerly called NOD2. CARD15 means caspase-associated recruitment domain containing protein 15, while NOD2 refers to nucleotide oligomerisation domain 2 or NOTCH protein domain.

826. The disease-related gene of IBD1 on chromosome 16 is?
   N Engl J Med. 2002;347:417
   A. NOD-1
   B. NOD-2
   C. NOD-3
   D. NOD-4

The IBD1 locus encodes NOD2 (nucleotide-binding oligomerization domain also designated CARD 15 or caspase recruitment domain protein 15) found in approximately one-half of patients with CD.

827. Which of the following syndromes is associated with NOD2 mutation?
   Harrison's 20th Ed. Chapter 362 Page 2613
   A. Muckle-Wells syndrome (MWS)
   B. Blau's syndrome
   C. Syndrome of pyogenic arthritis with pyoderma gangrenosum and acne (PAPA)
   D. Schnitzler's syndrome

Blau's syndrome is caused by mutations in CARD15 (also known as NOD2), which regulates nuclear factor-κB activation. Blau's syndrome is characterized by granulomatous dermatitis, uveitis and arthritis. Distinct CARD15 variants predispose to Crohn's disease.

828. Intracellular NOD1 and NOD2 proteins are best related to?
   N Engl J Med. 2002;347:417
   A. FoxP3 transcription factor
   B. Antitumor necrosis factor
   C. Pattern-recognition proteins
   D. All of the above

Pattern-recognition proteins that are important for sensing microbes include the intracellular NOD1 and NOD2 proteins which recognize discrete fragments of bacterial peptidoglycan.

829. Which of the following IBD subtype has its loci on chromosome 16?
   N Engl J Med. 2002;347:417, Indian J Gastroenterol. 2008;27:8-11
   A. IBD 6
   B. IBD 7
   C. IBD 8
   D. IBD 9

IBD loci are on chromosomes 16q12 (IBD1), 12q13 (IBD2), 6p13 (IBD3), 14q11 (IBD4), 5q31-33 (IBD5), 19p13 (IBD6), 1p36 (IBD7), 16p (IBD8), 3p (IBD9). Three alleles of the NOD2/CARD15 gene on chromosome 16 have been found in ~one-half of patients with CD.

830. CARD15 is constitutively expressed in?
   N Engl J Med. 2002;347:417
   A. Paneth cells
   B. Parietal or oxyntic cells
   C. G cells
   D. D cells

Paneth cells are specialized epithelial cells selectively expressed in ileum, located mainly in crypts in close proximity to epithelial stem cells. Paneth cells secrete antibacterial substances. Main antimicrobial factors secreted by Paneth cell include lysozyme, phospholipase A2, trypsin, alpha-defensins & angiogenins.

831. CARD15 protein is expressed in the cytoplasm of?
   N Engl J Med. 2002;347:417
   A. Peripheral blood monocytes
   B. Paneth cells
   C. Dendritic cells
   D. All of the above

CARD15 (caspase activation and recruitment domain) is expressed by intestinal epithelial cells (Paneth cells, monocytes, macrophages & dendritic cells).

832. Which of the following is false about CARD15 protein?
   N Engl J Med. 2002;347:417
   A. CARD15 was formerly called NOD1
   B. Intracellular recognition protein for bacterial components
   C. Activates nuclear factor kappa B pathway
   D. Gain-of-function mutations are associated with CD

CARD15 protein acts as an intracellular recognition protein for bacterial components such as peptidoglycans and activates nuclear factor kappa B pathway which regulates apoptosis and inflammation. Loss-of-function mutations in CARD15 are highly associated with CD.

833. Signaling adaptor protein MyD88 is related to which of the following?
   N Engl J Med. 2002;347:417
   A. Goblet cells
   B. Paneth cells
   C. Enteroendocrine cell
   D. All of the above

Paneth cells directly sense the presence of a microbiota through expression of the signaling adaptor protein MyD88, which helps transduce signals to host cells upon recognition of microbial products through Toll-like receptors (TLRs). This recognition drives expression of antibacterial products (the lectin RegIIIγ) that act to prevent microbial translocation across the gut mucosal barrier.

834. Which of the following stimulates Paneth cells to produce RegIII-γ?
   N Engl J Med. 2002;347:417
   A. Porphyromonas asaccharolytica
   B. B. fragilis
   C. Prevotella bivia
   D. B. thetaiotaomicron

B. thetaiotaomicron stimulates Paneth cells to produce RegIII-γ, a bactericidal lectin that can result in killing of gram-positive bacteria.

835. Which of the following is an anti-inflammatory bacterial species?
   Harrison's 20th Ed. Chapter 319 Page 2261
   A. Faecalibacterium prausnitzii
   B. Eggerthella lenta
   C. Ruminococcus gnavus
   D. All of the above

Faecalibacterium prausnitzii belongs to anti-inflammatory bacterial species. Ruminococcus gnavus belongs to pro-inflammatory bacterial species. Digoxin is inactivated by the human gut bacterium Eggerthella lenta.

836. **Which of the following bacterial species prevents growth impairment?**
Harrison's 20th Ed. Chapter 459 Page 3385

A. Faecalibacterium prausnitzii
B. Ruminococcus gnavus
C. Clostridium nexile
D. All of the above

Investigators have identified five bacterial species (Faecalibacterium prausnitzii, Ruminococcus gnavus, Clostridium nexile, Clostridium symbiosum, and Dorea formicigenerans) that when administered together as a "cocktail" were able to prevent growth impairments.

837. **Lack of immune responsiveness of gut mucosal immune system to dietary antigens is best related to?**
Harrison's 20th Ed. Chapter 319 Page 2261

A. Intestinal tolerance
B. Gastric tolerance
C. Oral tolerance
D. All of the above

The gut mucosal immune system is normally unreactive to luminal contents due to oral (mucosal) tolerance. In IBD this suppression of inflammation is altered, leading to uncontrolled inflammation.

838. **Which of the following is an anti-inflammatory cytokine?**
Harrison's 20th Ed. Chapter 319 Page 2261

A. IL-10
B. IL-35
C. Transforming growth factor β (TGF-β)
D. All of the above

In IBD, suppression of inflammation is altered, leading to uncontrolled inflammation.

839. **Which of the following is related to regulation of responses to commensal bacteria?**
Harrison's 20th Ed. Chapter 319 Page 2261

A. XBP1
B. Mucus glycoproteins
C. Nuclear factor-κB (NF-κB)
D. All of the above

840. **In unstimulated cells, NF-κB is found in?**
N Engl J Med. 1997;336:1067

A. Nucleus
B. Cytoplasm
C. Cell membrane
D. All of the above

NF-κB (nuclear factor kappa-light-chain-enhancer of activated B cells) is located in the cytosol complexed with the inhibitory protein IκB.

841. **In unstimulated cells, NF-κB remains bound to?**
N Engl J Med. 1997;336:1067

A. G-κB
B. H-κB
C. I-κB
D. J-κB

In unstimulated cells, the NF-κB dimers are sequestered in cytoplasm by a family of inhibitors, called IκB (Inhibitor of κB). Activation of NF-κB is initiated by signal-induced degradation of IκB which occurs via activation of a kinase called the IκB kinase (IKK). With degradation of IκB inhibitor, NF-κB complex is freed to enter the nucleus where it activates expression of genes that have DNA-binding sites for NF-κB leading to physiological responses like inflammatory or immune response, cell survival response, cellular proliferation and activating expression of its own repressor, IκB. IκB then re-inhibits NF-κB (auto feedback loop).

842. **Which of the following can activate NF-κB?**
N Engl J Med. 1997;336:1067

A. Cytokines
B. Activators of protein kinase C
C. Viruses
D. All of the above

NF-κB is a rapidly acting primary transcription factor found in all cell types. It is activated through TLR-4 by cytokines, activators of protein kinase C, bacteria / viruses, stress, UV.

843. **CD4+ T helper (T_H) cell that promotes inflammation is?**
Harrison's 20th Ed. Chapter 319 Page 2261

A. T_H1 cells
B. T_H2 cells
C. T_H17 cells
D. All of the above

CD4+ T helper (T_H) cells that promote inflammation are of three major types namely T_H1 cells, T_H2 cells and T_H17 cells.

844. **Which of the following is a type of CD4+ T cell?**
Harrison's 20th Ed. Chapter 319 Page 2261

A. T_H1 cells
B. T_H2 cells
C. T_H17 cells
D. All of the above

CD4+ T cells are of three major types : T_H1 cells, T_H2 cells and T_H17 cells.

845. **T_H2 of CD4+ T cells produce all except?**
Harrison's 20th Ed. Chapter 319 Page 2261

A. Interferon-γ (IFN-γ)
B. Interleukin-4 (IL-4)
C. Interleukin-5 (IL-5)
D. Interleukin-13 (IL-13)

CD4+ T cells are composed of Th1 cells, that produce interferon-gamma (IFN-γ), and Th2 cells that produce interleukin-4, IL-5 and IL-13.

846. **Interferon (IFN) gamma is secreted by which of the following?**
Harrison's 20th Ed. Chapter 319 Page 2261

A. T_H1 cells
B. T_H2 cells
C. T_H17 cells
D. All of the above

T_H1 cells secrete interferon (IFN) gamma, T_H2 cells secrete IL-4, IL-5, IL-13, and T_H17 cells secrete IL-17, IL-21.

847. **Which of the following cells induce transmural granulomatous inflammation that resembles CD?**
Harrison's 20th Ed. Chapter 319 Page 2261

A. T_H1 cells
B. T_H2 cells
C. T_H17 cells
D. All of the above

T_H1 cells induce transmural granulomatous inflammation that resembles CD.

848. Which of the following cells induce superficial mucosal inflammation resembling UC?
Harrison's 20th Ed. Chapter 319 Page 2261

A. T_H1 cells
B. T_H2 cells
C. T_H17 cells
D. All of the above

T_H2 cells, & related natural killer T cells that secrete IL-13 induce superficial mucosal inflammation resembling UC. T_H17 cells may be responsible for neutrophilic recruitment.

849. The T_H1 cytokine pathway is initiated by?
Harrison's 20th Ed. Chapter 319 Page 2262

A. IL-4
B. IL-6
C. IL-12
D. IL-23

The T_H1 cytokine pathway is initiated by IL-12. IL-4 and IL-23, together with IL-6 and TGF-beta, induce T_H2 and T_H17 cells, respectively.

850. Which of the following is also called "lymphotoxin"?
Harrison's 20th Ed. Chapter 343 Page 2482

A. TNF-α
B. TNF-β
C. IFN-α
D. IFN-γ

Tumor-necrosis factor-beta (TNF-β) is also known as lymphotoxin.

851. Levels of which of the following is elevated in IBD?
N Engl J Med. 2009;361:2066-78

A. Tumor necrosis factor α (TNF-α)
B. Interleukin-1β
C. Interferon-γ
D. All of the above

Levels of tumor necrosis factor α (TNF-α), interleukin-1β, interferon-γ, and cytokines of the interleukin-23–Th17 pathway are elevated in IBD.

852. Which of the following is not a probiotic?
Harrison's 20th Ed. Chapter 317 Page 2234

A. Lactobacillus spp.
B. Bifidobacterium spp.
C. Campylobacter spp.
D. Saccharomyces spp.

Salmonella sp., Shigella sp., Campylobacter sp., Clostridium difficile are pathogens that may initiate IBD by triggering an inflammatory response. While Faecalibacterium prausnitzii, Lactobacillus, Bifidobacterium and Saccharomyces boulardii are probiotics that may inhibit inflammation.

853. What proportion of UC patients have involvement of whole colon?
Harrison's 20th Ed. Chapter 319 Page 2262

A. 10%
B. 20%
C. 30%
D. 40%

~40-50% of UC patients have disease limited to rectum & rectosigmoid, 30-40% have disease extending beyond sigmoid but not involving whole colon. 20% have a total colitis.

854. Backwash ileitis occurs when which part of colon is involved in UC?
Harrison's 20th Ed. Chapter 319 Page 2262

A. Ascending colon
B. Transverse colon
C. Descending colon
D. Whole colon

UC is a mucosal disease that almost always involves rectum and extends proximally to involve colon in continuity without areas of uninvolved mucosa. When "whole colon" is involved, inflammation extends 1-2 cm into terminal ileum in 10–20% of patients. This is called backwash ileitis.

855. Psychosocial factors can contribute to worsening of symptoms in following illnesses except?
Harrison's 20th Ed. Chapter 319 Page 2262

A. Malabsorption syndrome
B. Fibromyalgia
C. Amyotrophic lateral sclerosis
D. Bipolar mood disorder

856. Which of the following statements about pathology of Ulcerative colitis (UC) is false?
Harrison's 20th Ed. Chapter 319 Page 2262

A. Mucosal disease involving rectum and colon
B. Proximal spread occurs in continuity
C. Sandpaper like appearance of mucosa reflects severe inflammation
D. Inflammatory polyps (pseudopolyps) are due to epithelial regeneration

In UC, with "mild inflammation" mucosa is erythematous & has a fine granular surface that looks like sandpaper.

857. Which of the following statements about pathology of Ulcerative colitis (UC) is false?
Harrison's 20th Ed. Chapter 319 Page 2262

A. Limited to mucosa & superficial submucosa
B. Crypt architecture of colon is preserved
C. Basal lymphoplasmacytosis suggests chronicity
D. Cryptitis and crypt atrophy

UC process is limited to mucosa and superficial submucosa, with deeper layers unaffected except in fulminant disease. Histologic features that suggest chronicity are that crypt architecture of colon is distorted and presence of basal plasma cells and multiple basal lymphoid aggregates.

858. Which of the following statements about pathology of Crohn's disease (CD) is false?
Harrison's 20th Ed. Chapter 319 Page 2262

A. Can affect any part of gastrointestinal tract
B. Terminal ileum involved in 90% of patients
C. Rectum is always involved in CD
D. Segmental with skip areas

Unlike UC, which almost always involves the rectum, the rectum is often spared in CD.

859. Which of the following statements about pathology of Crohn's disease (CD) is false?
Harrison's 20th Ed. Chapter 319 Page 2262

A. Perirectal fistulas, abscesses & anal stenosis common
B. Never involves liver & pancreas
C. Transmural process
D. "Cobblestone" appearance on endoscopy

In CD, granulomas are seen in lymph nodes, mesentery, peritoneum, liver & pancreas.

860. Which of the following statements is false?
Harrison's 20th Ed. Chapter 319 Page 2262

A. CD is a transmural process
B. Between lesions, mucosa is histologically normal
C. Thickening of the colon wall
D. None of the above

861. "Cobblestone mucosa" in CD is mainly seen in?
Harrison's 20th Ed. Chapter 319 Page 2262

A. Sigmoid colon
B. Transverse colon
C. Ileum
D. Rectum

Unlike UC, CD is a transmural process. CD is segmental with skip areas in the midst of diseased intestine. In CD, stellate ulcerations fuse longitudinally & transversely to demarcate islands of mucosa that are histologically normal. This "cobblestone" appearance is characteristic of CD, endoscopically and by barium radiography. Oral mucosal lesions in CD include aphthous stomatitis & "cobblestone" lesions of the buccal mucosa.

862. Which of the following statements about pathology of Crohn's disease (CD) is false?
Harrison's 20th Ed. Chapter 319 Page 2263

A. Earliest lesions are aphthoid ulcerations & focal crypt abscesses
B. Caseating granulomas in all bowel wall layers common
C. Granulomas can be seen in liver & pancreas
D. Granulomas can be seen in lymph nodes, mesentery, peritoneum

In CD, earliest lesions are aphthoid ulcerations & focal crypt abscesses with loose aggregations of macrophages, forming "noncaseating" granulomas in all layers of bowel wall.

863. In CD, "creeping fat" is the term given to?
Harrison's 20th Ed. Chapter 319 Page 2263

A. Excessive enlargement of omentum
B. Necrosis of omentum
C. Projections of thickened mesentery encasing bowel
D. Fatty adhesions

Projections of thickened mesentery encase the bowel is termed as "creeping fat".

864. Which of the following is a feature of UC?
Harrison's 20th Ed. Chapter 319 Page 2263

A. Bowel wall thickening
B. Cobblestoning
C. Pseudopolyps
D. Skip areas in the midst of diseased intestine

865. Which of the following is not a major symptom of UC?
Harrison's 20th Ed. Chapter 319 Page 2263

A. Rectal bleeding
B. Constipation
C. Crampy abdominal pain
D. Tenesmus

The major symptoms of UC are diarrhea, rectal bleeding, tenesmus, passage of mucus, and crampy abdominal pain. Other symptoms in moderate to severe disease include anorexia, nausea, vomiting, fever, and weight loss. With proctitis or proctosigmoiditis, proximal transit slows, which may account for the constipation commonly seen in patients with distal disease.

866. Which of the following statements about clinical features of Ulcerative colitis (UC) is false?
Harrison's 20th Ed. Chapter 319 Page 2263

A. Tenesmus is a major symptom
B. Severity of symptoms do not correlate with extent of disease
C. Constipation seen in patients with distal disease
D. Diarrhea is often nocturnal and/or postprandial

Severity of symptoms correlates with the extent of disease.

867. Which of the following is not a manifestion severe UC?
Harrison's 20th Ed. Chapter 319 Page 2263 Table 319-4

A. Bowel movements 4-6/day
B. Mean body temperature >37.5°C
C. Mean pulse rate > 90 / minute
D. ESR > 30 mm in first hour

In severe UC, bowel movements are >6 per day.

868. In severe ulcerative colitis, number of bowel movements per day is?
Harrison's 20th Ed. Chapter 319 Page 2263 Table 319-4

A. 2 – 3
B. 3 – 4
C. 4 – 5
D. > 6

869. Which of the following about investigative features of Ulcerative colitis (UC) is false?
Harrison's 20th Ed. Chapter 319 Page 2263

A. CRP levels may rise in active disease
B. Orosomucoid levels may rise in active disease
C. Leukocytosis is a specific indicator of disease activity
D. Proctitis or proctosigmoiditis rarely cause rise in CRP

In UC, leukocytosis occurs but is not a specific indicator of disease activity. Proctitis or proctosigmoiditis rarely causes a rise in CRP.

870. Which of the following is a highly sensitive & specific marker for detecting intestinal inflammation?
Harrison's 20th Ed. Chapter 319 Page 2263

A. Fecal lactoferrin
B. Fecal transferrin
C. Fecal hemolysin
D. Fecal reactin

Fecal lactoferrin is a highly sensitive and specific marker of fecal leukocytes and for detecting intestinal inflammation, tested by latex agglutination & enzyme-linked immunosorbent assays.

871. Which of the following about fecal calprotectin is false?
Harrison's 20th Ed. Chapter 319 Page 2263

A. Levels correlate well with histologic inflammation
B. Predict relapses
C. Detects pouchitis
D. None of the above

Fecal calprotectin levels correlate well with histologic inflammation, predict relapses, and detect pouchitis.

872. **Which of the following is fecal marker of GI tract inflammation?**
Clinical and Experimental Gastroenterology 2016:9 21–29

A. Lactoferrin
B. S100A12
C. M2-PK
D. All of the above

Fecal marker of GI tract inflammation include calprotectin, lactoferrin, S100A12, polymorphonuclear elastase, and M2-PK, which is an isoform of pyruvate kinase expressed by rapidly dividing cells.

873. **Which of the following is false about "fecal calprotectin"?**
Harrison's 20th Ed. Chapter 319 Page 2263

A. Neutrophilic cytosolic protein
B. Resistant to colonic bacterial degradation
C. Formerly called L1 protein
D. None of the above

874. **Which of the following is false about "fecal calprotectin"?**
Clinical and Experimental Gastroenterology 2016:9 21–29

A. Calcium binding
B. Has antimicrobial properties
C. Predict relapses in IBD
D. None of the above

Fecal Calprotectin is a neutrophilic cytosolic protein, first isolated from granulocytes by Fagerhol and named L1 protein. It was renamed calprotectin upon identification of its calcium binding, antimicrobial properties and resistance to colonic bacterial degradation. Calprotectin, although present in blood, enters bowel lumen as part of an inflammatory process. It is positive in stools of IBD and colorectal cancer patients. Fecal calprotectin & lactoferrin is useful in predicting impending clinical relapse in CD & UC patients.

875. **Which of the following statements about complications of Ulcerative colitis (UC) is false?**
Harrison's 20th Ed. Chapter 319 Page 2264

A. Toxic megacolon means a transverse colon with diameter > 6 cm, with loss of haustration
B. Toxic megacolon can be triggered by electrolyte abnormalities and narcotics
C. In toxic colitis and severe ulcerations, bowel may perforate without first dilating
D. UC patients never develop anal fissures, perianal abscesses

UC patients occasionally develop anal fissures, perianal abscesses, or hemorrhoids, but occurrence of extensive perianal lesions should suggest CD.

876. **Which of the following statements about clinical features of Crohn's disease (CD) is false?**
Harrison's 20th Ed. Chapter 319 Page 2264

A. Can be of fibrostenotic-obstructing or penetrating-fistulous pattern
B. Most common site of inflammation is caecum
C. Presentation may mimic acute appendicitis
D. Radiographic "string sign" refers to narrowed intestinal lumen

In CD, the most common site of inflammation is terminal ileum.

877. **Which of the following is not a feature of pain in CD?**
Harrison's 20th Ed. Chapter 319 Page 2264

A. Colicky
B. Precedes defecation
C. Relieved by defecation
D. Continues after defecation

Pain is colicky, precedes and is relieved by defecation.

878. **Right lower quadrant abdominal inflammatory mass in CD is composed of?**
Harrison's 20th Ed. Chapter 319 Page 2264

A. Inflamed bowel
B. Adherent and indurated mesentery
C. Enlarged abdominal lymph nodes
D. All of the above

Abdominal mass in CD is composed of inflamed bowel, adherent and indurated mesentery, and enlarged abdominal lymph nodes.

879. **Radiographic "string sign" of a narrowed intestinal lumen in CD is due to?**
Harrison's 20th Ed. Chapter 319 Page 2264

A. Edema of bowel wall
B. Bowel wall thickening
C. Fibrosis of bowel wall
D. All of the above

Transmural inflammation of CD causes decreased luminal diameter & limited distensibility. Radiographic "string sign" represents long areas of circumferential inflammation & fibrosis causing long segments of luminal narrowing. Edema, bowel wall thickening & fibrosis of bowel wall account for the radiographic "string sign" of a narrowed intestinal lumen.

880. **Factors recognized to exacerbate CD include?**
Am J Gastroenterol 2009; 104:465-483

A. Intercurrent infections
B. Cigarette smoking
C. Non-steroidal anti-inflammatory drugs
D. All of the above

Factors recognized to exacerbate CD include intercurrent infections (both upper respiratory tract & enteric infections, including C. difficile), cigarette smoking & non-steroidal anti-inflammatory drugs.

881. **Which of the following statements about clinical features of Crohn's disease (CD) is false?**
Harrison's 20th Ed. Chapter 319 Page 2264

A. Pneumaturia may be present
B. Fecaluria may be present
C. Enterocutaneous fistulas may be present
D. Enterocholedocal fistulas may be present

Severe inflammation of ileocecal region may lead to microperforation and fistula formation to adjacent bowel, skin, urinary bladder, to abscess cavity in mesentery, or vagina.

882. **In Crohn's disease (CD), intestinal malabsorption can cause all except?**
Harrison's 20th Ed. Chapter 319 Page 2264

A. Hyperoxaluria
B. Hypocalcemia
C. Hypomagnesemia
D. Hypokalemia

In CD, intestinal malabsorption can cause anemia, hypoalbuminemia, hypocalcemia, hypomagnesemia, coagulopathy, hyperoxaluria, vitamin D deficiency and vitamin B_{12} deficiency.

883. Diarrhea in active CD is caused by?
Harrison's 20th Ed. Chapter 319 Page 2264

A. Bacterial overgrowth
B. Bile-acid malabsorption
C. Intestinal inflammation
D. All of the above

Causes of diarrhea in active CD include bacterial overgrowth in obstructive stasis or fistulization, bile-acid malabsorption due to diseased or resected terminal ileum & intestinal inflammation with decreased water absorption, increased secretion of electrolytes and decreased rectal compliance.

884. Which of the following about CD is false?
Harrison's 20th Ed. Chapter 319 Page 2265

A. Epigastric pain
B. *H. pylori* negative gastritis
C. Second part of duodenum more commonly involved than bulb
D. None of the above

885. Which of the following statements about investigations of Crohn's disease (CD) is false?
Harrison's 20th Ed. Chapter 319 Page 2265

A. Elevated ESR
B. Elevated CRP
C. Leucopenia
D. Hypoalbuminemia

Laboratory abnormalities in CD include elevated ESR & CRP, hypoalbuminemia, anemia & leukocytosis.

886. Which of the following about endoscopic features of Crohn's disease (CD) is false?
Harrison's 20th Ed. Chapter 319 Page 2265

A. Rectal sparing
B. Aphthous ulcerations & skip lesions
C. Fistulas
D. None of the above

Endoscopic features of CD include rectal sparing, aphthous ulcerations, fistulas, and skip lesions.

887. Earliest macroscopic findings of colonic CD is?
Harrison's 20th Ed. Chapter 319 Page 2265

A. Aphthous ulcers
B. Longitudinal stellate, serpiginous, & linear ulcers
C. Fistulas
D. Polyps

Earliest macroscopic findings of colonic CD are aphthous ulcers which are small, multiple ulcers separated by normal intervening mucosa.

888. Which out of the following is the first-line test for evaluation of suspected CD and its complications?
Harrison's 20th Ed. Chapter 319 Page 2265

A. USG
B. MRI
C. CT enterography
D. Endoscopy

CT enterography permits visualization of entire small bowel for inflammation associated with CD by displaying mural hyperenhancement, interloop sinus tracts, mesenteric fat stranding, engorged vasa recta and perienteric inflammatory changes. MRI may superior for demonstrating pelvic lesions like ischiorectal abscesses.

889. Which of the following statements about complications of Crohn's disease (CD) is false?
Harrison's 20th Ed. Chapter 319 Page 2265

A. Serosal adhesions common
B. Free perforation common in duodenum
C. Systemic glucocorticoid therapy increase risk of intraabdominal & pelvic abscesses
D. Perianal disease common

Perforation occur usually in ileum but occasionally in jejunum.

890. Which of the following antibody reactivity to antigens is associated with CD?
Harrison's 20th Ed. Chapter 319 Page 2266

A. Bacterial flagellin (CBir1)
B. Outer membrane porin C (OmpC)
C. Bacterial sequence I2 (anti-I2)
D. All of the above

Presence of antibody reactivity to antigens like oligomannan (ASCA, anti-Saccharomyces cerevisiae antibody) is seen in CD. Antibodies associated with CD include antibodies to bacterial proteins (Omp-C and I2), flagellin (CBir1) and bacterial carbohydrates, including laminaribioside (ALCA), chitobioside (ACCA) and mannobioside (SMCA).

891. Autoantibody found in cases of UC is?
Harrison's 20th Ed. Chapter 319 Page 2266

A. Anti dsDNA
B. cANCA
C. pANCA
D. Antimitochondrial

pANCA positivity is found in about 60 – 70% of UC patients and 5 – 10% of CD patients.

892. Which of the following statements about serological diagnosis of IBD is false?
Harrison's 20th Ed. Chapter 319 Page 2266

A. pANCA (+) in 5-10% of UC & 60-70% of CD patients
B. 5-15% of I° relatives of UC patients are pANCA (+)
C. pANCA positivity is associated with pancolitis, early surgery, and primary sclerosing cholangitis
D. pANCA in CD is associated with colonic disease

pANCA positivity is found in about 60–70% of UC patients and 5–10% of CD patients.

893. Which of the following about ASCA in IBD is false?
Harrison's 20th Ed. Chapter 319 Page 2266

A. ASCA is associated with large bowel CD
B. 60–70% of CD, 10–15% of UC patients are ASCA (+)
C. ASCA positivity is associated with increased & early CD complications
D. Saccharomyces cerevisiae is Brewer's or Baker's yeast

The presence of both Anti-Saccharomyces cerevisiae antibodies (ASCA) IgG and IgA is highly specific for the presence of Crohn's disease. ASCA is the most sensitive serologic marker of Crohn's disease. Saccharomyces cerevisiae is Brewer's or Baker's yeast.

894. Which of the following about serology of CD is false?
Harrison's 20th Ed. Chapter 319 Page 2266

A. Omp C (+) patients more likely to have internal perforating disease
B. I_2 (+) patients more likely to have fibrostenosing disease

C. Anti-CBir1 expression is associated with small-bowel disease, fibrostenosing, and internal penetrating disease
D. None of the above

Omp C–positive patients are more likely to have internal perforating disease; and I₂ positive patients are more likely to have fibrostenosing disease. Anti-Cbir1 expression is associated with small-bowel disease, fibrostenosing, and internal penetrating disease.

895. Cases of IBD that cannot be categorized as UC or CD are termed?
Harrison's 20th Ed. Chapter 319 Page 2266

A. Indeterminate colitis
B. Lymphocytic colitis
C. Diversion colitis
D. Collagenous colitis

Cases of IBD that cannot be categorized as UC or CD are called indeterminate colitis. IBD cases cannot be distinguished between UC & CD in ~15% of cases.

896. Which of the following is independently associated with disabling CD after 5 years?
Harrison's 20th Ed. Chapter 319 Page 2266

A. Age at diagnosis below 40 years
B. ASCA positivity
C. pANCA positivity
D. Rectal involvement

Features of CD that have been shown to be independently associated with subsequent disabling CD after 5 years are initial requirement for glucocorticoid use, age at diagnosis below 40 years and presence of perianal disease at diagnosis.

897. All of the following are true for CD except?
Harrison's 20th Ed. Chapter 319 Page 2267 Table 319-5

A. Abdominal mass
B. pANCA positivity
C. Response to antibiotics
D. Recurrence after surgery

898. Which of the following can mimic the endoscopic appearance of severe UC?
Harrison's 20th Ed. Chapter 319 Page 2266

A. Herpes simplex infection
B. Yersinia enterocolitica infection
C. Campylobacter colitis
D. Mycobacterium avium-intracellulare complex infection

Campylobacter colitis can mimic the endoscopic appearance of severe UC and can cause a relapse of established UC.

899. Which of the following can cause watery diarrhea?
Harrison's 20th Ed. Chapter 319 Page 2266

A. Salmonella
B. Shigella
C. C. difficile
D. All of the above

Apart from above three, the main symptom in Collagenous colitis is chronic watery diarrhea.

900. Which of the following can cause proctitis?
Harrison's 20th Ed. Chapter 319 Page 2266

A. Gonorrhea
B. Chlamydia
C. Syphilis
D. All of the above

Gonorrhea, Chlamydia, and syphilis can cause proctitis.

901. CMV infection occurs least commonly in?
Harrison's 20th Ed. Chapter 319 Page 2267

A. Esophagus
B. Small intestine
C. Colon
D. Rectum

902. Herpes simplex infection occurs most commonly in?
Harrison's 20th Ed. Chapter 319 Page 2267

A. Oropharynx
B. Anorectum
C. Perianal areas
D. All of the above

903. Parasitic infections that mimic IBD include all except?
Harrison's 20th Ed. Chapter 319 Page 2267

A. Necator americanus
B. Trichuris trichiura
C. Strongyloides stercoralis
D. Enterobius vermicularis

Parasitic infections that may mimic IBD include hookworm (Necator americanus), whipworm (Trichuris trichiura), Strongyloides stercoralis, Isospora belli and Entamoeba histolytica.

904. Mucosal abnormalities in diverticular-associated colitis are limited to?
Harrison's 20th Ed. Chapter 319 Page 2268

A. Caecum
B. Ascending colon
C. Transverse colon
D. Sigmoid and descending colon

Diverticular-associated colitis is similar to CD, but mucosal abnormalities are limited to the sigmoid and descending colon.

905. Patients of ischemic colitis usually present with sudden onset of pain in?
Harrison's 20th Ed. Chapter 319 Page 2268

A. Epigastrium
B. Periumbilical region
C. Right lower quadrant
D. Left lower quadrant

Patients of ischemic colitis usually present with sudden onset of left lower quadrant pain, urgency to defecate and the passage of bright red blood per rectum. Endoscopic examination often demonstrates a normal-appearing rectum and a sharp transition to an area of inflammation in the descending colon and splenic flexure.

906. Which of the following is typical of effects of radiotherapy on the GI tract?
Harrison's 20th Ed. Chapter 319 Page 2268

A. Abscesses
B. Mucus fistula
C. Telangiectasia
D. Ulceration

Flexible sigmoidoscopy reveals mucosal granularity, friability, numerous telangiectasias and occasionally discrete ulcerations.

907. Use of which of the following drugs can mimic IBD?
Harrison's 20th Ed. Chapter 319 Page 2268

A. Azathioprine
B. Mycophenolate mofetil
C. Cyclosporine
D. Rituximab

Use of ipilimumab, mycophenolate mofetil (MMF) & entanercept can mimic IBD.

908. Ipilimumab-induced colitis is typically treated with?
Harrison's 20th Ed. Chapter 319 Page 2268

A. Rituximab
B. Infliximab
C. Tacrolimus
D. Belatacept

Ipilimumab-induced colitis is typically treated with glucocorticoids or infliximab.

909. Patients with inflammatory bowel disease are at risk for?
N Engl J Med. 2009;361:2066-78

A. Primary sclerosing cholangitis
B. Ankylosing spondylitis
C. Psoriasis
D. All of the above

Patients with IBD are at risk for primary sclerosing cholangitis, ankylosing spondylitis, and psoriasis.

910. Which of the following is false about collagenous colitis?
Harrison's 20th Ed. Chapter 319 Page 2268

A. Increased subepithelial collagen deposition
B. Male to female ratio is 9:1
C. Most patients present in 6th or 7th decades
D. Main symptom is chronic watery diarrhea

Female to male ratio is 9:1.

911. Sertraline is a risk factor for which of the following?
Harrison's 20th Ed. Chapter 319 Page 2268

A. Diversion colitis
B. Collagenous colitis
C. Lymphocytic colitis
D. All of the above

912. The frequency of celiac disease is increased in which of the following?
Harrison's 20th Ed. Chapter 319 Page 2268

A. Diversion colitis
B. Collagenous colitis
C. Lymphocytic colitis
D. All of the above

The frequency of celiac disease is increased in lymphocytic colitis and ranges from 9 to 27%.

913. Which of the following is false about Erythema nodosum (EN) in IBD?
Harrison's 20th Ed. Chapter 319 Page 2268

A. Correlate with bowel activity
B. Develop after onset of bowel symptoms
C. Concomitant active peripheral arthritis
D. None of the above

EN occurs in ~15% of CD and 10% of UC patients. Attacks correlate with bowel activity, develop after onset of bowel symptoms, and frequently have concomitant active peripheral arthritis.

914. Which of the following is false about Erythema nodosum?
Harrison's 20th Ed. Chapter 319 Page 2268

A. Erythematous tender nodules
B. 1-5 cm in diameter
C. Found on anterior surface of lower legs and arms
D. None of the above

Lesions of EN are hot, red, tender nodules measuring 1 to 5 cm in diameter and found on anterior surface of lower legs, ankles, calves, thighs and arms.

915. Which of the following is false about Pyoderma gangrenosum (PG) in IBD?
Harrison's 20th Ed. Chapter 319 Page 2268

A. May occur years before onset of bowel symptoms
B. Independent of the bowel disease
C. Respond poorly to colectomy
D. None of the above

PG occurs years before the onset of bowel symptoms, is independent of bowel disease & respond poorly to colectomy, usually associated with severe disease.

916. Which of the following is false about Pyoderma gangrenosum (PG)?
Harrison's 20th Ed. Chapter 319 Page 2268

A. Found on dorsal surface of feet and legs
B. Usually begins as a macule
C. May be single or multiple
D. Difficult to treat

PG usually begins as a pustule and then spreads concentrically to rapidly undermine healthy skin.

917. Dermatologic manifestations of IBD include all except?
Harrison's 20th Ed. Chapter 319 Page 2268

A. Erythema nodosum (EN)
B. Pyoderma gangrenosum (PG)
C. Pyoderma vegetans
D. Erythema marginatum

918. Dermatologic manifestations of IBD include all except?
Harrison's 20th Ed. Chapter 319 Page 2268

A. Pyostomatitis vegetans
B. Alopecia
C. Perianal skin tags
D. Psoriasis

919. Which of the following skin lesions is most frequent in CD?
Harrison's 20th Ed. Chapter 319 Page 2268

A. Erythema nodosum (EN)
B. Pyoderma gangrenosum (PG)
C. Psoriasis
D. Perianal skin tags

Perianal skin tags are found in 75 – 80% of patients with CD, especially those with colon involvement.

920. Which of the following is sometimes associated with Crohn's disease?
Harrison's 20th Ed. Chapter 55 Page 359

A. Epidermolysis bullosa acquisita (EBA)
B. Dermatitis herpetiformis (DH)
C. Pemphigoid gestationis (PG)
D. Mucous membrane pemphigoid (MMP)

921. Peripheral arthritis that develops in IBD patients involves which of the following joints?
Harrison's 20th Ed. Chapter 319 Page 2268

A. Small joints of upper & lower extremities
B. Large joints of upper & lower extremities
C. Small joints of upper extremity
D. Small joints of lower extremity

Peripheral arthritis of IBD patients is asymmetric, polyarticular and migratory and affects large joints of upper and lower extremities.

922. Rheumatologic manifestations of IBD include all except?
Harrison's 20th Ed. Chapter 319 Page 2269

A. Peripheral arthritis
B. Ankylosing spondylitis (AS)
C. Osteopetrosis
D. Sacroiliitis

923. Rheumatologic manifestations of IBD include all except?
Harrison's 20th Ed. Chapter 319 Page 2269

A. Hypertrophic osteoarthropathy
B. Pelvic/femoral osteomyelitis
C. Relapsing polychondritis
D. Osteitis

924. Which of the following skeletal disease occurs equally in UC and CD?
Harrison's 20th Ed. Chapter 319 Page 2269

A. Peripheral arthritis
B. Ankylosing spondylitis (AS)
C. Sacroiliitis
D. All of the above

Symmetric sacroiliitis occurs equally in UC & CD. Peripheral arthritis and ankylosing spondylitis are more common in CD than UC.

925. Ocular manifestations of IBD include all except?
Harrison's 20th Ed. Chapter 319 Page 2269

A. Conjunctivitis
B. Anterior uveitis / iritis
C. Episcleritis
D. Retinitis

Ocular manifestations of IBD include conjunctivitis, anterior uveitis/iritis, and episcleritis.

926. Which of the following is false about ocular complications in IBD?
Harrison's 20th Ed. Chapter 319 Page 2269

A. Uveitis may be found during periods of remission
B. May develop in IBD patients following bowel resection
C. Episcleritis is a benign disorder more common in Crohn's colitis
D. None of the above

927. Common hepatobiliary manifestations of IBD include all except?
Harrison's 20th Ed. Chapter 319 Page 2269

A. Hepatic steatosis
B. Pancreatitis
C. Cholelithiasis
D. Primary sclerosing cholangitis (PSC)

Pancreatitis is a rare extraintestinal manifestation of IBD and results from duodenal fistulas, ampullary CD, gallstones, PSC, autoimmune pancreatitis and primary CD of the pancreas.

928. All are complications of UC except?
Harrison's 20th Ed. Chapter 319 Page 2269

A. Hemorrhage
B. Malignant change
C. Intusucception
D. Polyposis

929. Urologic manifestations of IBD include all except?
Harrison's 20th Ed. Chapter 319 Page 2269

A. Calculi
B. Ureteral obstruction
C. Ileal bladder fistulas
D. Glomerulonephritis

930. Hypercoagulable state in IBD is due to all except?
Harrison's 20th Ed. Chapter 319 Page 2269

A. Reactive thrombocytosis
B. Increased fibrinopeptide A, factor V, VIII & fibrinogen
C. Decreased thromboplastin generation
D. Antithrombin III deficiency

In IBD, risk of venous & arterial thrombosis increases even when disease is not active due to abnormalities of platelet-endothelial interaction, hyperhomocysteinemia, alterations in coagulation cascade, impaired fibrinolysis, involvement of tissue factor-bearing microvesicles, disruption of normal coagulation system by autoantibodies, vasculitides and genetic predisposition.

931. Cardiopulmonary manifestations of IBD include all except?
Harrison's 20th Ed. Chapter 319 Page 2269

A. Endocarditis / Myocarditis
B. Pleuropericarditis
C. Interstitial lung disease (ILD)
D. Obstructive lung disease

In IBD, cardiopulmonary manifestations include endocarditis, myocarditis, pleuropericarditis, & ILD.

932. Most common extraintestinal pulmonary complication of IBD is?
Harrison's 20th Ed. Chapter 319 Page 2269

A. ILD
B. Pneumonitis
C. Malignancy
D. Obstructive lung disease

933. Which of the following studies is related to patients of IBD?
Harrison's 20th Ed. Chapter 319 Page 2276

A. CESAME study
B. IDEAL trial
C. TONIC study
D. BLOOM study

In the prospective observational CESAME study in a cohort of IBD patients in France, the standardized incidence ratios of colorectal cancer were 2.2 for all IBD patients and 7.0 for patients with long-standing extensive colitis (both Crohn's and UC).

934. Risk of colorectal cancer in patients with IBD is relatively small during the initial?
Harrison's 20th Ed. Chapter 319 Page 2276

A. 2 years
B. 5 years
C. 10 years
D. 20 years

Risk of colorectal cancer in patients with IBD is relatively small during initial 10 years of the disease, but increases at a rate of ~0.5-1% per year. Cancer may develop in 8-30% of patients after 25 years of disease. The risk is higher in younger patients with pancolitis.

935. Role of sulfasalazine is not clear in which of the following?
Harrison's 20th Ed. Chapter 319 Page 2270

A. Inducing remission in UC
B. Maintaining remission in UC
C. Inducing remission in CD
D. Maintaining remission in CD

Sulfasalazine and other 5-ASA agents are effective at inducing and maintaining remission in UC with limited role in inducing remission in CD but no clear role in maintenance of CD. The most convincing evidence for use of sulfasalazine is treatment of active CD involving colon.

936. Which of the following is commonly referred to as sulphasalazine (SASP)?
Mediators of Inflammation. 1992;1:151-165

A. Salicylazosulphanilamide
B. Salicylazosulphapyridine
C. Salicylazosulphaguanidine
D. Salicylazosulphasuxidine

Salicylazosulphapyridine is also referred to as sulphasalazine (SASP) and consisting of 5-aminosalicylic acid (5-ASA) and sulphapyridine (SP) joined together by a diazo bond.

937. Enzymatic oxidation of arachidonic acid gives rise to?
Mediators of Inflammation. 1992;1:151-165

A. Prostaglandins & thromboxanes by cyclooxygenase pathway
B. Leukotrienes & intermediate hydroxyeicosatetraenoic acids (HETEs) from lipoxygenase pathway
C. Lipoxins
D. All of the above

938. Which of the following is a functional receptor mediating aminosalicylate activities in IBD?
World Journal of Gastroenterology. 2011;17(2):197-206

A. Steroidogenic factor 1 (SF1)
B. Peroxisome proliferator activated receptor-γ (PPAR-γ)
C. Retinoic acid receptor (RAR)
D. All of the above

PPAR-γ is the key receptor for 5-ASA that mediates its main effects in the colon Activation of PPAR-γ can antagonize nuclear factor κB (NFκB) action in macrophages resulting in downregulation of proinflammatory cytokines.

939. Very high expression levels of PPAR-γ are found in?
World Journal of Gastroenterology. 2011;17(2):197-206

A. Colonic epithelium
B. Macrophages, lymphocytes
C. Hepatocytes
D. Skeletal muscle

940. Nuclear receptor PPAR-γ controls expression of regulatory genes in?
World Journal of Gastroenterology. 2011;17(2):197-206

A. Lipid metabolisms
B. Insulin sensitization
C. Inflammation
D. All of the above

PPAR-γ is an essential nuclear receptor that controls expression of regulatory genes in lipid metabolisms, insulin sensitization, inflammation, and cell proliferation.

941. PPAR-γ interferes with inflammatory pathways by interactions with which of the following transcription factors?
World Journal of Gastroenterology. 2011;17(2):197-206

A. Nuclear factor kappa B (NF-κB)
B. Activating protein-1 (AP-1)
C. Signal transducer and activator of transcription (STAT)
D. All of the above

PPAR-γ interferes with inflammatory pathways by interactions with transcription factors like nuclear factor kappa B (NF-κB), activating protein-1 (AP-1), signal transducer and activator of transcription (STAT), and nuclear factor-activated T cell (NFAT).

942. Which of the following is critical in colonic steady state PPAR-γ expression through Toll-like receptor (TLR)?
Journal of Advances in Internal Medicine. 2012;01(1):33-38

A. Polyunsaturated fatty acids intake
B. Eicosanoids
C. Lipopolysaccharide (LPS) of Gram negative bacteria
D. Lipopolysaccharide (LPS) of Gram positive bacteria

Lipopolysaccharide (LPS) of Gram negative bacteria is critical in colonic steady state PPAR-γ expression through Toll-like receptor (TLR).

943. Which of the following is a dual acting PPAR-α/γ agonist?
Journal of Advances in Internal Medicine. 2012;01(1):33-38

A. Trogliazone
B. Rosiglitazone
C. Pioglitazone
D. Glitazar

Glitazar is a dual acting PPAR-α/γ agonist used for oral treatment for insulin resistance related glucose & lipid abnormalities associated with T2DM & metabolic syndrome.

944. Name of the bond linking the sulfa and 5-ASA moieties in Sulfasalazine is?
Harrison's 20th Ed. Chapter 319 Page 2270

A. Azo bond
B. Thio bond
C. Tau bond
D. Conn bond

Sulphasalazine (SASP) consists of 5-aminosalicylic acid (5-ASA) and sulphapyridine (SP) joined together by a diazo bond. Sulfasalazine is broken down in colon by bacterial azo reductases. They cleave the azo bond linking the sulfa and 5-ASA moieties.

945. Which of the following about sulphasalazine (SASP) is false?
Mediators of Inflammation. 1992;1:151-165

A. SASP acts as a pro-drug
B. Sulphapyridine (SP) acts as a carrier
C. 5-ASA is the active moiety
D. None of the above

Sulfasalazine, the azo-bonded 5-ASA prodrug, undergoes metabolism by bacterial azoreductase enzymes in colonic lumen to release the active 5-ASA moiety and the therapeutically inactive sulfapyridine. 5-ASA acts on and is metabolised by intestinal epithelial cells.

946. Sulfasalazine intolerable side effects are attributable to?
Harrison's 20th Ed. Chapter 319 Page 2270

A. Sulfapyridine moiety
B. Sulfasialic moiety
C. Sulfaphenol moiety
D. All of the above

Allergic reactions or intolerable side effects of sulfasalazine are attributable to sulfapyridine moiety.

947. With sulfasalazine therapy, which of the following should be supplemented?
Harrison's 20th Ed. Chapter 319 Page 2270

A. Iron
B. Folic acid
C. Vitamin B_{12}
D. Pyridoxine

Sulfasalazine can also impair folate absorption, and patients should be given folic acid supplements.

948. Which of the following is a folic acid antagonist?
N Engl J Med. 2000;343:1608-14

A. Trimethoprim
B. Triamterene
C. Carbamazepine
D. All of the above

949. Which of the following is a folic acid antagonist?
N Engl J Med. 2000;343:1608-14

A. Phenytoin
B. Phenobarbital
C. Primidone
D. All of the above

Folic acid antagonists include trimethoprim, triamterene, carbamazepine, phenytoin, phenobarbital, and primidone. These folic acid antagonists affect various enzymes in folate metabolism, impair absorption of folate, or increase degradation of folate.

950. Which of the following is a dihydrofolate reductase inhibitor?
N Engl J Med. 2000;343:1608-14

A. Methotrexate
B. Sulfasalazine
C. Pyrimethamine
D. All of the above

Dihydrofolate reductase inhibitors include aminopterin, methotrexate, sulfasalazine, pyrimethamine, triamterene, and trimethoprim, which displace folate from the enzyme and thereby block conversion of folate to its more active metabolites.

951. Use of folic acid antagonists in early pregnancy may increase the risk of?
N Engl J Med. 2000;343:1608-14

A. Cardiovascular defects
B. Oral clefts
C. Urinary tract defects
D. All of the above

Use of folic acid antagonists in early pregnancy may increase the risk of cardiovascular defects, oral clefts, and urinary tract defects.

952. Hypersensitivity reactions to sulfasalazine include all except?
Harrison's 20th Ed. Chapter 319 Page 2270

A. Hepatitis
B. Thrombocytosis
C. Worsening of colitis
D. Reversible sperm abnormalities

Hypersensitivity reactions of sulfasalazine include rash, fever, hepatitis, agranulocytosis, hypersensitivity pneumonitis, pancreatitis, worsening of colitis and reversible sperm abnormalities.

953. Most common adverse effect reported with 5-ASA agents is?
Gastroenterology & Hepatology. 2008; 4(11), Supplement 24:5

A. Headache
B. Skin rash
C. Constipation
D. Teeth discoloration

The most common adverse effects reported with 5-ASA agents include headaches and GI symptoms such as diarrhea, gas, and nausea.

954. Which out of the following mesalamine formulation has ethylcellulose coating?
Harrison's 20th Ed. Chapter 319 Page 2270

A. Asacol
B. Balsalazide
C. Claversal
D. Pentasa

Pentasa is a mesalamine formulation that has an ethylcellulose coating to allow water absorption into small beads containing mesalamine.

955. Which of the following is a pH-independent formulation mesalamine formulation to deliver 5-ASA?
Gastroenterology & Hepatology. 2008; 4(11), Supplement 24:5

A. Asacol
B. Lialda
C. Pentasa
D. All of the above

Lialda consists of a core of lipophilic & hydrophilic matrices (multimatrix core, MMX) enclosed within a pH-dependent coating. Like Asacol, pH-dependent coating delays release of mesalamine until the tablet is exposed to a pH of 7 or greater. Pentasa is a controlled-released, pH-independent formulation containing microspheres of 5-ASA enclosed within a moisture-sensitive, methylcellulose, semipermeable membrane.

956. Which of the following is a azo-bonded prodrugs of 5-ASA?
Gastroenterology & Hepatology. 2008; 4(11), Supplement 24:5
- A. Sulfasalazine
- B. Olsalazine
- C. Balsalazide
- D. All of the above

Olsalazine & balsalazide are prodrugs that deliver 5-ASA to colon without using a sulfapyridine carrier.

957. Which of the following is composed of two 5-ASA radicals linked by an azo bond?
Harrison's 20th Ed. Chapter 319 Page 2270
- A. Asacol
- B. Balsalazide
- C. Claversal
- D. Olsalazine

Olsalazine is composed of two 5-ASA radicals linked by an azo bond, which is split in colon by bacterial reduction and two 5-ASA molecules are released. Balsalazide links 5-ASA via a diazo bond to an inactive carrier molecule, 4-aminobenzoyl-β-alanine.

958. 5-ASA agents act within what period of time?
Harrison's 20th Ed. Chapter 319 Page 2270
- A. 6-12 hours
- B. 1-7 days
- C. 2-4 weeks
- D. 4-6 weeks

As a general rule, 5-ASA agents act within 2-4 weeks.

959. Which of the following about budesonide is false?
Harrison's 20th Ed. Chapter 319 Page 2271
- A. Released entirely in colon
- B. Has minimal to no glucocorticoid side effects
- C. No taper is required
- D. None of the above

Budesonide is useful in UC. It is released entirely in colon and has minimal to no glucocorticoid side effects. Dose is 9 mg/day for 8 weeks, and no taper is required.

960. Which of the following is false regarding treatment of IBD?
Harrison's 20th Ed. Chapter 319 Page 2271
- A. Antibiotics have no role in treatment of active or quiescent UC
- B. Glucocorticoids useful in maintenance therapy in UC & CD
- C. 5-ASA effective in inducing remission in UC & CD
- D. 5-ASA useful in maintaining remission in UC

Glucocorticoids play no role in maintenance therapy in UC or CD. 5-ASA is effective in inducing remission in UC & CD & maintaining remission in UC. Its role in remission maintenance in CD is not established. Topical 5-ASA therapy is more effective than topical steroid therapy in the treatment of distal UC.

961. Which of the following side effects of glucocorticoid therapy in IBD is not related to dose & duration of therapy?
Harrison's 20th Ed. Chapter 319 Page 2271
- A. Abdominal striae
- B. Subcapsular cataract
- C. Osteonecrosis
- D. Emotional disturbances

Most of these side effects of glucocorticoids, other than osteonecrosis, are related to dose and duration of therapy.

962. First line treatment in active inflammatory, fistulizing and perianal CD is?
Harrison's 20th Ed. Chapter 319 Page 2271
- A. 5-ASA
- B. Azathioprine
- C. Metronidazole
- D. Glucocorticoids

Metronidazole is effective in active inflammatory, fistulous, and perianal CD and may prevent recurrence after ileal resection.

963. First line treatment in active inflammatory, fistulizing and perianal CD is?
Harrison's 20th Ed. Chapter 319 Page 2271
- A. 5-ASA
- B. Azathioprine
- C. Ciprofloxacin
- D. Glucocorticoids

Both ciprofloxacin and metronidazole antibiotics can be used as first-line drugs for short periods of time in active inflammatory, fistulizing and perianal CD.

964. Achilles tendinitis and rupture is associated with which of the following medicines?
Harrison's 20th Ed. Chapter 319 Page 2271
- A. Azathioprine
- B. Glucocorticoids
- C. Ciprofloxacin
- D. Metronidazole

Ciprofloxacin has recently been associated with Achilles tendinitis and rupture.

965. Active end product of Azathioprine is?
Harrison's 20th Ed. Chapter 319 Page 2271
- A. 6-MP
- B. Thioinosinic acid
- C. Inosinic acid
- D. Thioguanic acid

Azathioprine is converted to 6-MP, which is metabolized to active end product, thioinosinic acid, an inhibitor of purine ribonucleotide synthesis and cell proliferation.

966. Which of the following is the end product of 6-MP metabolism?
Harrison's 20th Ed. Chapter 319 Page 2271
- A. 6-thymidine-mercaptopurine
- B. 6-methyl-mercaptopurine
- C. 6-propyl-mercaptopurine
- D. 6-ethyl-mercaptopurine

Azathioprine therapy adherence can be monitored by levels of 6-thioguanine & 6-methyl-mercaptopurine, end products of 6-MP metabolism. 1 in 300 individuals lacks thiopurine methyltransferase, the enzyme responsible for drug metabolism to inactive end-products (6-methylmercaptopurine).

967. Which of the following drugs is used for postoperative prophylaxis of CD?
Harrison's 20th Ed. Chapter 319 Page 2271
- A. 5-ASA
- B. Azathioprine
- C. Metronidazole
- D. Salicylates

6-MP or azathioprine is effective for postoperative prophylaxis of CD.

968. Which of the following statements about azathioprine use in IBD is false?
Harrison's 20th Ed. Chapter 319 Page 2271

   A. Pancreatitis as a side effect is completely reversible on stopping drug
   B. Thiopurine methyltransferase is the enzyme responsible for its metabolism
   C. No increased risk of cancer in IBD patients chronically taking azathioprine
   D. Leukopenia is dose-related and delayed

IBD patients treated with azathioprine/6-MP are at a fourfold increased risk of developing a lymphoma due to medications, underlying disease, or both.

969. Methotrexate (MTX) inhibits which of the following?
Harrison's 20th Ed. Chapter 319 Page 2271

   A. Dihydrofolate reductase
   B. HMG-CoA reductase
   C. Trypanothione reductase
   D. Fumarate reductase

Methotrexate (MTX) inhibits dihydrofolate reductase, resulting in impaired DNA synthesis. Additional anti-inflammatory properties may be related to decreased IL-1 production.

970. Potential toxicities of Methotrexate include all except?
Harrison's 20th Ed. Chapter 319 Page 2271

   A. Leukopenia
   B. Hepatic fibrosis
   C. Hypersensitivity pneumonitis
   D. Cholelithiasis

Potential toxicities of MTX include leukopenia, hepatic fibrosis and hypersensitivity pneumonitis (rarely).

971. Which of the following drugs is a lipophilic peptide?
Harrison's 20th Ed. Chapter 319 Page 2271

   A. Azathioprine
   B. Methotrexate
   C. Cyclosporine
   D. Tacrolimus

Cyclosporine (CSA) is a lipophilic peptide with inhibitory effects on both the cellular and humoral immune systems.

972. Cyclosporine (CSA) acts by inhibition of?
Harrison's 20th Ed. Chapter 319 Page 2271

   A. IL-1
   B. IL-2
   C. IFN-α
   D. All of the above

973. Cyclosporine (CSA) binds to?
Harrison's 20th Ed. Chapter 319 Page 2271

   A. Cyclocysteine
   B. Cyclopurine
   C. Cyclophilin
   D. Cycloserine

974. CSA inhibits which of the following?
Harrison's 20th Ed. Chapter 319 Page 2271

   A. Calcitriol
   B. Calcineurin
   C. Osteocalcin
   D. Calcitonin

CSA blocks production of IL-2 by T-helper lymphocytes. CSA binds to cyclophilin, and this complex inhibits calcineurin, a cytoplasmic phosphatase enzyme involved in activation of T cells. CSA also indirectly inhibits B cell function by blocking helper T cells.

975. Which of the following about cyclosporine is false?
Harrison's 20th Ed. Chapter 307 Page 2128 Table 307-3

   A. Forms trimolecular complex with cyclophilin & calcineurin
   B. Blocks cytokine IL-2 production
   C. Stimulates TGF-β production
   D. None of the above

976. Blood levels of cyclosporine should be maintained between?
Harrison's 20th Ed. Chapter 319 Page 2271

   A. 50 and 50 ng/mL
   B. 50 and 150 ng/mL
   C. 150 and 350 ng/mL
   D. 350 and 550 ng/mL

Blood levels of cyclosporine should be maintained between 150 and 350 ng/mL.

977. Severe UC patients that are refractory to IV glucocortcoids, should be treated with?
Harrison's 20th Ed. Chapter 319 Page 2271

   A. IV Cyclosporine
   B. Oral cyclosporine
   C. Azathioprine
   D. 6 Mercaptopurine

CSA is given intravenously in severe UC that is refractory to intravenous glucocorticoids.

978. Which of the following is not a side effect of cyclosporine therapy?
Harrison's 20th Ed. Chapter 319 Page 2271

   A. Hypertension
   B. Gingival hyperplasia
   C. Alopecia
   D. Paresthesias

Creatinine elevation, hypertension, gingival hyperplasia, hypertrichosis, paresthesias, tremors, headaches, electrolyte abnormalities and seizures are common side effects of cyclosporine therapy.

979. Seizures may complicate cyclosporine therapy if there is?
Harrison's 20th Ed. Chapter 319 Page 2271

   A. Hypocholesterolemia
   B. Hypercholesterolemia
   C. Hypertriglyceridemia
   D. All of the above

Seizures may complicate CSA therapy if the patient is hypomagnesemic or if serum cholesterol levels are <120 mg/dL.

980. Opportunistic infection that commonly occurs with cyclosporine therapy is?
Harrison's 20th Ed. Chapter 319 Page 2271

A. Pneumocystis carnii infection
B. M. tuberculosis infection
C. Klebsiella infection
D. Pseudomonas infection

Opportunistic infections, most often Pneumocystis carinii pneumonia, may occur with CSA combination immunosuppressive treatment.

981. Tacrolimus has immunomodulatory properties similar to?
Harrison's 20th Ed. Chapter 319 Page 2271

A. Methotrexate
B. Cyclosporine
C. Mycophenolate mofetil
D. Thalidomide

Tacrolimus is a macrolide antibiotic with immunomodulatory properties similar to CSA.

982. Which of the following drugs is a macrolide antibiotic?
Harrison's 20th Ed. Chapter 319 Page 2271

A. Azathioprine
B. Methotrexate
C. Cyclosporine
D. Tacrolimus

Tacrolimus is a macrolide antibiotic, 100 times as potent as CSA. It is not dependent on bile or mucosal integrity for absorption.

983. First biologic therapy approved for CD & UC is?
Harrison's 20th Ed. Chapter 319 Page 2272

A. Adalimumab
B. Infliximab
C. Natalizumab
D. Etanercept

The first biologic therapy approved for Crohn's disease & UC was infliximab.

984. Infliximab is?
Harrison's 20th Ed. Chapter 319 Page 2272

A. IgG_1 chimeric monoclonal antibody against TNF-α
B. IgG_1 fully human monoclonal antibody against TNF-α
C. IgG_4 chimeric monoclonal antibody against TNF-α
D. P75 TNF receptor fusion protein

Infliximab is a chimeric mouse-human monoclonal antibody against TNF-α. It blocks TNF in serum and at cell surface and lyses TNF-producing macrophages & T cells.

985. Which of the following trials evaluated infliximab in CD?
Harrison's 20th Ed. Chapter 319 Page 2272

A. PRECISE II
B. ACCENT I
C. CHARM
D. GEMINI I

The ACCENT I (A Crohn's Disease Clinical Trial Evaluating Infliximab in a New Long-Term Treatment Regimen) study showed that of the patients who experience an initial response, 40% will maintain remission for at least 1 year with repeated infusions of infliximab every 8 weeks.

986. Which of the following trials evaluated infliximab in CD?
Harrison's 20th Ed. Chapter 319 Page 2272

A. ACCENT I
B. ACCENT II
C. SONIC
D. All of the above

987. Adalimumab is a?
Harrison's 20th Ed. Chapter 319 Page 2272

A. IgG_1 chimeric monoclonal antibody against TNF
B. IgG_1 recombinant human monoclonal antibody against TNF
C. IgG_4 chimeric monoclonal antibody against TNF
D. P75 TNF receptor fusion protein

Less immunogenic than Infliximab, Adalimumab is a recombinant human monoclonal IgG1 antibody containing only human peptide sequences. Adalimumab binds TNF and neutralizes its function by blocking the interaction between TNF and its cell-surface receptor.

988. Anti-TNF monoclonal antibody useful in treatment of moderate to severely active CD in patients is?
Harrison's 20th Ed. Chapter 319 Page 2272

A. Infliximab
B. Adalimumab
C. Certolizumab pegol
D. All of the above

Anti-TNF monoclonal antibodies, infliximab, adalimumab, certolizumab pegol and golimumab are effective in the treatment of moderate to severely active CD in patients who have not responded despite complete & adequate therapy with a corticosteroid or an immunosuppressive agent.

989. Infusion reaction that occur with Infliximab therapy is due to?
Harrison's 20th Ed. Chapter 319 Page 2272

A. Antibody to Infliximab
B. Concurrent Methotrexate therapy
C. Anti ds-DNA antibody
D. Antinuclear factor

The development of antibodies to infliximab (ATI) is associated with an increased risk of infusion reactions and a decreased response to treatment.

990. Which one of the following is considered to be useful additional therapy with treatment of CD with Infliximab?
Harrison's 20th Ed. Chapter 319 Page 2272

A. Oral steroids
B. 5-ASA
C. Azathioprine
D. Elemental diet

If infliximab is used episodically for flares, concomitant immunosuppression with AZA, 6-MP or methotrexate in therapeutic doses is recommended to reduce clinical consequences of immunogenicity of chimeric antibodies. SONIC (Study of Biologic and Immunomodulator-Naïve Patients with Crohn's Disease) Trial compared infliximab plus azathioprine, infliximab alone and azathioprine alone in moderate-to-severe Crohn's disease with infliximab plus azathioprine group showing best results and no greater adverse events.

991. Risk of which of the following is increased with anti-TNF therapy?
Harrison's 20th Ed. Chapter 319 Page 2272

A. Non-Hodgkin's Lymphoma (NHL)
B. Hepatosplenic T Cell Lymphoma (HSTCL)
C. Melanoma
D. All of the above

992. Infliximab is not useful in?
Harrison's 20th Ed. Chapter 319 Page 2272
A. Crohn's disease
B. Rheumatoid arthritis
C. Ankylosing spondilitis
D. Primary sclerosing cholangitis

993. Which one of the following specifically blocks Integrin-α₄ and prevents lymphocyte trafficking to the intestine in IBD?
Harrison's 20th Ed. Chapter 319 Page 2273
A. Anti IL-12 P40 antibody
B. Anti-gamma interferon
C. Natalizumab
D. Basiliximab

Humanized monoclonal antibody to alpha-4 integrin - Natalizumab inhibits lymphocyte trafficking and is effective in treatment of moderate to severely active CD who have had an inadequate response or are unable tolerate conventional CD therapies and anti-TNF monoclonal antibody therapy.

994. Natalizumab is a?
Harrison's 20th Ed. Chapter 319 Page 2273
A. IgG₁ chimeric monoclonal antibody against TNF
B. IgG₁ recombinant human monoclonal antibody against TNF
C. Recombinant humanized IgG₄ antibody against α4 integrin
D. P75 TNF receptor fusion protein

Natalizumab is a recombinant humanized immunoglobulin G4 antibody against α4 integrin that is effective in the induction and maintenance of remission in CD patients.

995. Natalizumab causes progressive multifocal leukoencephalopathy (PML) by reactivation of which virus?
Harrison's 20th Ed. Chapter 319 Page 2273, Am J Gastroenterol 2009; 104:465.483
A. Hepatitis B
B. Human JC polyoma virus
C. Hepatitis C
D. Cytomegalovirus (CMV)

Natalizumab reactivates the human John Cunningham (JC) polyoma virus, which can lead to progressive multifocal leukoencephalopathy (PML). It is not used in combination with any immunosuppressant medications.

996. Which of the following provides gut-selective immunosuppression?
Harrison's 20th Ed. Chapter 319 Page 2273
A. Natalizumab
B. Vedolizumab
C. Ustekinumab
D. Tofacitinib

Vedolizumab is a leukocyte trafficking inhibitor. It does not cross the blood-brain barrier. It is a monoclonal antibody directed against α4β7 integrin specifically and has the ability to convey gut-selective immunosuppression.

997. Which of the following biologic therapy agents blocks the biologic activity of IL-12 & IL-23?
Harrison's 20th Ed. Chapter 319 Page 2273
A. Natalizumab
B. Vedolizumab
C. Ustekinumab
D. All of the above

Ustekinumab is a fully human IgG1 monoclonal antibody that blocks the biologic activity of IL-12 & IL-23.

998. Which of the following is a infliximab biosimilar?
Harrison's 20th Ed. Chapter 319 Page 2273
A. CT-P12
B. CT-P13
C. CT-P14
D. CT-P15

Biosimilars are biological products that are replicas of their innovator biopharmaceuticals, developed after patent expiration and are submitted for separate marketing approval. Biosimilars should not be considered as "biological generics". Infliximab biosimilar CT-P13 is approved & available for use.

999. Which of the following is an oral inhibitor of Janus kinases 1?
Harrison's 20th Ed. Chapter 319 Page 2273
A. Ozanimod
B. Tofacitinib
C. Tocilizumab
D. Omalizumab

1000. Which of the following causes peripheral lymphocyte sequestration?
Harrison's 20th Ed. Chapter 319 Page 2273
A. Ozanimod
B. Tofacitinib
C. Tocilizumab
D. Omalizumab

Ozanimod is an oral agonist of the sphingosine-1-phosphate receptor subtypes 1 and 5 that causes peripheral lymphocyte sequestration.

1001. Which of the following is false about ileoanal J pouch anastomosis (IPAA)?
Harrison's 20th Ed. Chapter 319 Page 2273
A. Most frequent complication is pouchitis
B. Ileum serves as a neorectum
C. Contraindicated in CD
D. None of the above

1002. Which of the following is false in females with IBD?
Harrison's 20th Ed. Chapter 319 Page 2275
A. Normal fertility rates in quiescent IBD
B. Fallopian tubes scarred by inflammatory process of CD, especially on right side
C. Fallopian tubes scarred by inflammatory process of CD, especially on left side
D. Dyspareunia common

Fallopian tubes can be scarred by inflammatory process of CD, especially on right side because of the proximity of terminal ileum.

1003. In IBD, which of following drugs is safe for use in pregnancy?
Harrison's 20th Ed. Chapter 319 Page 2275
A. Sulfasalazine
B. Mesalamine
C. Balsalazide
D. All of the above

Sulfasalazine, mesalamine, and balsalazide are safe for use in pregnancy and nursing, but additional folate supplementation must be given with sulfasalazine. Topical 5-ASA agents are also safe during pregnancy and nursing. Glucocorticoids are generally safe for use during pregnancy.

1004. The safe antibiotics to use for short periods in pregnant CD patients are all except?
Harrison's 20th Ed. Chapter 319 Page 2275

A. Ampicillin
B. Cephalosporin
C. Ciprofloxacin
D. Metronidazole

Safest antibiotics in CD in pregnancy for weeks, not months are ampicillin and cephalosporin. Metronidazole can be used in the second or third trimester. Ciprofloxacin causes cartilage lesions and should be avoided.

1005. In treatment of IBD with pregnancy, which of the following drugs is contraindicated?
Harrison's 20th Ed. Chapter 319 Page 2275

A. 6-Mercaptopurine
B. Azathioprine
C. Methotrexate
D. Cyclosporine

Methotrexate is contraindicated in pregnancy and nursing. 6-MP and azathioprine pose minimal or no risk during pregnancy. In severe IBD treated with IV CSA during pregnancy, 80% of pregnancies were successfully completed without development of renal toxicity, congenital malformations, or developmental defects.

1006. In pregnancy, exacerbation in Crohn's disease is seen in?
Harrison's 20th Ed. Chapter 466 Page 3444

A. First trimester
B. Second and third trimesters
C. Postpartum period
D. All of the above

1007. In pregnancy, exacerbation in Ulcerative colitis is seen in?
Harrison's 20th Ed. Chapter 466 Page 3444

A. First trimester
B. Second trimester
C. Third trimester
D. All of the above

Crohn's disease may be associated with exacerbations in the second and third trimesters. Ulcerative colitis is associated with disease exacerbations in first trimester & during early postpartum period.

1008. Patients with CD have an increased risk of developing which of the following cancers?
Harrison's 20th Ed. Chapter 319 Page 2275

A. Non-Hodgkin's lymphoma
B. Hodgkin's lymphoma
C. Bronchogenic carcinoma
D. Carcinoma cervix

1009. Patients with CD have an increased risk of developing which of the following cancers?
Harrison's 20th Ed. Chapter 319 Page 2275

A. Hodgkin's lymphoma
B. Endometrial carcinoma
C. Bronchogenic carcinoma
D. Squamous cell cancers

Patients with CD may have an increased risk of non-Hodgkin's lymphoma, leukemia, and myelodysplastic syndromes. Severe chronic, complicated perianal disease in CD patients may be associated with an increased risk of cancer in lower rectum and anal canal (squamous cell cancers).

1010. Mucosal ulcerations of the gut resembling Crohn's disease can be seen in?
Harrison's 20th Ed. Chapter 357 Page 2590

A. Sjogren's syndrome
B. Behcet's syndrome
C. Hypereosinophilic syndrome
D. All of the above

In Behcet's syndrome, gastrointestinal involvement is seen more frequently in patients from Japan and consists of mucosal ulcerations of the gut, resembling Crohn's disease.

1011. Rectal biopsy findings of which of the following resemble those in Crohn's disease?
Harrison's 20th Ed. Chapter 131 Page 989

A. Herpes
B. Lymphogranuloma venereum (LGV)
C. Chancroid
D. Donovanosis

In LGV, rectal biopsy typically shows crypt abscesses, granulomas and giant cells - findings resembling those in Crohn's disease.

1012. Presentation of which of the following may mimic that of ulcerative colitis or Crohn's disease?
Harrison's 20th Ed. Chapter 162 Page 1186

A. Shigella-induced dysentery
B. Cholera
C. Campylobacter enteritis
D. Salmonella gastroenteritis

Presentation of Campylobacter enteritis may mimic that of ulcerative colitis or Crohn's disease.

1013. Before making a diagnosis of IBD, which of the following infections should be ruled out?
Harrison's 20th Ed. Chapter 162 Page 1186

A. Campylobacter
B. Arcobacter
C. Helicobacter
D. All of the above

Presentation of Campylobacter enteritis may mimic UC or CD. As Campylobacter enteritis is much more common than UC and CD among young adults, a diagnosis of IBD should not be made until Campylobacter infection has been ruled out.

1014. Ulcerative colitis and Crohn's disease may be complicated by?
Harrison's 20th Ed. Chapter 438 Page 3214

A. SLE
B. Sjogren's syndrome
C. GBS
D. All of the above

Ulcerative colitis and Crohn's disease may be complicated by GBS, CIDP, generalized axonal sensory or sensorimotor polyneuropathy, small-fiber neuropathy or mononeuropathy.

1015. Which of the following seronegative arthropathies is strongly associated with HLA-B27 histocompatibility antigen?
Harrison's 20th Ed. Chapter 355 Page 2573

A. Ankylosing spondylitis
B. Psoriatic arthritis
C. Arthritides associated with ulcerative colitis
D. All of the above

Seronegative arthropathies like ankylosing spondylitis, reactive arthritis, psoriatic arthritis and arthritides associated with ulcerative colitis and regional enteritis are all strongly associated with the HLA-B27 histocompatibility antigen.

Irritable Bowel Syndrome

1016. Which of the following is a criteria for the diagnosis of Irritable Bowel Syndrome (IBS)?
Harrison's 20th Ed. Chapter 320 Page 2276

A. Paris
B. Rome
C. Helsinki
D. Warsaw

Rome IV criteria is useful for the diagnosis of IBS.

1017. In which year, Rome III criteria for diagnosis of IBS was updated to Rome IV?
Harrison's 20th Ed. Chapter 320 Page 2276

A. 2012
B. 2014
C. 2016
D. 2018

In 2016, the Rome III criteria for the diagnosis of IBS were updated to Rome IV. Rome II criteria for diagnosis of IBS was revised in 2006.

1018. Which of the following is not included in the Rome IV criteria for the diagnosis of IBS?
Harrison's 20th Ed. Chapter 320 Page 2276 Table 320-1

A. Recurrent abdominal pain related to defecation
B. Recurrent abdominal pain related to nausea & vomiting
C. Recurrent abdominal pain with change in frequency of stool
D. Recurrent abdominal pain with change in form of stool

Rome IV diagnostic criteria for IBS includes recurrent abdominal pain at least 1 day per week in the last 3 months associated with two or more of the following-related to defecation, associated with change in frequency of stool and associated with a change in form or appearance of stool. Painless diarrhea or constipation are not included in the criteria.

1019. Which of the following is a key symptom for the diagnosis of IBS?
Harrison's 20th Ed. Chapter 320 Page 2276

A. Abdominal pain
B. Frequency of stool
C. Form (appearance) of stool
D. Feeling of incomplete bowel movement and bloating

1020. Which of the following is not included in the criteria for the diagnosis of IBS?
Harrison's 20th Ed. Chapter 320 Page 2276

A. Painless diarrhea or constipation
B. Feeling of incomplete bowel movement
C. Passing mucus in stool
D. All of the above

Abdominal pain is a key symptom for the diagnosis of IBS. Supportive symptoms that are not part of the diagnostic criteria include defecation straining, urgency or a feeling of incomplete bowel movement, passing mucus and bloating.

1021. IBS symptoms often overlap with which of the following functional disorders?
Harrison's 20th Ed. Chapter 320 Page 2276

A. Fibromyalgia
B. Headache
C. Genitourinary symptoms
D. All of the above

IBS symptoms have a tendency to come & go over time and often overlap with other functional disorders such as fibromyalgia, headache, backache and genitourinary symptoms.

1022. Which of the following about IBS is false?
Harrison's 20th Ed. Chapter 320 Page 2276

A. Most patients have their first symptoms before 45 years
B. Women make up to 80% of severe IBS patients
C. Rome II criteria for diagnosis of IBS was revised in 2006
D. None of the above

1023. Which of the following about abdominal pain in IBS is false?
Harrison's 20th Ed. Chapter 320 Page 2276

A. Sleep deprivation is usual
B. Exacerbated by eating
C. Improved by passage of flatus or stools
D. Worsens during the premenstrual & menstrual phases

Sleep deprivation is unusual and abdominal pain is almost uniformly present only during waking hours.

1024. Which of the following is a prerequisite clinical feature of IBS?
Harrison's 20th Ed. Chapter 320 Page 2276

A. Abdominal pain
B. Alteration in bowel habits
C. Gas and Flatulence
D. Dyspepsia

1025. Abdominal pain in IBS is exacerbated by?
Harrison's 20th Ed. Chapter 320 Page 2276

A. Eating
B. Emotional stress
C. During premenstrual & menstrual phases in female patients
D. All of the above

1026. Which of the following is the most consistent clinical feature in IBS?
Harrison's 20th Ed. Chapter 320 Page 2277

A. Abdominal pain or discomfort
B. Alteration in bowel habits
C. Gas and Flatulence
D. Dyspepsia

Abdominal pain or discomfort is a prerequisite clinical feature of IBS. While, alteration in bowel habits is the most consistent clinical feature in IBS.

1027. Which of the following is rare in IBS?
Harrison's 20th Ed. Chapter 320 Page 2276

A. Malnutrition
B. Weight loss
C. Sleep deprivation
D. All of the above

1028. Which of the following about diarrhea in IBS is false?
Harrison's 20th Ed. Chapter 320 Page 2277

A. Small volume
B. Nocturnal
C. Aggravated by emotional stress
D. Aggravated by eating

Nocturnal diarrhea or steatorrheal stools do not occur in IBS and malabsorption or weight loss does not occur. Stool volume >200–300 mL/day argues against IBS.

1029. Which of the following IBS subgroup is most prevalent?
Harrison's 20th Ed. Chapter 320 Page 2277

A. IBS-diarrhea predominant (IBS-D)
B. IBS-constipation predominant (IBS-C)
C. IBS-mixed (IBS-M)
D. None of the above

On the basis of the predominant bowel habit, IBS has been categorized into one of the following subgroups: IBS with diarrhea (more common in men), IBS with constipation (more common in women), and IBS with mixed bowel habits. Each group accounts for about one third of all patients.

1030. What percentage of IBS patients change subtypes over 1 year?
Harrison's 20th Ed. Chapter 320 Page 2277

A. 25%
B. 50%
C. 75%
D. 100%

75% of IBS patients change subtypes and 29% switch between IBS-C and IBS-D over 1 year.

1031. Which of the following is false in IBS patients?
Harrison's 20th Ed. Chapter 320 Page 2277

A. Impaired transit of intestinal gas loads
B. Impaired tolerance of intestinal gas loads
C. Gas reflux from distal to more proximal intestine
D. None of the above

1032. Motor abnormalities under stimulated conditions in IBS are seen in?
Harrison's 20th Ed. Chapter 320 Page 2277

A. Transverse colon
B. Descending colon
C. Sigmoid colon
D. All of the above

Colonic myoelectrical & motor activity under "unstimulated" conditions do not show consistent abnormalities in IBS. IBS patients exhibit increased rectosigmoid motor activity for up to 3 hours after eating.

1033. Which of the following myoelectrical and motor abnormality is seen in IBS under stimulated conditions?
Harrison's 20th Ed. Chapter 320 Page 2277

A. Increased rectosigmoid motor activity
B. Prolonged distention-evoked contractile activity
C. Increased peak amplitude of high-amplitude propagating contractions (HAPCs)
D. All of the above

1034. In IBS, postprandial pain is temporally related to entry of food bolus into which of the following?
Harrison's 20th Ed. Chapter 320 Page 2277

A. Stomach
B. Duodenum
C. Jejunum
D. Cecum

Postprandial pain is temporally related to entry of the food bolus into cecum in IBS.

1035. Which of the following lower the thresholds for the first sensation of gas, discomfort & pain in IBS patients?
Harrison's 20th Ed. Chapter 320 Page 2277

A. Carbohydrates
B. Proteins
C. Lipids
D. Water

Lipids lower the thresholds for the first sensation of gas, discomfort and pain in IBS patients. Thus, postprandial symptoms in IBS patients are explained by a nutrient-dependent exaggerated sensory component of the gastrocolonic response. Afferent pathway disturbances in IBS are selective for visceral innervation with sparing of somatic pathways.

1036. In IBS, mechanisms responsible for visceral hypersensitivity may be?
Harrison's 20th Ed. Chapter 320 Page 2277

A. Recruitment of "silent" nociceptors
B. Spinal hyperexcitability
C. Neuroplasticity
D. All of the above

1037. Brain region concerned with attention processes & response selection is?
Harrison's 20th Ed. Chapter 320 Page 2278

A. Amygdala
B. Mid-cingulate cortex
C. Perigenual anterior cingulated cortex
D. Hippocampus

Mid-cingulate cortex is a region in brain that is concerned with attention processes & response selection. This region shows greater activation in IBS patients. Modulation of this region produces changes in subjective unpleasantness of pain. Also, in IBS patients there occurs preferential activation of the prefrontal lobe that increases alertness.

1038. Which of the following is the most important risk factor for developing post-infectious IBS?
Harrison's 20th Ed. Chapter 320 Page 2278

A. Toxicity of infecting bacterial strain
B. Smoking
C. Prolonged duration of initial illness
D. Depression

Risk factors for developing postinfectious IBS include, in order of importance, prolonged duration of initial illness, toxicity of infecting bacterial strain, smoking, mucosal markers of inflammation, female gender, depression, hypochondriasis and adverse life events in the preceding 3 months.

1039. Which of the following protects against post-infectious IBS?
Harrison's 20th Ed. Chapter 320 Page 2278

A. Age > 60 years
B. Treatment with antibiotics
C. Presence of mucosal markers of inflammation
D. Female sex

Age older than 60 years might protect against post-infectious IBS.

1040. **Microbe involved in the initial infection of post-infectious IBS is?**
Harrison's 20th Ed. Chapter 320 Page 2278
- A. Campylobacter
- B. Salmonella
- C. Shigella
- D. All of the above

Microbes involved in the initial infection of post-infectious IBS are Campylobacter, Salmonella & Shigella.

1041. **Functional Bowel Disorder Severity Index (FBDSI) was developed and published by?**
Gastroenterology 2016;150:1262
- A. Talley
- B. Eswaran
- C. Drossman
- D. Mayer

1042. **Which of the following is a nonselective cation channel expressed in nociceptive neurons?**
Harrison's 20th Ed. Chapter 320 Page 2278
- A. TRPV 1
- B. TRPV 2
- C. TRPV 3
- D. TRPV 4

TRPV 1 is a nonselective cation channel expressed in nociceptive neurons and are central to the initiation & persistence of visceral hypersensitivity.

1043. **TRPV stands for?**
Harrison's 20th Ed. Chapter 320 Page 2278
- A. Transient receptor potential cation channel
- B. Terminal receptor potential cation channel
- C. Total receptor potential cation channel
- D. Timed receptor potential cation channel

TRPV4 stands for transient receptor potential cation channel subfamily V, member 4. TRPV5 and TRPV6 are calcium transporters expressed by intestinal epithelia whose expression is controlled principally by $1,25(OH)_2D$.

1044. **TRP channels are cellular sensors involved in?**
Br J Pharmacol. 2014;171(10):2474-2507
- A. Nociception
- B. Taste perception
- C. Thermosensation
- D. All of the above

TRP channels are cellular sensors involved in nociception, taste perception, thermosensation, mechano- and osmolarity sensing.

1045. **Which of the following is a member of the TRP channels?**
Br J Pharmacol. 2014;171(10):2474-2507
- A. TRPC (Canonical)
- B. TRPV (Vanilloid)
- C. TRPM (Melastatin)
- D. All of the above

TRP channels comprise 28 members and are divided into six subfamilies: TRPC (Canonical), TRPV (Vanilloid), TRPM (Melastatin), TRPP (Polycystin), TRPML (Mucolipin) and TRPA (Ankyrin).

1046. **Which of the following is a TRP channelopathy?**
Br J Pharmacol. 2014;171(10):2474-2507
- A. Focal segmental glomerular sclerosis (FSGS)
- B. ADPKD
- C. Scapuloperoneal spinal muscular atrophy
- D. All of the above

'TRP channelopathies' include focal segmental glomerular sclerosis (FSGS), ADPKD and scapuloperoneal spinal muscular atrophy.

1047. **In healthy adults, 80% of the identified fecal microbiota belong to phyla?**
BMC Microbiology 2009;9:123
- A. Bacteroidetes
- B. Firmicutes
- C. Actinobacteria
- D. All of the above

In healthy adults, 80% of the identified fecal microbiota can be classified into three dominant phyla: Bacteroidetes, Firmicutes and Actinobacteria. They predominantly influence human nutrition & metabolism.

1048. **Firmicutes best relate to?**
BMC Microbiology 2009;9:123
- A. Prevotella
- B. Bifidobacterium
- C. Clostridium
- D. All of the above

The Firmicutes include a large number of genera that belong to Clostridium clusters IV and XIV. Some prominent members being Eubacterium, Faecalibacterium, Roseburia & Ruminococcus.

1049. **Which of the following is false in IBS patients?**
Harrison's 20th Ed. Chapter 320 Page 2278
- A. Decreased Bifidobacterium proportion
- B. Decreased Lactobacillus proportion
- C. Increased ratio of Firmicutes : Bacteroidetes
- D. None of the above

1050. **Which of the following pathways is abnormal in IBS?**
Harrison's 20th Ed. Chapter 320 Page 2278
- A. Serotonin
- B. Dopamine
- C. Norepinephrine
- D. All of the above

1051. **Which of the following is the rate-limiting enzyme in enterochromaffin cell 5-HT biosynthesis?**
Harrison's 20th Ed. Chapter 320 Page 2278
- A. Tryptophan hydroxylase 1
- B. Tryptophan hydroxylase 2
- C. Tryptophan hydroxylase 3
- D. Tryptophan hydroxylase 4

Tryptophan hydroxylase 1 (TPH1) is the rate-limiting enzyme in enterochromaffin cell 5-HT biosynthesis.

1052. **Which of the following is a diagnostic criteria for IBS?**
Harrison's 20th Ed. Chapter 320 Page 2278
- A. Manning's criteria
- B. Barbara's criteria
- C. Mayer's criteria
- D. Talley's criteria

1053. Which of the following argue against the diagnosis of IBS?
Harrison's 20th Ed. Chapter 320 Page 2279

A. Appearance for the first time in old age
B. Persistent diarrhea after a 48 hour fast
C. Nocturnal diarrhea or steatorrheal stools
D. All of the above

Appearance of the disorder for the first time in old age, progressive course from time of onset, persistent diarrhea after a 48-hour fast, and presence of nocturnal diarrhea or steatorrheal stools argue against the diagnosis of IBS.

1054. Which of the following argue against the diagnosis of IBS?
Harrison's 20th Ed. Chapter 320 Page 2279

A. Anemia
B. Presence of leukocytes or blood in stool
C. Stool volume > 200 - 300 mL/day
D. All of the above

Laboratory features that argue against IBS include evidence of anemia, elevated sedimentation rate, presence of leukocytes or blood in stool and stool volume >200-300 mL/day.

1055. Which of the following abnormality is pathognomonic of IBS?
Harrison's 20th Ed. Chapter 320 Page 2279

A. Abdominal pain
B. Abdominal bloating
C. Alteration in bowel habits
D. None of the above

IBS is a disorder for which no pathognomonic abnormality has been identified.

1056. Painful constipation is a major complaint in which of the following?
Harrison's 20th Ed. Chapter 320 Page 2279

A. Acute intermittent porphyria
B. Hypothyroidism
C. Hypoparathyroidism
D. All of the above

Painful constipation is a major complaint in acute intermittent porphyria and lead poisoning.

1057. Which of the following is a FODMAP?
Harrison's 20th Ed. Chapter 320 Page 2279

A. Lactose
B. Fructose
C. Sorbitol
D. All of the above

FODMAP stands for fermentable oligosaccharides, disaccharides, monosaccharides and polyols such as lactose, fructose or sorbitol. FODMAPs are poorly absorbed by the small intestine and fermented by bacteria in colon to produce gas and osmotically active carbohydrates. A diet low in FODMAPs has been shown to be helpful in IBS patients.

1058. Fiber can exacerbate which of the following?
Harrison's 20th Ed. Chapter 320 Page 2280

A. Bloating
B. Flatulence
C. Diarrhea
D. All of the above

Fiber can exacerbate bloating, flatulence, constipation and diarrhea.

1059. In IBS, the best time to give antispasmodics for postprandial pain is?
Harrison's 20th Ed. Chapter 320 Page 2280

A. 30 minutes before meals
B. Along with meals
C. Immediately following meals
D. 1 hour after meals

Antispasmodics are most effective when prescribed in anticipation of predictable pain. To inhibit gastrocolic reflex and postprandial pain, antispasmodics are given 30 minutes before meals.

1060. Which of the following is an antidiarrheal agent?
Harrison's 20th Ed. Chapter 320 Page 2280

A. Loperamide
B. Paregoric
C. Cholestyramine
D. All of the above

1061. Which of the following antibiotic is useful for the treatment of IBS?
Harrison's 20th Ed. Chapter 320 Page 2281

A. Neomycin
B. Amoxycillin
C. Azithromycin
D. Levofloxacin

Neomycin and nonabsorbed oral antibiotic Rifaximin are useful in IBS.

1062. Which of the following about rifaximin is false?
Harrison's 20th Ed. Chapter 320 Page 2281

A. Oral drug
B. Nonsystemic, broad-spectrum antibiotic
C. Not absorbed
D. None of the above

Rifaximin is a minimally absorbed oral antimicrobial agent that is concentrated in gastrointestinal tract. It has broad-spectrum in vitro activity against gram-positive, gram-negative aerobic and anaerobic enteric bacteria, and has a low risk of inducing bacterial resistance.

1063. Which of the following probiotics has shown significant benefit in IBS patients?
Harrison's 20th Ed. Chapter 320 Page 2281

A. Faecalibacterium prausnitzii
B. Bifidobacterium breve
C. Taenia suis
D. All of the above

Probiotics naturally alter the gut flora. Bifidobacterium breve, B. longum and Lactobacillus acidophilus species showed significant improvement in the composite score for IBS.

1064. Alosetron was withdrawn from the market due to the increased incidence of?
Harrison's 20th Ed. Chapter 320 Page 2282

A. Depression & suicidal tendency
B. Dyslipidemia
C. Ischemic colitis
D. Myocardial infarction

Alosetron is a 5-HT3 receptor antagonist that reduces perception of painful visceral stimulation in IBS. Alosetron was withdrawn from the market due to the increased incidence of ischemic colitis.

1065. **Which of the following is a 5-HT4 receptor antagonist?**
Harrison's 20th Ed. Chapter 320 Page 2282
   A. Alosetron
   B. Rifaximin
   C. Tegaserod
   D. Lubiprostone

Tegaserod is a 5-HT4 receptor agonist that exhibits prokinetic activity by stimulating peristalsis.

1066. **Tegaserod was withdrawn from the market due to increased incidence of?**
Harrison's 20th Ed. Chapter 320 Page 2282
   A. Seizure events
   B. Cardiovascular events
   C. Hematologic diathesis
   D. Depression & suicidal tendency

1067. **Which of the following is a chloride channel activator?**
Harrison's 20th Ed. Chapter 320 Page 2282
   A. Alosetron
   B. Rifaximin
   C. Tegaserod
   D. Lubiprostone

1068. **Which of the following about Lubiprostone is false?**
Harrison's 20th Ed. Chapter 320 Page 2282
   A. Bicyclic fatty acid
   B. Stimulates Cl⁻ channels in intestinal epithelial cells
   C. Oral administration
   D. None of the above

Lubiprostone is a bicyclic fatty acid that stimulates chloride channels in the apical membrane of intestinal epithelial cells. Chloride secretion induces passive movement of sodium & water into bowel lumen & improves bowel function in constipation-predominant IBS patients. Alosetron is a 5-HT3 receptor antagonist. Rifaximin is a non-absorbed oral antibiotic. Tegaserod is a 5-HT4 receptor agonists.

1069. **Which of the following about Linaclotide is false?**
Harrison's 20th Ed. Chapter 320 Page 2282
   A. Guanylate cyclase-C (GC-C) agonist
   B. Action mediated by cGMP
   C. Minimally absorbed
   D. None of the above

Novel agents that induce secretion or intestinal secretagogues are lubiprostone (chloride channel activator) and linaclotide (a guanylate cyclase C agonist).

1070. **Which of the following is an osmotic laxative?**
Harrison's 20th Ed. Chapter 42 Page 268
   A. Magnesium salts
   B. Lactulose
   C. Polyethylene glycol
   D. All of the above

Osmotic laxatives are magnesium salts, lactulose, sorbitol and polyethylene glycol.

Mesenteric Vascular Insufficiency

1071. Mesenteric circulation consists of?
N Engl J Med. 2016;374:959-68

- A. Celiac artery
- B. Superior mesenteric artery
- C. Inferior mesenteric artery
- D. All of the above

Three primary vessels contributing to mesenteric circulation are the celiac artery (foregut), superior mesenteric artery (midgut), and inferior mesenteric artery (hindgut). They are interconnect through collateral networks between visceral & nonvisceral circulations. These interconnections ensure that the loss of a single vessel does not lead to catastrophic malperfusion of the viscera.

1072. Which of the following is a category of intestinal ischemia?
Harrison's 20th Ed. Chapter 322 Page 2291

- A. Arterioocclusive mesenteric ischemia (AOMI)
- B. Nonocclusive mesenteric ischemia (NOMI)
- C. Mesenteric venous thrombosis (MVT)
- D. All of the above

Arterial obstruction, the most common cause of mesenteric ischemia, has both acute and chronic forms.

1073. Risk factors for acute intestinal arterial ischemia include?
Harrison's 20th Ed. Chapter 322 Page 2291

- A. Atrial fibrillation
- B. Recent myocardial infarction
- C. Valvular heart disease
- D. All of the above

Risk factors for acute intestinal arterial ischemia include atrial fibrillation, recent myocardial infarction, valvular heart disease, and recent cardiac or vascular catheterization.

1074. "Intestinal angina" best applies to?
Harrison's 20th Ed. Chapter 322 Page 2291

- A. Arterioocclusive mesenteric ischemia (AOMI)
- B. Nonocclusive mesenteric ischemia (NOMI)
- C. Mesenteric venous thrombosis (MVT)
- D. All of the above

1075. Nonocclusive mesenteric ischemia is seen in?
Harrison's 20th Ed. Chapter 322 Page 2292

- A. Patients receiving high-dose vasopressor infusions
- B. Patients presenting with cardiogenic or septic shock
- C. Cocaine overdose
- D. All of the above

The mesenteric circulation is a high-resistance vascular bed in which impaired regional perfusion owing to vasospasm can develop. The resulting ischemia is referred to as nonocclusive mesenteric ischemia.

1076. Mesenteric venous thrombosis is associated with?
Harrison's 20th Ed. Chapter 322 Page 2292

- A. Antithrombin III deficiency
- B. Polycythemia vera
- C. Carcinoma
- D. All of the above

Mesenteric venous thrombosis is associated with the presence of a hypercoagulable state like protein C or S deficiency, antithrombin III deficiency, polycythemia vera, and carcinoma.

1077. Which of the following is a watershed area within the colonic blood supply and common location for intestinal ischemia?
Harrison's 20th Ed. Chapter 322 Page 2292

- A. Matsumoto point
- B. Griffiths' point
- C. Wyers point
- D. Mitchell point

1078. Which of the following is a watershed area within the colonic blood supply and common location for intestinal ischemia?
Harrison's 20th Ed. Chapter 322 Page 2292

- A. Shih point
- B. Sudeck's point
- C. Hsu point
- D. Sise point

Collateral vessels within small bowel meet within duodenum & bed of pancreas. Collateral vessels within colon meet at splenic flexure & descending/sigmoid colon. These watershed areas are inherently at risk for decreased blood flow and are known as Griffiths' point and Sudeck's point respectively and are the most common locations for colonic ischemia.

1079. Nationality of Jean Riolan was?

- A. French
- B. German
- C. Spanish
- D. Portugese

Arch of Riolan is named after Jean Riolan, French anatomist (1580–1657). It connects the proximal superior mesenteric artery (SMA) or one of its primary branches (middle colic artery) to the proximal inferior mesenteric artery (IMA) or one of its primary branches and runs close to the root of the mesentery.

1080. Emboli originating from heart preferentially lodge in?
Harrison's 20th Ed. Chapter 322 Page 2292

- A. Superior mesenteric artery
- B. Inferior mesenteric artery
- C. Celiac trunk
- D. Arc of Riolan

In >75% of cases, emboli originate from heart & preferentially lodge in superior mesenteric artery (SMA) just distal to the origin of middle colic artery.

1081. "Pain out of proportion to examination," with an epigastric bruit is indicative of?
N Engl J Med. 2016;374:959-68

- A. Acute mesenteric ischemia
- B. Chronic mesenteric ischemia
- C. Mesenteric venous thrombosis
- D. Nonocclusive mesenteric ischemia

1082. Patients with chronic mesenteric ischemia can present as?
N Engl J Med. 2016;374:959-68

A. Postprandial pain
B. Early satiety
C. Weight loss
D. Any of the above

Patients with chronic mesenteric ischemia can present with abdominal pain, postprandial pain, nausea or vomiting, early satiety, diarrhea or constipation & weight loss. Abdominal pain 30 to 60 minutes after eating is common and is often self-treated with food restriction ("food fear" or sitophobia), resulting in weight loss.

1083. Postprandial pain is a feature of?
N Engl J Med. 2016;374:959-68

A. Peptic ulcer disease
B. Pancreatitis
C. Irritable bowel syndrome
D. All of the above

Postprandial pain may be associated with biliary disease, peptic ulcer disease, pancreatitis, diverticular disease, gastric reflux, irritable bowel syndrome, and gastroparesis.

1084. Which of the following is an ominous pathological findings in patients with mesenteric ischemia?
N Engl J Med. 2016;374:959-68

A. Pneumatosis
B. Free intraabdominal air
C. Portal venous gas
D. All of the above

1085. Progressive thrombosis of at least how many major vessels supplying intestine is required for chronic intestinal angina?
Harrison's 20th Ed. Chapter 322 Page 2292

A. One
B. Two
C. Three
D. Four

Progressive thrombosis of at least two of the major vessels supplying the intestine is required for the development of chronic intestinal angina.

1086. Mortality rate in intestinal ischemia is?
Harrison's 20th Ed. Chapter 322 Page 2292

A. > 10%
B. > 20%
C. > 30%
D. > 50%

The most critical factor influencing outcomes in patients with mesenteric ischemia is the speed of diagnosis and intervention.

1087. Which of the following is a feature of intestinal ischemia?
Harrison's 20th Ed. Chapter 322 Page 2292

A. Thumbprinting
B. Pneumatosis intestinalis
C. Air within the portal venous system
D. All of the above

Features of intestinal ischemia include bowel-wall edema ("thumbprinting"), air within the bowel wall (pneumatosis intestinalis) and within the portal venous system.

1088. The gold standard for confirmation of acute mesenteric arterial occlusion is?
Harrison's 20th Ed. Chapter 322 Page 2292

A. Mesenteric angiography
B. Duplex ultrasound
C. Magnetic resonance angiography
D. Abdominal spiral CT

Gold standard for confirmation of mesenteric arterial occlusion is mesenteric angiography. Duplex ultrasound evaluation of the mesenteric vessels is used as a screening test for patients with symptoms suggestive of chronic mesenteric ischemia.

1089. Which of the following is spared in superior mesenteric artery (SMA) occlusion?
Harrison's 20th Ed. Chapter 322 Page 2293

A. Jejunum
B. Terminal ileum
C. Caecum
D. Ascending colon

In SMA occlusion, where embolus usually lies just proximal to the origin of middle colic artery, proximal jejunum is often spared while remainder of the small bowel up to transverse colon becomes ischemic.

1090. Markers for intestinal ischemia include all except?
Harrison's 20th Ed. Chapter 322 Page 2293

A. D-dimer
B. Glutathione S-transferase
C. UDP-glucuronosyltransferase
D. Platelet-activating factor (PAF)

Markers for intestinal ischemia include D-dimer, glutathione S-transferase, platelet-activating factor (PAF), and mucosal pH monitoring.

1091. Which of the following is associated with the best prognosis?
Harrison's 20th Ed. Chapter 322 Page 2294

A. Arterioocclusive mesenteric ischemia (AOMI)
B. Nonocclusive mesenteric ischemia (NOMI)
C. Mesenteric venous thrombosis (MVT)
D. All of the above

1092. Which of the following is not a feature of chronic mesenteric angina?
Harrison's 20th Ed. Chapter 322 Page 2294

A. Abdominal cramping & pain following ingestion of meal
B. Weight loss
C. Constipation
D. Chronic diarrhea

Patients of chronic intestinal ischemia (intestinal angina) presents with abdominal cramping and pain following ingestion of a meal, weight loss and chronic diarrhea. Abdominal pain without weight loss is not chronic mesenteric angina.

Approach to the Patient with Liver Disease

1093. The liver weighs about?
Harrison's 20th Ed. Chapter 329 Page 2332
- A. 0.5 - 1.0 kg
- B. 1.0 - 1.5 kg
- C. 1.5 - 2.0 kg
- D. 2.0 - 2.5 kg

1094. The liver represents what percentage of lean body mass?
Harrison's 20th Ed. Chapter 329 Page 2332
- A. 0.5 - 1.0%
- B. 1.0 - 1.5%
- C. 1.5 - 2.5%
- D. 2.5 - 3.5%

The liver is the largest organ of body, weighing 1–1.5 kg & representing 1.5-2.5% of the lean body mass.

1095. The contribution of blood supply to liver from hepatic artery and portal vein is?
Harrison's 20th Ed. Chapter 329 Page 2332
- A. 50% and 50% respectively
- B. 40% and 60% respectively
- C. 60% and 40% respectively
- D. 20% and 80% respectively

Liver receives a dual blood supply, ~20% of blood flow is oxygen-rich blood from hepatic artery and 80% is nutrient-rich blood from the portal vein arising from stomach, intestines, pancreas & spleen.

1096. From a metabolic perspective, the functional unit of liver is?
Diseases of liver & biliary system, Sheila Sherlock 9th Ed. 1
- A. Hepatic lobule
- B. Hepatic acinus
- C. Portal lobule
- D. All of the above

1097. Which of the following statements is false?
Diseases of liver & biliary system, Sheila Sherlock 9th Ed. 1
- A. Shape of hepatic lobule is polygonal
- B. Shape of portal lobule is triangular
- C. Shape of hepatic acinus is elliptical
- D. None of the above

1098. Which of the following statements is true?
Diseases of liver & biliary system, Sheila Sherlock 9th Ed. 1
- A. Central vein is at the center of hepatic acinus
- B. Central vein is at the center of hepatic lobule
- C. Central vein is at the center of portal lobule
- D. All of the above

1099. Which of the following hepatic zones is most oxygenated?
Diseases of liver & biliary system, Sheila Sherlock 9th Ed. 1
- A. Zone 1
- B. Zone 2
- C. Zone 3
- D. All of the above

Hepatic zone 3 is least oxygenated.

1100. Right lobe of liver is about how many times bigger than the left lobe?
Diseases of liver & biliary system, Sheila Sherlock 9th Ed. 1
- A. 2 times
- B. 4 times
- C. 6 times
- D. 8 times

1101. Pressure in the free hepatic vein is about?
Diseases of liver & biliary system, Sheila Sherlock 9th Ed. 1
- A. 3 mm Hg
- B. 6 mm Hg
- C. 9 mm Hg
- D. 12 mm Hg

1102. All are true regarding hepatic venous system except?
Diseases of liver & biliary system, Sheila Sherlock 9th Ed. 1
- A. Hepatic venous blood in ~67% saturated with oxygen
- B. Hepatic venous blood is usually sterile
- C. Hepatic veins are seven in number
- D. Hepatic veins begin as zone 3 veins

1103. Blood of caudate lobe of liver drains into?
Diseases of liver & biliary system, Sheila Sherlock 9th Ed. 1
- A. Right hepatic vein
- B. Left hepatic vein
- C. Middle hepatic vein
- D. Inferior vena cava

1104. Right & left lobes of liver are separated inferiorly by?
Diseases of liver & biliary system, Sheila Sherlock 9th Ed. 1
- A. Falciform ligament
- B. Fissure for ligamentum venosum
- C. Fissure for ligamentum teres
- D. All of the above

The right and left lobes of liver are separated anteriorly by falciform ligament, posteriorly by fissure for ligamentum venosum and inferiorly by fissure for ligamentum teres.

1105. Capacity of gallbladder is about?
Diseases of liver & biliary system, Sheila Sherlock 9th Ed. 3
- A. 20 ml
- B. 30 ml
- C. 40 ml
- D. 50 ml

Gallbladder is a pear shaped bag, ~9 cm long with a capacity of about 50 ml.

1106. Rokitansky-Aschoff sinuses are related to which of the following organs?

Diseases of liver & biliary system, Sheila Sherlock 9th Ed. 4

A. Liver
B. Pancreas
C. Gallbladder
D. Intestine

Rokitansky-Aschoff sinuses are branching evaginations from the lumen into the mucosa and muscularis of the gallbladder.

1107. Which of the following is not a cell type in liver?

Harrison's 20th Ed. Chapter 329 Page 2332

A. Hepatocyte
B. Rho cells
C. Kupffer cells
D. Ito cells

Hepatocytes constitute two-thirds of mass of liver. The remaining cell types are Kupffer cells (RE system), stellate (Ito or fat-storing) cells, endothelial cells and blood vessels, bile ductular cells and supporting structures.

1108. Portal areas from which zone of the hepatic acinus?

Harrison's 20th Ed. Chapter 329 Page 2332

A. Zone 1
B. Zone 2
C. Zone 3
D. Zone 4

Functionally, liver is organized into acini. Hepatic arterial and portal venous blood enter acinus from portal areas (zone 1) and flow through the sinusoids to terminal hepatic veins (zone 3). Intervening hepatocytes constitute zone 2.

1109. "Central veins" in liver are also called?

Harrison's 20th Ed. Chapter 329 Page 2332

A. Terminal hepatic veins
B. Terminal portal veins
C. Terminal sinusoidal veins
D. All of the above

Blood from portal areas is distributed through sinusoids, passing from zone 1 to zone 3 of acinus and draining into terminal hepatic veins ("central veins").

1110. In hepatic acinus, secreted bile flows in which of the following direction?

Harrison's 20th Ed. Chapter 329 Page 2332

A. Zone 1 to zone 3
B. Zone 3 to zone 1
C. Zone 1 to zone 2
D. Zone 2 to zone 1

In hepatic acinus, secreted bile flows in a counter current pattern from zone 3 to zone 1.

1111. Which of the following is false about subendothelial space of Disse?

Harrison's 20th Ed. Chapter 329 Page 2332

A. Plasma is in direct contact with hepatocytes
B. Lined by basolateral side of the hepatocyte
C. Stellate cells are located in it
D. None of the above

The plasma is in direct contact with hepatocytes in the subendothelial space of Disse.

1112. Kupffer cells are best described as?

Harrison's 20th Ed. Chapter 329 Page 2332

A. Peripheral T lymphocytes
B. Circulating B lymphocytes
C. Fixed macrophages
D. None of the above

Kupffer cells lie within sinusoidal vascular space & represent largest group of fixed macrophages in body.

1113. Hepatocytes produce which of the following?

Harrison's 20th Ed. Chapter 329 Page 2332

A. Cholesterol
B. Lecithin
C. Phospholipids
D. All of the above

Hepatocytes produce bile and its carriers i.e. bile acids, cholesterol, lecithin, phospholipids.

1114. Liver regulates which of the following nutrients?

Harrison's 20th Ed. Chapter 329 Page 2332

A. Glycogen
B. Cholesterol
C. Amino acids
D. All of the above

1115. Which out of the following is the more liver-specific symptom?

Harrison's 20th Ed. Chapter 329 Page 2333

A. Nausea
B. Bloating
C. Poor appetite
D. Malaise

Constitutional symptoms of liver disease include fatigue, weakness, nausea, poor appetite, and malaise. More liver-specific symptoms include jaundice, dark urine, light stools, itching, abdominal pain, and bloating.

1116. Most common & most characteristic symptom of liver disease is?

Harrison's 20th Ed. Chapter 329 Page 2333

A. Fatigue
B. Nausea
C. Poor appetite
D. Itching

Fatigue is the most common & most characteristic symptom of liver disease. It typically arises after activity or exercise & is rarely present or severe in the morning after adequate rest. Fatigue in liver disease is often intermittent and variable in severity from hour to hour and day to day.

1117. Severe right upper quadrant pain ("liver pain") is most typical of all except?

Harrison's 20th Ed. Chapter 329 Page 2333

A. Gallbladder disease
B. Liver abscess
C. Severe veno-occlusive disease
D. Acute hepatitis

Right upper quadrant severe pain is most typical of gallbladder disease, liver abscess, and severe veno-occlusive disease but is an occasional accompaniment of acute hepatitis.

1118. Which of the following is the most reliable marker of severity of liver disease?
Harrison's 20th Ed. Chapter 329 Page 2333

A. Jaundice
B. Serum albumin
C. Prothrombin time
D. Hepatic enzymes

Jaundice is the hallmark symptom of liver disease & perhaps the most reliable marker of severity.

1119. Jaundice without dark urine indicates which of the following?
Harrison's 20th Ed. Chapter 329 Page 2333

A. Hemolytic anemia
B. Gilbert's syndrome
C. Crigler-Najjar syndrome
D. All of the above

Jaundice without dark urine indicates indirect (unconjugated) hyperbilirubinemia and is typical of hemolytic anemia, Gilbert's syndrome and Crigler-Najjar syndrome.

1120. In Gilbert's syndrome, jaundice is more noticeable after which of the following?
Harrison's 20th Ed. Chapter 329 Page 2333

A. Fasting
B. Overnight sleep
C. Exposure to sun
D. All of the above

In Gilbert's syndrome, jaundice is more noticeable after fasting and with stress.

1121. Which of the following statements about hepatitis C is false?
Harrison's 20th Ed. Chapter 329 Page 2333

A. Sexual exposure is a rare mode of spread
B. Maternal-infant transmission occurs
C. No means of prevention of vertical spread
D. None of the above

Vertical spread of hepatitis C occurs uncommonly. Sexual exposure is a common mode of spread of hepatitis B and hepatitis C.

1122. Single most common risk factor for hepatitis C is?
Harrison's 20th Ed. Chapter 329 Page 2333

A. Blood transfusion
B. Injection drug use
C. Maternal-infant transmission
D. Sexual exposure

Injection drug use is now the single most common risk factor for hepatitis C.

1123. Screening for antibody to hepatitis B & C was introduced in?
Harrison's 20th Ed. Chapter 329 Page 2333

A. 1982 & 1990 respectively
B. 1984 & 1991 respectively
C. 1986 & 1992 respectively
D. 1988 & 1993 respectively

Screening for antibody to hepatitis B core antigen was introduced 1986 and for hepatitis C in 1992.

1124. An average drink representing how many grams of alcohol?
Harrison's 20th Ed. Chapter 329 Page 2334

A. 5 - 10 grams
B. 8 - 12 grams
C. 11 - 15 grams
D. 15 - 19 grams

An average drink representing 11–15 grams of alcohol.

1125. What quantity of alcohol consumption per day is associated with an increased rate of alcoholic liver disease in men?
Harrison's 20th Ed. Chapter 329 Page 2334

A. 10 to 25 grams
B. 25 to 33 grams
C. 33 to 45 grams
D. 45 to 62 grams

1126. What quantity of alcohol consumption per day is associated with an increased rate of alcoholic liver disease in women?
Harrison's 20th Ed. Chapter 329 Page 2334

A. 10 to 22 grams
B. 22 to 30 grams
C. 33 to 45 grams
D. 45 to 62 grams

Alcohol consumption associated with an increased rate of alcoholic liver disease is probably more than 22–30 gram per day in women and 33–45 gram in men.

1127. Alcoholism is usually defined by the?
Harrison's 20th Ed. Chapter 329 Page 2334

A. Amount of alcohol
B. Type of alcohol
C. Consequences of alcohol intake
D. All of the above

Alcoholism is usually defined by behavioral patterns & consequences of alcohol intake, not by the amount.

1128. Of the following, which is considered the more serious & advanced form of alcoholism?
Harrison's 20th Ed. Chapter 329 Page 2334

A. Abuse
B. Binge
C. Dependence
D. All of the above

Abuse is defined by a repetitive pattern of drinking alcohol that has adverse effects on social, family, occupational or health status. Dependence is defined by alcohol-seeking behavior, despite its adverse effects. Dependence is considered the more serious & advanced form of alcoholism.

1129. CAGE questionnaire is used for?
Harrison's 20th Ed. Chapter 329 Page 2334 Table 329-2

A. Sexual behaviour
B. Cigarette smoking
C. Alcohol dependence & abuse
D. None of the above

One "yes" response of the four questions in CAGE questionnaire should raise suspicion of an alcohol use problem, and more than one is a strong indication that alcohol abuse or dependence exists.

1130. **In CAGE questionnaire, "C" refers to?**
Harrison's 20th Ed. Chapter 329 Page 2334 Table 329-2

   A. Continuous
   B. Cut
   C. Craving
   D. Constant

C = Cut, A = Annoyed, G = Guilty, E = Eyeopener. One "yes" response should raise suspicion of an alcohol use problem, and more than one is a strong indication that abuse or dependence exists.

1131. **Which of the following is an inherited liver disease?**
Harrison's 20th Ed. Chapter 329 Page 2334

   A. Wilson's disease
   B. Hemochromatosis
   C. a_1 antitrypsin (a1AT) deficiency
   D. All of the above

1132. **Which of the following is an inherited pediatric liver disease?**
Harrison's 20th Ed. Chapter 329 Page 2334

   A. Familial intrahepatic cholestasis
   B. Benign recurrent intrahepatic cholestasis
   C. Alagille syndrome
   D. All of the above

1133. **Which of the following mutations is typical of genetic hemochromatosis?**
Harrison's 20th Ed. Chapter 329 Page 2334

   A. 167delT
   B. G1896A
   C. H63D
   D. FIC1

C282Y & H63D mutations in HFE gene are typical of genetic hemochromatosis.

1134. **Which of the following statements is false?**
Harrison's 20th Ed. Chapter 329 Page 2334

   A. Muscle wasting is a sign of advanced liver disease
   B. Palmar erythema occurs in acute liver disease
   C. Jaundice may be detectable with S. bilirubin <2.5 mg/dL
   D. None of the above

Signs of advanced liver disease include muscle wasting, ascites, edema, bruising, dilated abdominal veins, hepatic fetor, asterixis, mental confusion, stupor, and coma. During recovery phase, jaundice may be detectable with S. bilirubin <2.5 mg/dL. Spider angiomata & palmar erythema occur in both acute & chronic liver disease.

1135. **Which of the following best relates to asterixis?**
Harrison's 20th Ed. Chapter 428 Page 3138

   A. Action myoclonus
   B. Negative myoclonus
   C. Dystonia
   D. Paroxysmal dyskinesia

Negative myoclonus consists of a brief loss of muscle activity, exemplified by asterixis in hepatic failure.

1136. **Asterixis is seen in which of the following?**
Harrison's 20th Ed. Chapter 300 Page 2071

   A. Hepatic encephalopathy
   B. Hypercapnia
   C. Uremia
   D. All of the above

Asterixis is not specific to liver disease but also appears in encephalopathy from other causes like hypercapnia, uremia or drug intoxication. Unilateral asterixis indicates structural disease in the contralateral brain.

1137. **Which of the following about spider angiomata is false?**
Harrison's 20th Ed. Chapter 329 Page 2334

   A. Occur in acute & chronic liver disease
   B. Occur during pregnancy
   C. Occur only on arms, face & upper torso
   D. None of the above

Spider angiomata occur only on the arms, face, and upper torso. Spider angiomata and palmar erythema occur in both acute and chronic liver disease and are prominent in cirrhosis, but they can occur in normal individuals and are frequently present during pregnancy.

1138. **The nature of vessel involved in spider angiomata is?**
Harrison's 20th Ed. Chapter 329 Page 2334

   A. Artery
   B. Arteriole
   C. Vein
   D. Capillary

Spider angiomata are superficial, tortuous arterioles & fill from center outwards & can be pulsatile. Spider telangiectasia has three components: (1) central arteriole ("body" of the spider) that can be seen to pulsate when compressed slightly with a glass slide; (2) multiple radiating "legs"; and (3) surrounding erythema, which may encompass the entire lesion or only its central portion. After blanching, returning blood fills central arteriole first before traveling to the peripheral tips of each leg.

1139. **Spiders are most numerous on?**
Harrison's 20th Ed. Chapter 329 Page 2334

   A. Face
   B. Palms
   C. Soles
   D. Scalp

Spiders are most numerous on face & neck, followed by shoulders, thorax, arms, and hands. They are rare on palms, scalp, and below the umbilicus. This peculiar distribution may reflect the neurohormonal properties of the microcirculation, because it is similar to the distribution of where blushing is most intense.

1140. **Acquired vascular spiders are associated with?**
Harrison's 20th Ed. Chapter 329 Page 2334

   A. Liver disease
   B. Pregnancy
   C. Malnutrition
   D. All of the above

Acquired vascular spiders are associated with liver disease, pregnancy and malnutrition. Vascular spiders were first described by the English physician Erasmus Wilson in 1867.

1141. **Marked hepatomegaly is typical of?**
Harrison's 20th Ed. Chapter 329 Page 2334

   A. Cirrhosis
   B. Sinusoidal obstruction syndrome
   C. Alcoholic hepatitis
   D. All of the above

Marked hepatomegaly is typical of cirrhosis, sinusoidal obstruction syndrome, infiltrative disorders (amyloidosis, metastatic, or primary cancers of the liver) and alcoholic hepatitis.

1142. Most reliable physical finding in examining the liver is?
Harrison's 20th Ed. Chapter 329 Page 2334

A. Size
B. Shape
C. Tenderness
D. Liver edge

Most reliable physical finding in examining the liver is hepatic tenderness.

1143. Foetor hepaticus best relates to?
Harrison's 20th Ed. Chapter 337 Page 2413

A. Vaptan
B. Mercaptan
C. Mercaptoethane
D. Mercaptoethanesulfonate

1144. Foetor hepaticus best relates to?
Br J Gen Pract. 2012;62(605):652-653

A. Dimethylformamide
B. Dimethylarginine
C. Dimethyl disulphide
D. Dimethyltryptamine

Foetor hepaticus is a feature of severe liver disease; a sweet & musty smell both on breath and in urine. It is caused by excretion of dimethyl disulphide & methyl mercaptan (CH_3SH), arising from an excess of methionine.

1145. In chronic liver disease, encephalopathy is triggered by?
Harrison's 20th Ed. Chapter 329 Page 2335

A. Infection
B. Constipation
C. Use of narcotic analgesics
D. All of the above

In chronic liver disease, encephalopathy is triggered by gastrointestinal bleeding, over-diuresis, uremia, dehydration, electrolyte imbalance, infection, constipation, or use of narcotic analgesics.

1146. Which of the following is a test of mental status in hepatic encephalopathy?
Harrison's 20th Ed. Chapter 329 Page 2335

A. Trail-making test
B. Comparison of signatures
C. Drawing abstract objects
D. All of the above

Mental status examination for hepatic encephalopathy include trail-making test, drawing abstract objects or comparison of a signature to previous ones.

1147. Which of the following is false about trail-making test?
Harrison's 20th Ed. Chapter 329 Page 2335

A. Series of 10 numbered circles
B. Normal time for connect-the-dot test is 15-30 seconds
C. Considerable delay means early hepatic encephalopathy
D. None of the above

Mental status examination by trail-making test consists of a series of 25 numbered circles that the patient is asked to connect as rapidly as possible using a pencil. Normal range for connect-the-dot test is 15-30 seconds. Delay means early hepatic encephalopathy.

1148. Which of the following is not a feature of hepatopulmonary syndrome?
Harrison's 20th Ed. Chapter 329 Page 2335

A. Hypoxemia
B. Pulmonary arteriovenous shunting
C. Orthodeoxia
D. Hypercarbia

Hepatopulmonary syndrome is defined by the triad of liver disease, hypoxemia and pulmonary arteriovenous shunting. It is characterized by platypnea and orthodeoxia, representing shortness of breath and oxygen desaturation that occur upon assuming an upright position.

1149. Slate-gray pigmentation to the skin also occurs with?
Harrison's 20th Ed. Chapter 329 Page 2335

A. Primary biliary cirrhosis
B. Sclerosing cholangitis
C. Xanthelasma
D. Hemochromatosis

A slate-gray pigmentation of the skin occurs in hemochromatosis, if iron levels are high for a prolonged period.

1150. Mucocutaneous vasculitis with palpable purpura is typical of?
Harrison's 20th Ed. Chapter 329 Page 2335

A. Primary biliary cirrhosis
B. Primary hepatocellular carcinoma
C. Cryoglobulinemia of chronic hepatitis C
D. Wilsons disease

Mucocutaneous vasculitis with palpable purpura on lower extremities is typical of cryoglobulinemia of chronic hepatitis C.

1151. Kayser-Fleischer rings are a finding in?
Harrison's 20th Ed. Chapter 329 Page 2335

A. Primary biliary cirrhosis
B. Primary hepatocellular carcinoma
C. Wilson's disease
D. Hemochromatosis

Kayser-Fleischer rings occur in Wilson's disease also called hepatolenticular degeneration/ Westphal-Strumpell disease/Westphal pseudosclerosis. Bernhard Kayser and Bruno Fleischer were German ophthalmologists.

1152. Which of the following statements about Kayser-Fleischer ring is false?
Br J Ophthalmol 2002;86:114

A. Found in 95% of patients of Wilson's disease
B. All patients with KF rings have neurological manifestations
C. Density of a KF ring correlates with severity of WD
D. None of the above

K-F-like ring has been reported in many other conditions like cryptogenic cirrhosis, chronic active hepatitis, neonatal hepatitis, primary biliary cirrhosis, cholestatic cirrhosis, hepatocellular disorders (when bilirubin rises acutely above 20mg/dl), alcoholic liver disease, galactosialidosis, schistosoma infection, multiple myeloma and intraocular foreign body containing copper.

1153. The color of Kayser-Fleischer ring is?
Harrison's 20th Ed. Chapter 329 Page 2335

A. Yellow-red
B. Yellow-green
C. Golden-brown
D. Green-brown

Kayser-Fleischer rings consist of a golden-brown copper pigment deposited in Descemet's membrane at the periphery of the cornea—sclero-corneal junction. It may regress or disappear when systemic condition is well treated. It is usually bilateral & appears initially superiorly at 10 to 2 o'clock position, then inferiorly and later becomes circumferential.

1154. Wilson's disease is due to defect in?
Harrison's 20th Ed. Chapter 408 Page 2982

A. ATP6B gene
B. ATP7B gene
C. ATP8B gene
D. ATP9B gene

Wilson disease is an autosomal recessive disorder caused by mutations in the ATP7B gene, a membrane-bound copper-transporting ATPase. ATP7B facilitates the transfer of copper into Golgi apparatus where it combines with ceruloplasmin. Failure of this process leads to instability and decreased half life of ceruloplasmin and paradoxical ceruloplasmin deficiency. Free circulating copper accumulates in liver cytosol resulting in hepatocyte degeneration and cirrhosis. Other hepatic conditions as listed above that prevent elimination of copper, or intraocular foreign bodies containing copper, lead to elevated free copper concentrations and K-F ring.

1155. Wilson's disease can produce a cataract described as?
Harrison's 20th Ed. Chapter 408 Page 2983

A. Christmas tree
B. Palm tree
C. Sunflower
D. Rose flower

Sunflower cataracts & Kayser-Fleischer rings (copper deposits in the outer rim of cornea) are seen in Wilson's disease.

1156. Testing for P-ANCA is for the diagnosis of which of the following?
Harrison's 20th Ed. Chapter 329 Page 2335 Table 329-3

A. Primary biliary cirrhosis
B. Primary sclerosing cholangitis
C. Autoimmune hepatitis
D. Nonalcoholic steatohepatitis

1157. Most common causes of chronic liver disease is?
Harrison's 20th Ed. Chapter 329 Page 2335

A. Chronic hepatitis C
B. Alcoholic liver disease
C. Chronic hepatitis B
D. Autoimmune hepatitis

Most common causes of chronic liver disease in general order of frequency are chronic hepatitis C, alcoholic liver disease, nonalcoholic steatohepatitis, chronic hepatitis B, autoimmune hepatitis, sclerosing cholangitis, primary biliary cirrhosis, hemochromatosis, and Wilson disease.

1158. Liver biopsy plays an important role in the diagnosis of?
Harrison's 20th Ed. Chapter 329 Page 2335

A. Autoimmune hepatitis
B. Primary biliary cholangitis
C. Nonalcoholic and alcoholic steatohepatitis
D. All of the above

Liver biopsy plays an important role in the diagnosis of autoimmune hepatitis, primary biliary cholangitis, nonalcoholic & alcoholic steatohepatitis and Wilson disease.

1159. γ-glutamyl transpeptidase (γGT) best relates to?
Harrison's 20th Ed. Chapter 329 Page 2335

A. Serum alanine aminotransferase (ALT)
B. Serum aspartate aminotransferase (AST)
C. Serum alkaline phosphatase (AlkP)
D. Serum bilirubin

γ-glutamyl transpeptidase (γGT) estimation helps to define whether alkaline phosphatase (AlkP) elevations are due to liver disease.

1160. ERCP is more valuable in evaluating which of the following?
Harrison's 20th Ed. Chapter 329 Page 2336

A. Pancreatitis
B. Primary sclerosing cholangitis
C. Choledocholithiasis
D. Fatty liver

ERCP is more valuable in evaluating ampullary lesions and primary sclerosing cholangitis.

1161. Which of the following liver cells is the primary source of extracellular matrix?
N Engl J Med. 2015;372:1138-49

A. Kupffer cell
B. Hepatic stellate cell
C. Endothelial cell
D. All of the above

Hepatic stellate cells appear to be the primary source of extracellular matrix. Stellate cell is pericyte-like, undergoing transformation into myofibroblast in response to injury.

1162. Hepatic stellate cells or HSCs are also called?
Biomarker Insights. 2012;7:105-117

A. Vitamin A-storing cells
B. Lipocytes
C. Ito cells
D. All of the above

1163. Vitamin A is stored in the cytoplasm of Hepatic stellate cells (HSCs) as?
Biomarker Insights. 2012;7:105-117

A. Retinyl sialate
B. Retinyl palmitate
C. Retinyl stearate
D. Retinyl fumarate

Hepatic stellate cells (HSCs) are the key fibrogenic cells and their 'activation' is the dominant event in fibrogenesis. Activation of HSCs refers to conversion of quiescent, vitamin A-storing cells into proliferative, fibrogenic & contractile myofibroblasts which can synthesize & secrete large amounts of fibril-forming collagens, particularly collagen type I and III. HSCs, also called vitamin A-storing cells, lipocytes, interstitial cells, fat-storing cells, Ito cells, exist in the space between parenchymal cells & sinusoidal endothelial cells of hepatic lobule, and store 80% of vitamin A in the whole body as retinyl palmitate in lipid droplets in the cytoplasm.

1164. Which of the following is the major stimulus for HSCs to synthesize extracellular matrix (ECM)?
Biomarker Insights. 2012;7:105-117

A. TNF-α
B. TGF-β
C. IL-6
D. INF-γ

TGF-β is the major stimulus for HSCs to synthesize ECM. Platelet-derived growth factor (PDGF), mainly produced by Kupffer cells, is a potent fibrogenic growth factor known to synergize with TGF-β.

1165. Normal AST/ALT ratio in healthy subjects is?
Biomarker Insights. 2012;7:105-117

A. 0.4
B. 0.6
C. 0.8
D. 1.0

Ratio of AST to ALT tends to increase with advancing stages of fibrosis from ~0.8 in healthy subjects. A ratio of more than 1 suggests the presence of cirrhosis.

1166. Which of the following variable is used in calculating AST-to-platelet ratio index (APRI)?
Harrison's 20th Ed. Chapter 329 Page 2337, Biomarker Insights. 2012;7:105-117

A. AST value
B. Upper limit of normal range of AST
C. Platelet count
D. All of the above

The AST-to-platelet ratio index (APRI) is calculated as (AST/upper limit of normal range)/platelet count (10^9/L) × 100.

1167. Which of the following is a serum biochemical marker associated with hepatic fibrosis?
Harrison's 20th Ed. Chapter 329 Page 2337 Table 329-4

A. Alpha-2-macroglobulin
B. Apolipoprotein A1
C. Haptoglobin
D. All of the above

The fibrotest is a composite of five serum biochemical markers i.e. alpha-2-macroglobulin, apolipoprotein A1, haptoglobin, γ-glutamyl transpeptidase, and bilirubin associated with hepatic fibrosis.

1168. Which of the following is a numerical scales for grading activity in chronic liver disease?
Harrison's 20th Ed. Chapter 329 Page 2337

A. METAVIR
B. Knodell histology activity index
C. Ishak fibrosis scale
D. All of the above

Numerical scales for grading activity in chronic liver disease, the most commonly used are the METAVIR, Knodell histology activity index, Ishak fibrosis scale (modified Knodell score) and International Association for Study of the Liver system.

1169. Stage F4 on the METAVIR fibrosis score means?
N Engl J Med. 2014;371:2375-82

A. No fibrosis
B. Portal fibrosis without septa
C. Fibrosis consistent with compensated cirrhosis
D. Fibrosis consistent with decompensated cirrhosis

METAVIR fibrosis score for chronic hepatitis ranges from F0 to F4, with F0 indicating no fibrosis and F4 fibrosis consistent with compensated cirrhosis. F0 (no fibrosis), F1 (portal fibrosis without septa), F2 (portal fibrosis with few septa), F3 (numerous septa without cirrhosis) and F4 (cirrhosis). Also, A0 (No activity), A1 (Mild activity), A2 (Moderate activity) and A3 (Severe activity).

1170. METAVIR stands for?
N Engl J Med. 2014;371:2375-82

A. Meta-analysis of Histological Data in Viral Hepatitis
B. Meta-analysis of Histological Data in Virology
C. Meta-analysis of Histological Data in Viral diseases
D. Meta-analysis of Histological Data in Viral infections

1171. Which of the following is activated on the surface of stellate cells triggering fibrogenesis?
N Engl J Med. 2015;372:1138-49

A. Toll-like receptor 1 (TLR1)
B. Toll-like receptor 2 (TLR2)
C. Toll-like receptor 3 (TLR3)
D. Toll-like receptor 4 (TLR4)

A pathway that is unique to liver involves toll-like receptor 4 (TLR4) that is activated on surface of stellate cells by intestinal bacterial LPS derived from gut, triggering cell activation & fibrogenesis. TLR4 expression is associated with portal inflammation & fibrosis in patients with fatty liver disease.

1172. Which of the following is often the first indication of worsening fibrosis in liver cirrhosis?
Harrison's 20th Ed. Chapter 329 Page 2337

A. Mild elevations of bilirubin
B. Prolongation of prothrombin time
C. Slight decreases in serum albumin
D. Mild thrombocytopenia

Noninvasive tests that suggest advanced liver fibrosis include mild elevations of bilirubin, prolongation of prothrombin time, slight decreases in serum albumin, and mild thrombocytopenia (which is often the first indication of worsening fibrosis).

1173. Which of the following is not a factor in Child-Pugh classification of cirrhosis liver?
Harrison's 20th Ed. Chapter 329 Page 2337

A. Serum bilirubin
B. SGPT
C. Ascites
D. Hepatic encephalopathy

Factors included in Child-Pugh classification of cirrhosis liver are serum bilirubin, serum albumin, prothrombin time, ascites & hepatic encephalopathy.

1174. Child-Pugh score can predict which of the following?
Harrison's 20th Ed. Chapter 329 Page 2337

A. Bleeding from varices
B. Spontaneous bacterial peritonitis
C. Need for liver transplantation
D. All of the above

Child-Pugh score is a reliable predictor of bleeding from varices, spontaneous bacterial peritonitis and need for liver transplantation.

1175. Decompensation indicates cirrhosis with a Child-Pugh score of?
Harrison's 20th Ed. Chapter 329 Page 2337 Table 329-4

A. 4
B. 5
C. 6
D. 7

The Child-Pugh score is calculated by adding the scores of the five factors and can range from 5 to 15. Child-Pugh class is either A (a score of 5 to 6), B (7 to 9), or C (10 or above). Decompensation indicates cirrhosis with a Child-Pugh score of 7 or more (Class B).

1176. MELD score is used for?
Harrison's 20th Ed. Chapter 329 Page 2337

A. Assessing bleeding from varices
B. Assessing hepatocellular carcinoma
C. Assessing spontaneous bacterial peritonitis
D. Assessing need for liver transplantation

Model for end-stage liver disease (MELD) score is used for assessing the need for liver transplantation.

1177. **Variables for calculation of MELD score include all except?**

Harrison's 20th Ed. Chapter 329 Page 2337

A. Prothrombin time
B. Serum bilirubin
C. Blood urea
D. Serum creatinine

MELD score is a prospectively derived scoring system calculated using three noninvasive variables—prothrombin time (INR), serum bilirubin and serum creatinine.

1178. **System similar to MELD used for children below the age of 12 is termed?**

Harrison's 20th Ed. Chapter 329 Page 2337

A. CELD
B. SELD
C. PELD
D. KELD

System similar to MELD using bilirubin, INR, serum albumin, age, and nutritional status is used for children below the age of 12 is PELD.

Evaluation of Liver Function

1179. Which of the following liver function tests do not measure liver function at all?
Harrison's 20th Ed. Chapter 330 Page 2338

A. S. Bilirubin
B. S. Aminotransferases
C. S. Albumin
D. Prothrombin time

Aminotransferases or alkaline phosphatase do not measure liver function at all.

1180. Upper limit of normal for conjugated bilirubin is?
Harrison's 20th Ed. Chapter 330 Page 2338

A. 0.2 mg/dL
B. 0.3 mg/dL
C. 0.4 mg/dL
D. 0.5 mg/dL

The most frequently reported upper limit of normal for conjugated bilirubin is 0.3 mg/dL. If the direct-acting fraction is <15% of the total, all bilirubin can be considered to be indirect.

1181. Which of the following statements is false?
Harrison's 20th Ed. Chapter 330 Page 2338

A. Elevation of unconjugated bilirubin is rarely due to liver disease
B. Conjugated hyperbilirubinemia almost always implies liver or biliary tract disease
C. Rate-limiting step in bilirubin metabolism is bilirubin conjugation
D. In most liver diseases, both conjugated & unconjugated bilirubin are elevated

The rate-limiting step in bilirubin metabolism is not conjugation of bilirubin, but transport of conjugated bilirubin into bile canaliculi.

1182. Which of the following about liver functions is false?
Harrison's 20th Ed. Chapter 330 Page 2338

A. Increased unconjugated bilirubin is rarely due to liver disease
B. Conjugated hyperbilirubinemia almost always implies liver or biliary tract disease
C. In most liver diseases, both conjugated & unconjugated bilirubin are elevated
D. None of the above

1183. Isolated elevation of unconjugated bilirubin is seen in?
Harrison's 20th Ed. Chapter 330 Page 2338

A. Hemolytic disorders
B. Crigler-Najjar syndrome
C. Gilbert's syndrome
D. All of the above

Isolated elevation of unconjugated bilirubin is seen in hemolytic disorders, Crigler-Najjar & Gilbert's syndromes.

1184. Total serum bilirubin correlates with poor outcomes in?
Harrison's 20th Ed. Chapter 330 Page 2338

A. Alcoholic hepatitis
B. Autoimmune hepatitis
C. Hepatocellular carcinome
D. All of the above

Total serum bilirubin correlates with poor outcomes in alcoholic hepatitis.

1185. In isolated unconjugated hyperbilirubinemia, of the total bilirubin, the direct bilirubin is?
Harrison's 20th Ed. Chapter 330 Page 2338

A. < 15%
B. < 20%
C. < 25%
D. < 30%

In isolated unconjugated hyperbilirubinemia, serum bilirubin is elevated but direct bilirubin is <15%.

1186. In liver disease, rate-limiting step in bilirubin metabolism is?
Harrison's 20th Ed. Chapter 330 Page 2338

A. Entry of bilirubin in hepatocyte
B. Conjugation of bilirubin in hepatocyte
C. Transport of conjugated bilirubin into bile canaliculi
D. All of the above

Rate-limiting step in bilirubin metabolism is not conjugation of bilirubin, but transport of conjugated bilirubin into the bile canaliculi.

1187. Total serum bilirubin correlates with poor outcomes in?
Harrison's 20th Ed. Chapter 330 Page 2338

A. Viral hepatitis
B. Alcoholic hepatitis
C. Drug-induced liver disease
D. All of the above

Serum bilirubin serves as a prognostic marker in viral hepatitis, alcoholic hepatitisin MELD score, drug-induced liver disease indicates more severe injury.

1188. Bilirubin found in urine is?
Harrison's 20th Ed. Chapter 330 Page 2338

A. Unconjugated
B. Conjugated
C. Unconjugated + conjugated
D. All of the above

Unconjugated bilirubin always binds to albumin in serum and is not filtered by kidney. Therefore, any bilirubin found in urine is conjugated bilirubin and bilirubinuria implies the presence of liver disease.

1189. Which of the following may give a false-positive reading with Ictotest tablet?
Harrison's 20th Ed. Chapter 330 Page 2338

A. Barbiturates
B. Phenothiazines
C. Antacids
D. NSAIDs

Phenothiazines may give a false-positive reading with Ictotest tablet.

1190. **Which of the following is true in patients recovering from jaundice?**
Harrison's 20th Ed. Chapter 330 Page 2338

   A. Urine bilirubin clears prior to serum bilirubin
   B. Serum bilirubin clears prior to urine bilirubin
   C. Urine and serum bilirubin clear simultaneously
   D. Any of the above

In patients recovering from jaundice, the urine bilirubin clears prior to the serum bilirubin.

1191. **Aspartate aminotransferase (AST) found in all except?**
Harrison's 20th Ed. Chapter 330 Page 2339

   A. Skeletal muscle
   B. Kidneys
   C. Spleen
   D. Lungs

1192. **Aspartate aminotransferase (AST) not found in?**
Harrison's 20th Ed. Chapter 330 Page 2339

   A. Leukocytes
   B. Erythrocytes
   C. Platelets
   D. All of the above

1193. **Least concentration of AST is in?**
Harrison's 20th Ed. Chapter 330 Page 2339

   A. Brain
   B. Erythrocytes
   C. Lungs
   D. Pancreas

AST is found in liver, cardiac muscle, skeletal muscle, kidneys, brain, pancreas, lungs, leukocytes, & erythrocytes in decreasing order of concentration.

1194. **Aminotransferase level elevation up to what level are considered nonspecific?**
Harrison's 20th Ed. Chapter 330 Page 2339

   A. 100 U/L
   B. 200 U/L
   C. 300 U/L
   D. 400 U/L

1195. **Elevation of aminotransferases to >1000 U/L occurs in which of the following disorders?**
Harrison's 20th Ed. Chapter 330 Page 2339

   A. Viral hepatitis
   B. Ischemic liver injury
   C. Toxin or drug-induced liver injury
   D. All of the above

Aminotransferase levels of up to 300 U/L are nonspecific and may be found in any type of liver disorder. Aminotransferases levels of >1000 U/L occur in disorders associated with extensive hepatocellular injury like viral hepatitis, ischemic liver injury, and toxin or drug induced liver injury.

1196. **What AST : ALT ratio is highly suggestive of alcoholic liver disease?**
Harrison's 20th Ed. Chapter 330 Page 2339

   A. > 1.5:1
   B. > 2:1
   C. > 2.5:1
   D. > 3:1

An AST:ALT ratio >2:1 is suggestive while a ratio >3:1 is highly suggestive of alcoholic liver disease.

1197. **Which of the following about alcoholic liver disease is false?**
Harrison's 20th Ed. Chapter 330 Page 2339

   A. AST rarely > 300 U/L
   B. ALT often normal
   C. Increase in IgA levels
   D. None of the above

AST in alcoholic liver disease is rarely >300 U/L and ALT is often normal. Increases in IgA levels occur in alcoholic liver disease.

1198. **Which of the following about aminotransferases is false?**
Harrison's 20th Ed. Chapter 330 Page 2339

   A. Aminotransferases are present in serum in low concentrations
   B. Liver cell necrosis not required for release of aminotransferases
   C. Absolute elevation of aminotransferases is of no prognostic significance in acute hepatocellular disorders
   D. None of the above

1199. **Low serum ALT in alcoholic liver disease is due to alcohol-induced deficiency of?**
Harrison's 20th Ed. Chapter 330 Page 2339

   A. Pyridoxal sulphate
   B. Pyridoxal phosphate
   C. Pyridoxal gluconate
   D. Pyridoxal chloride

A low level of ALT in the serum is due to an alcohol-induced deficiency of pyridoxal phosphate.

1200. **Which of the following enzymes is elevated in cholestasis?**
Harrison's 20th Ed. Chapter 330 Page 2340

   A. Alkaline phosphatase
   B. 5'-nucleotidase
   C. Gamma glutamyl transpeptidase (GGT)
   D. All of the above

Alkaline phosphatase, 5'-nucleotidase & GGT are usually elevated in cholestasis.

1201. **Which of the following is located in endoplasmic reticulum of hepatocytes?**
Harrison's 20th Ed. Chapter 330 Page 2340

   A. Alkaline phosphatase
   B. 5'-nucleotidase
   C. Gamma glutamyl transpeptidase (GGT)
   D. All of the above

Alkaline phosphatase and 5'-nucleotidase are found in or near the bile canalicular membrane of hepatocytes, while GGT is located in the endoplasmic reticulum and in bile duct epithelial cells. Serum 5'-nucleotidase or GGT are rarely elevated in conditions other than liver disease.

1202. Elevated heat-stable fraction of serum alkaline phosphatase suggests its origin from?
Harrison's 20th Ed. Chapter 330 Page 2340

A. Liver
B. Bone
C. Placenta
D. Intestine

Elevated heat-stable fraction of serum alkaline phosphatase strongly suggests its placental or tumor source. Bone alkaline phosphatase is most susceptible to inactivation by heat.

1203. Individuals of which of the following blood group can have an elevation of serum alkaline phosphatase after eating a fatty meal?
Harrison's 20th Ed. Chapter 330 Page 2340

A. A
B. B
C. AB
D. All of the above

Individuals with blood types O & B can have an elevation of serum alkaline phosphatase after eating a fatty meal due to influx of intestinal alkaline phosphatase into the blood.

1204. In cholestatic liver disorders, alkaline phosphatase elevations are how many times greater than normal?
Harrison's 20th Ed. Chapter 330 Page 2340

A. 2 times
B. 3 times
C. 4 times
D. None of the above

Alkaline phosphatase elevations greater than four times normal occur primarily in cholestatic liver disorders, infiltrative liver diseases and Paget's disease.

1205. Conditions causing isolated elevations of serum alkaline phosphatase include all except?
Harrison's 20th Ed. Chapter 330 Page 2340

A. Hodgkin's disease
B. Inflammatory bowel disease
C. Hypothyroidism
D. Congestive heart failure

Isolated elevations of serum alkaline phosphatase is seen in Hodgkin's disease, diabetes, hyperthyroidism, CHF, amyloidosis and inflammatory bowel disease. Simultaneous measurement of serum 5'-nucleotidase or GGT enzymes helps to differentiate liver disease from others.

1206. Which of the following is not a cause of intrahepatic cholestasis?
Harrison's 20th Ed. Chapter 330 Page 2340

A. Drug-induced hepatitis
B. Sclerosing cholangitis
C. Primary biliary cirrhosis
D. Alcohol-induced steatohepatitis

Intrahepatic cholestasis is due to drug-induced hepatitis, primary biliary cirrhosis, rejection of transplanted livers and alcohol-induced steatohepatitis.

1207. Serum albumin is synthesized by?
Harrison's 20th Ed. Chapter 330 Page 2340

A. Hepatocyte
B. Kidney
C. Intestinal epithelial cells
D. All of the above

Serum albumin is synthesized exclusively by hepatocytes.

1208. Serum albumin has a half-life of?
Harrison's 20th Ed. Chapter 330 Page 2340

A. 18 to 20 days
B. 28 to 35 days
C. 35 to 45 days
D. > 60 days

1209. What proportion of albumin is degraded per day?
Harrison's 20th Ed. Chapter 330 Page 2340

A. 2%
B. 4%
C. 6%
D. 8%

Serum albumin has a half-life of 18 to 20 days with approximately 4% degraded per day.

1210. Minimal changes in the serum albumin are seen in?
Harrison's 20th Ed. Chapter 330 Page 2340

A. Viral hepatitis
B. Drug-related hepatotoxicity
C. Obstructive jaundice
D. All of the above

Minimal changes in the serum albumin are seen in acute liver conditions such as viral hepatitis, drug-related hepatotoxicity and obstructive jaundice.

1211. Albumin synthesis is inhibited by?
Harrison's 20th Ed. Chapter 330 Page 2340

A. Serum interleukin 1
B. Cholecystokinin
C. Lipase
D. All of the above

Prolonged increases in levels of serum cytokines IL-1 &/or tumor necrosis factor inhibit albumin synthesis.

1212. Which of the following serum globulins is not produced by hepatocytes?
Harrison's 20th Ed. Chapter 330 Page 2340

A. Alpha globulin
B. Beta globulin
C. Gamma globulin
D. All of the above

Gamma globulins (immunoglobulins) are produced by B lymphocytes and alpha and beta globulins are produced in hepatocytes.

1213. Which of the following statements is false?
Harrison's 20th Ed. Chapter 330 Page 2340

A. Gamma globulins are increased in chronic liver disease
B. IgG levels increase in autoimmune hepatitis
C. IgM levels increase in primary biliary cirrhosis
D. None of the above

In cirrhosis, increased serum gamma globulin concentration is due to increased synthesis of antibodies, some directed against intestinal bacteria because cirrhotic liver fails to clear bacterial antigens. Diffuse polyclonal increases in IgG levels are common in autoimmune hepatitis. Increases in IgM levels are common in primary biliary cirrhosis, while increases in IgA levels occur in alcoholic liver disease.

1214. Which of the following blood clotting factors is not made by hepatocytes?

Harrison's 20th Ed. Chapter 330 Page 2340

A. II
B. V
C. VIII
D. X

With the exception of factor VIII (produced by vascular endothelial cells), blood clotting factors are made exclusively in hepatocytes.

1215. Serum half-life of factor VII is?

Harrison's 20th Ed. Chapter 330 Page 2340

A. 6 hours
B. 24 hours
C. 48 hours
D. 72 hours

Serum half life of factor VII is 6 hours.

1216. Serum half-life of fibrinogen is?

Harrison's 20th Ed. Chapter 330 Page 2340

A. 2 days
B. 3 days
C. 5 days
D. 7 days

Serum half life of fibrinogen is 5 days.

1217. Serum prothrombin time does not measure which of the following factor?

Harrison's 20th Ed. Chapter 330 Page 2340

A. II
B. V
C. IX
D. X

Serum prothrombin time collectively measures factors II, V, VII and X.

1218. Single best acute measure of hepatic synthetic function is?

Harrison's 20th Ed. Chapter 330 Page 2340

A. Serum albumin
B. Serum globulins
C. Clotting factors
D. Serum bilirubin

Because of their rapid turnover, measurement of the clotting factors is the single best acute measure of hepatic synthetic function.

1219. Biosynthesis of factors which of the following factors depends on vitamin K?

Harrison's 20th Ed. Chapter 330 Page 2340

A. II
B. IX
C. X
D. All of the above

Biosynthesis of factors II, VII, IX, and X depends on vitamin K.

1220. Which of the following play a role in detoxification of ammonia?

Harrison's 20th Ed. Chapter 330 Page 2341

A. Spleen
B. Pancreas
C. Striated muscle
D. Cartilage

Liver converts ammonia to urea which is excreted by kidneys. Striated muscles detoxify ammonia by combining it with glutamic acid to form glutamine.

1221. Which of the following tests is useful in diagnosing advanced liver fibrosis?

Harrison's 20th Ed. Chapter 330 Page 2341

A. Haptoglobin
B. Apolipoprotein A-I
C. α2-macroglobulin
D. All of the above

Haptoglobin, bilirubin, GGT, apolipoprotein A-I and α2-macroglobulin are used for diagnosing advanced fibrosis in patients with chronic hepatitis C, chronic hepatitis B, alcoholic liver disease and patients taking methotrexate for psoriasis.

1222. First test ordered in patients suspected of having Budd-Chiari syndrome is?

Harrison's 20th Ed. Chapter 330 Page 2341

A. Percutaneous biopsy of the liver
B. Ultrasonography with Doppler imaging
C. Magnetic resonance cholangiopancreatography (MRCP)
D. Computerized tomography (CT)

Ultrasound with Doppler imaging is the first test ordered in patients suspected of having Budd-Chiari syndrome.

1223. Which of the following about Gilbert's syndrome is false?

Harrison's 20th Ed. Chapter 330 Page 2341 Table 330-1

A. Healthy patient
B. Isolated, unconjugated hyperbilirubinemia
C. Absence of hemolysis
D. None of the above

1224. Which of the following is elevated in Gilbert's syndrome?

Harrison's 20th Ed. Chapter 330 Page 2341 Table 330-1

A. S. Aminotransferases
B. S. Alkaline phosphatase
C. Prothrombin time
D. None of the above

In Hemolysis/Gilbert's syndrome, aminotransferases, alkaline phosphatase, albumin and prothrombin time are normal. There is no bilirubinuria.

Hyperbilirubinemias

1225. Which of the following chemical structure represents bilirubin?
- A. $C_{30}H_{36}N_4O_6$
- B. $C_{31}H_{36}N_4O_6$
- C. $C_{32}H_{36}N_4O_6$
- D. $C_{33}H_{36}N_4O_6$

Word bilirubin comes from Latin bilis + ruber meaning red. Bilirubin a a reddish-yellow pigment $C_{33}H_{36}N_4O_6$ that is formed by the breakdown of heme (ferroprotoporphyrin IX). Chemical structure of biliverdin is $C_{33}H_{34}N_4O_6$.

1226. Which of the following contain four pyrrolic rings?
- A. Bilirubin
- B. Phycobilin
- C. Phytochrome
- D. All of the above

1227. Which of the following about biliverdin is true?
- A. Green tetrapyrrolic bile pigment
- B. Red tetrapyrrolic bile pigment
- C. Yellow tetrapyrrolic bile pigment
- D. Blue tetrapyrrolic bile pigment

1228. Which of the following about urobilinogen is true?
Harrison's 20th Ed. Chapter 45 Page 276
- A. Yellow tetrapyrrole
- B. Orange tetrapyrrole
- C. Green tetrapyrrole
- D. Colorless tetrapyrrole

Urobilinogens are colorless because each of the bridges connecting the pyrrole rings is saturated, and the conjugation of double bonds is limited to individual rings.

1229. Which of the following about Heme is true?
Harrison's 20th Ed. Chapter 57 Page 377
- A. Iron-chelated tetrapyrrole
- B. Zinc-chelated tetrapyrrole
- C. Iron-Zinc chelated tetrapyrrole
- D. All of the above

Heme is an iron-chelated tetrapyrrole or porphyrin. The most complex known tetrapyrrole is cobalt-containing cobalamin (vitamin B12).

1230. Term linear tetrapyrrole best relates to?
Harrison's 20th Ed. Chapter 409 Page 2987
- A. Uroporphyrinogen III
- B. Hydroxymethylbilane
- C. Coproporphyrinogen III
- D. 5-aminolevulinic acid

In contrast to cyclic tetrapyrroles, linear tetrapyrroles do not contain a tightly bound metal. Light-responsive regulatory systems utilize linear tetrapyrroles as cofactors.

1231. What proportion of bilirubin is derived from degradation of the hemoglobin of senescent red blood cells?
Harrison's 20th Ed. Chapter 331 Page 2342
- A. ~ 30 - 50%
- B. ~ 50 - 70%
- C. ~ 70 - 90%
- D. ~ 100%

About 70–90% of bilirubin is derived from degradation of the hemoglobin of senescent red blood cells. Rest comes from degradation of cytochromes and others.

1232. In a normal adult, what quantity of bilirubin is produced daily?
Front. Pharmacol. 2017;8:887
- A. 50 – 150 mg
- B. 200 – 300 mg
- C. 300 – 500 mg
- D. 500 – 7500 mg

Bilirubin (BR) is a tetrapyrrolic pigment found in plasma as an albumin-bound reversible complex. It is derived from catabolism of heme, released by hemoglobin (75%) and cytochromes (25%), with a daily production of about 200–300 mg. in a normal healthy adult.

1233. Glutathione-S-transferase (GST) is related to which of the following steps in bilirubin metabolism?
Harrison's 20th Ed. Chapter 331 Page 2342
- A. Hepatocellular uptake
- B. Intracellular binding
- C. Conjugation
- D. Biliary excretion

After hepatocellular uptake, bilirubin is kept in solution by binding to glutathione-S-transferases formerly called ligandins.

1234. Bilirubin-UDP-glucuronosyltransferase (UGT1A1) is related to which of the following steps in bilirubin metabolism?
Harrison's 20th Ed. Chapter 331 Page 2342
- A. Hepatocellular uptake
- B. Intracellular binding
- C. Conjugation
- D. Biliary excretion

Bilirubin is conjugated with one or two glucuronic acid moieties by a specific UDP-glucuronosyltransferase to form bilirubin mono- and diglucuronide, respectively.

1235. Aqueous insolubility of bilirubin is due to which of the following?
Harrison's 20th Ed. Chapter 331 Page 2342
- A. Internal phosphate bonding
- B. Internal hydrogen bonding
- C. Internal sulphate bonding
- D. Internal glucoronate bonding

Conjugation of bilirubin with glucuronic acid moieties disrupts internal hydrogen bonding that limits aqueous solubility of bilirubin & the resulting glucuronide conjugates are highly soluble in water.

1236. Which of the following are the four common exons that encode the shared carboxyl-terminal half of all UGT1 isoforms?
Harrison's 20th Ed. Chapter 331 Page 2342

A. Exons 1 - 4
B. Exons 2 - 5
C. Exons 3 - 6
D. Exons 4 - 7

Exons 2–5 are four common exons that encode the shared carboxyl-terminal half of all UGT1 isoforms. A mutation in exons 2–5 will alter all isoforms encoded by the UGT1 gene complex. Mutations in a first exon affect only a single isoform.

1237. UDP-glucuronosyltransferases (UGT) that conjugate bilirubin belong to which UGT family?
Harrison's 20th Ed. Chapter 331 Page 2342

A. UGT1
B. UGT2
C. UGT3
D. UGT4

UDP-glucuronosyltransferases (UGT) that conjugate bilirubin belong to the UGT1 family. Exon A1 and the four common exons, collectively designated the UGT1A1 gene, encode the physiologically critical enzyme bilirubin-UDP-glucuronosyltransferase (UGT1A1).

1238. Human UGT1 gene complex is on which of the following chromosomes?
Harrison's 20th Ed. Chapter 331 Page 2343 Figure 331-2

A. 2
B. 4
C. 6
D. 8

Human UGT1 gene complex is on chromosome 2. It contains at least 13 substrate-specific first exons (A1, A2, etc.). Since four of these are pseudogenes, nine UGT1 isoforms with differing substrate specificities are expressed. Mutations in a first exon affect only a single isoform. Those in exons 2–5 affect all enzymes encoded by the UGT1 complex.

1239. Multidrug resistance-associated protein 2 (MRP2) is related to which of the following steps in bilirubin metabolism?
Harrison's 20th Ed. Chapter 331 Page 2342

A. Hepatocellular uptake
B. Intracellular binding
C. Conjugation
D. Biliary excretion

Bilirubin mono- and diglucuronides are excreted across canalicular plasma membrane into bile canaliculus by ATP-dependent transport process mediated by a canalicular membrane protein called multidrug resistance-associated protein 2 (MRP2). Mutations of MRP2 result in Dubin-Johnson syndrome.

1240. Which of the following is false about urobilinogen?
Harrison's 20th Ed. Chapter 331 Page 2342

A. Made from unconjugated bilirubin in gut
B. Water-soluble
C. Colorless
D. Undergoes enterohepatic cycling

"Conjugated bilirubin" is converted by bacterial metabolism in gut to water-soluble colorless urobilinogen. Urobilinogen undergoes enterohepatic cycling. Urobilinogen not taken up by liver reaches systemic circulation, from which some is cleared by kidneys.

1241. Which of the following interrupts bilirubin enterohepatic cycling?
Harrison's 20th Ed. Chapter 331 Page 2343

A. Aluminum hydroxide
B. Magnesium sulphate
C. Calcium phosphate
D. Calcium carbonate

Oral administration of calcium phosphate with or without the lipase inhibitor orlistat may be an efficient means to interrupt bilirubin enterohepatic cycling.

1242. In response to hemolytic stress, bone marrow is capable of increasing erythrocyte production by?
Harrison's 20th Ed. Chapter 331 Page 2343

A. Two fold
B. Four fold
C. Six fold
D. Eight fold

In response to hemolytic stress, bone marrow is capable of a sustained eight fold increase in erythrocyte production.

1243. Hemolysis alone cannot result in a sustained hyperbilirubinemia of more than?
Harrison's 20th Ed. Chapter 331 Page 2343

A. ~ 2 mg/dL
B. ~ 4 mg/dL
C. ~ 6 mg/dL
D. ~ 8 mg/dL

Hemolysis alone cannot result in a sustained hyperbilirubinemia of more than ~ 4 mg/dL.

1244. Direct-reacting fraction is how much of total serum bilirubin in isolated hemolysis?
Harrison's 20th Ed. Chapter 331 Page 2343

A. ≤ 10%
B. ≤ 12%
C. ≤ 15%
D. ≤ 18%

Hemolysis results in pure unconjugated hyperbilirubinemia, with direct-reacting fraction being ≤15% of total serum bilirubin.

1245. Ineffective erythropoiesis is seen in all except?
Harrison's 20th Ed. Chapter 331 Page 2343

A. Thalassemia major
B. Congenital erythropoietic porphyria
C. Crigler-Najjar syndrome
D. Lead poisoning

In thalassemia major, megaloblastic anemias due to folate or vitamin B12 deficiency, congenital erythropoietic porphyria, lead poisoning, and congenital & acquired dyserythropoietic anemias, the fraction of total bilirubin production derived from ineffective erythropoiesis is increased, reaching as much as 70% of the total producing modest degrees of unconjugated hyperbilirubinemia.

1246. Which of the following produces hyperbilirubinemia due to decreased hepatic bilirubin uptake?
Harrison's 20th Ed. Chapter 331 Page 2343

A. Pregnanediol
B. Chloramphenicol
C. Gentamicin
D. Cholecystographic contrast agents

Apart from Gilbert's syndrome, flavaspidic acid, novobiocin, rifampin and cholecystographic contrast agents produce defects in bilirubin uptake. Pregnanediol, novobiocin, chloramphenicol, and gentamicin produce unconjugated hyperbilirubinemia by inhibiting UGT1A1 activity.

1247. Fetal bilirubin is cleared by?
Harrison's 20th Ed. Chapter 331 Page 2343

A. Fetal liver
B. Fetal kidney
C. Placenta
D. All of the above

Bilirubin produced by the fetus is cleared by the placenta and eliminated by the maternal liver.

1248. Most neonates develop mild unconjugated hyperbilirubinemia between days?
Harrison's 20th Ed. Chapter 331 Page 2343

A. 1 and 3 after birth
B. 2 and 5 after birth
C. 5 and 7 after birth
D. 7 and 10 after birth

Immediately after birth, due to incompletely developed hepatic physiologic processes like low levels of UGT1A1, undeveloped intestinal flora that convert bilirubin to urobilinogen, most neonates develop mild unconjugated hyperbilirubinemia between days 2 and 5 after birth.

1249. What are the peak levels of physiologic neonatal jaundice?
Harrison's 20th Ed. Chapter 331 Page 2343

A. 3 - 5 mg/dL
B. 5 - 10 mg/dL
C. 10 - 15 mg/dL
D. 15 - 20 mg/dL

Peak levels of physiologic neonatal jaundice are typically 5–10 mg/dL.

1250. Bilibubin levels of physiologic neonatal jaundice return to normal adult concentrations within?
Harrison's 20th Ed. Chapter 331 Page 2343

A. 1 week
B. 2 weeks
C. 3 weeks
D. 4 weeks

Bilibubin levels of physiologic neonatal jaundice return to normal adult concentrations within 2 weeks as mechanisms required for bilirubin disposition mature.

1251. Which of the following is false for bilirubin encephalopathy, or kernicterus?
Harrison's 20th Ed. Chapter 331 Page 2343

A. Rapidly rising unconjugated bilirubin concentration
B. Immature blood-brain barrier
C. Deposition in the basal ganglia
D. None of the above

A rapidly rising unconjugated bilirubin concentration, or absolute levels >20 mg/dL, exposed the infant to the at risk of bilirubin encephalopathy, or kernicterus.

1252. Which of the following drugs may produce unconjugated hyperbilirubinemia by inhibiting UGT1A1 activity?
Harrison's 20th Ed. Chapter 331 Page 2343

A. Pregnanediol
B. Chloramphenicol
C. Gentamicin
D. All of the above

Pregnanediol, novobiocin, chloramphenicol, atazanavir and gentamicin may produce unconjugated hyperbilirubinemia by inhibiting UGT1A1 activity.

1253. 'Breast milk jaundice' in neonates is due to presence of what in breast milk?
Harrison's 20th Ed. Chapter 331 Page 2343

A. Immunoglobulins
B. Proteins
C. Fatty acids
D. Carbohydrates

Bilirubin conjugation may be inhibited by certain fatty acids that are present in breast milk but not serum of mothers whose infants have excessive neonatal hyperbilirubinemia (breast milk jaundice).

1254. Lucey-Driscoll syndrome is related to?
Harrison's 20th Ed. Chapter 331 Page 2343

A. UGT1A1 inhibitor in breast milk
B. UGT1A1 inhibitor in maternal serum
C. Low UGT1A1 levels at birth
D. All of the above

In transient familial neonatal hyperbilirubinemia (Lucey-Driscoll syndrome) there is a UGT1A1 inhibitor in maternal serum.

1255. Which of the following about Crigler-Najjar Syndrome, Type I is false?
Harrison's 20th Ed. Chapter 331 Page 2344

A. Unconjugated hyperbilirubinemia of ~ 20-45 mg/dL
B. Appears in the neonatal period
C. Persists for life
D. Bilirubin is found in the urine

No bilirubin is found in the urine.

1256. Which of the following about Crigler-Najjar Syndrome, Type I is false?
Harrison's 20th Ed. Chapter 331 Page 2344

A. Normal serum aminotransferases
B. Normal alkaline phosphatase
C. No evidence of hemolysis
D. None of the above

1257. Which of the following is false about Crigler-Najjar Syndrome Type I?
Harrison's 20th Ed. Chapter 331 Page 2344

A. Unconjugated hyperbilirubinemia
B. Absent UGT1A1 activity in liver
C. Kernicterus common
D. Responds to phenobarbital

Crigler-Najjar Syndrome, Type I (CN-I) is characterized by unconjugated hyperbilirubinemia of ~20 to 45 mg/dL that appears in neonatal period and persists for life. Bilirubin glucuronides are absent from bile and there is no UGT1A1 activity in hepatic tissue. There is no response to phenobarbital or any enzyme inducer.

1258. Causative mutation is in the bilirubin-specific exon A1 of which variety of Crigler-Najjar Syndrome Type I?
Harrison's 20th Ed. Chapter 331 Page 2344

A. Crigler-Najjar syndrome Type IA
B. Crigler-Najjar syndrome Type IB
C. Crigler-Najjar syndrome Type IC
D. Crigler-Najjar syndrome Type ID

In Crigler-Najjar Syndrome Type IB, the defect is limited to bilirubin conjugation, and the causative mutation is in the bilirubin-specific exon A1.

1259. Which of the following is false about Crigler-Najjar Syndrome Type I?

Harrison's 20th Ed. Chapter 331 Page 2344

A. Rare (estimated prevalence = 0.6 - 1.0 per million)
B. Autosomal recessive pattern of inheritance
C. Estrogen glucuronidation is defective
D. Liver transplantation not helpful

In Crigler-Najjar Syndrome Type I, early liver transplantation remains the best hope to prevent brain injury and death.

1260. Crigler-Najjar Syndrome Type I (CN-I) differs from Crigler-Najjar Syndrome, Type II (CN-II) is which of the following?

Harrison's 20th Ed. Chapter 331 Page 2344

A. Average bilirubin concentrations are lower in CN-II
B. CN-II is infrequently associated with kernicterus
C. CN-II responds to phenobarbital
D. All of the above

Crigler-Najjar Syndrome Type II (CN-II) is characterized by marked unconjugated hyperbilirubinemia with normal conventional hepatic biochemical tests, hepatic histology and no hemolysis. Average bilirubin concentrations are lower in CN-II. CN-II is infrequently associated with kernicterus. Bile in CN-II contains bilirubin glucuronides mostly monoglucuronides. UGT1A1 in liver is present at reduced levels in CN-II and bilirubin concentrations fall with phenobarbital therapy.

1261. Which of the following is false about Gilbert's Syndrome?

Harrison's 20th Ed. Chapter 331 Page 2344

A. Conjugated hyperbilirubinemia
B. UGT1A1 activity - 10-35% of normal
C. Phenobarbital normalizes serum bilirubin
D. Aggravated by alcohol use

In Gilbert's Syndrome, UGT1A1 activity is typically reduced to 10 - 35% of normal, and bile pigments exhibit a characteristic increase in bilirubin monoglucuronides.

1262. Gilbert's Syndrome is a close clinical entity to which of the following?

Harrison's 20th Ed. Chapter 331 Page 2344

A. Crigler-Najjar syndrome Type I
B. Crigler-Najjar syndrome Type II
C. Lucey-Driscoll syndrome
D. Benign recurrent intrahepatic cholestasis (BRIC)

The clinical spectrum of Gilbert's Syndrome hyperbilirubinemia fades into that of CN-II at serum bilirubin concentrations of 5 - 8 mg/dL.

1263. Which of the following pigment is increased in hepatic histology of patients of Gilbert's Syndrome?

Harrison's 20th Ed. Chapter 331 Page 2345

A. Melanopsin
B. Lipofuscin
C. Hemosiderin
D. Oxidized homogentisic acid

1264. In GS, elevated bilirubin concentrations are associated with?

Harrison's 20th Ed. Chapter 331 Page 2345

A. Stress
B. Alcohol use
C. Reduced caloric intake
D. All of the above

In GS, elevated bilirubin concentrations particularly bilirubin monoglucuronides are associated with stress, fatigue, alcohol use, reduced caloric intake and intercurrent illness while increased caloric intake or administration of enzyme-inducing agents produces lower bilirubin levels.

1265. Which of the following drugs is glucuronidated specifically by bilirubin-UDP-glucuronosyltransferase?

Harrison's 20th Ed. Chapter 331 Page 2345

A. Estradiol benzoate
B. Acetaminophen
C. Tolbutamide
D. Irinotecan

In Gilbert's Syndrome, toxicity occurs upon administration of antitumor agent irinotecan (CPT-11) because its active metabolite (SN-38) is glucuronidated specifically by bilirubin-UDP-glucuronosyltransferase.

1266. Which of the following drugs used in HIV patients inhibits UGT1A1?

Harrison's 20th Ed. Chapter 331 Page 2345

A. Zidovudine
B. Indinavir
C. Enfuvirtide
D. All of the above

HIV protease inhibitors indinavir and atazanavir inhibit UGT1A1, resulting in hyperbilirubinemia that is most pronounced in patients with preexisting Gilbert's Syndrome.

1267. Which of the following are examples of familial defects in hepatic excretory function?

Harrison's 20th Ed. Chapter 331 Page 2345

A. Dubin-Johnson syndrome
B. Rotor syndrome
C. Benign recurrent intrahepatic cholestasis
D. All of the above

1268. Which of the following does not manifest as predominantly conjugated hyperbilirubinemia?

Harrison's 20th Ed. Chapter 331 Page 2345

A. Dubin-Johnson syndrome
B. Crigler-Najjar syndrome
C. Rotor syndrome
D. Benign recurrent intrahepatic cholestasis

1269. In Dubin-Johnson Syndrome, degree of hyperbilirubinemia may be increased by?

Harrison's 20th Ed. Chapter 331 Page 2345

A. Intercurrent illness
B. Oral contraceptive use
C. Pregnancy
D. All of the above

In Dubin-Johnson Syndrome, degree of hyperbilirubinemia may be increased by intercurrent illness, oral contraceptive use, and pregnancy.

1270. Liver is grossly black in appearance in which of the following?

Harrison's 20th Ed. Chapter 331 Page 2346

A. Dubin-Johnson syndrome
B. Rotor syndrome
C. Progressive familial intrahepatic cholestasis
D. Benign recurrent intrahepatic cholestasis (BRIC)

In DJS, due to accumulation in lysosomes of centrilobular hepatocytes of dark, coarsely granular pigment, liver is grossly black in appearance. This pigment is thought to be derived from epinephrine metabolites that are not excreted normally.

1271. Which of the following is false about Dubin-Johnson Syndrome?
Harrison's 20th Ed. Chapter 331 Page 2346

A. Conjugated hyperbilirubinemia
B. Bilirubinuria present
C. Liver grossly black
D. Pruritus common

DJS patients have normal serum & biliary bile acid concentrations & do not have pruritus.

1272. Dark, coarsely granular pigment in hepatocytes in Dubin-Johnson Syndrome disappears during?
Harrison's 20th Ed. Chapter 331 Page 2346

A. Enteric fever
B. Viral hepatitis
C. Malaria
D. All of the above

Dark, coarsely granular pigment in hepatocytes in Dubin-Johnson Syndrome disappears during bouts of viral hepatitis, only to reaccumulate slowly after recovery.

1273. Pigment producing grossly black liver in DJS is best related to?
Harrison's 20th Ed. Chapter 331 Page 2346

A. Tryptophan
B. Melanin
C. Epinephrine
D. Glutathione

A cardinal feature of DJS is the accumulation in the lysosomes of centrilobular hepatocytes of dark, coarsely granular pigment. As a result, liver is grossly black in appearance. This pigment is thought to be derived from epinephrine metabolites that are not excreted normally.

1274. Mutation in which of the following genes produce the Dubin-Johnson phenotype?
Harrison's 20th Ed. Chapter 331 Page 2346

A. ABCC2
B. NTCP
C. MRP2
D. FIC1

MRP2 is an ATP-dependent canalicular membrane transporter and mutations in the MRP2 gene produce the Dubin-Johnson phenotype, which has an autosomal recessive pattern of inheritance.

1275. In urine from Dubin-Johnson Syndrome patients, which is the predominant coproporphyrin isomer?
Harrison's 20th Ed. Chapter 331 Page 2346

A. Coproporphyrin isomer I
B. Coproporphyrin isomer II
C. Coproporphyrin isomer III
D. Coproporphyrin isomer IV

Naturally occurring coproporphyrin isomers are I and III. Normally, 75% of the coproporphyrin in urine is isomer III. In urine from DJS patients, total coproporphyrin content is normal, but >80% of the total is isomer I.

1276. Which of the following is typical of Dubin-Johnson Syndrome?
Harrison's 20th Ed. Chapter 331 Page 2346

A. Liver is grossly black in appearance
B. Gallbladder not visualized on oral cholecystography
C. Total urinary coproporphyrin excretion normal
D. All of the above

1277. Which of the following is an autosomal recessive disorder?
Harrison's 20th Ed. Chapter 331 Page 2346

A. Crigler-Najjar syndrome
B. Gilbert's syndrome
C. Rotor syndrome
D. All of the above

1278. Rotor Syndrome is clinically similar to?
Harrison's 20th Ed. Chapter 331 Page 2346

A. Dubin-Johnson syndrome
B. Crigler-Najjar syndrome
C. Gilbert's syndrome
D. Lucey-Driscoll syndrome

Rotor Syndrome is a benign, autosomal recessive disorder clinically similar to DJS.

1279. Which of the following is false about Rotor Syndrome?
Harrison's 20th Ed. Chapter 331 Page 2346

A. Conjugated hyperbilirubinemia
B. Gallbladder visualized on oral cholecystography
C. Liver normal in appearance
D. Total urinary coproporphyrin excretion normal

In Rotor syndrome, the gallbladder is visualized on oral cholecystography, in contrast to nonvisualization that is typical of DJS. Total urinary coproporphyrin excretion is substantially increased in Rotor syndrome, in contrast to the normal levels seen in DJS.

1280. Which of the following is related to transportation of bilirubin glucuronides into the portal circulation?
Harrison's 20th Ed. Chapter 331 Page 2346

A. MRP2
B. MRP3
C. Bilirubin-UDP-glucuronosyltransferase (UGT1A1)
D. All of the above

In addition to direct excretion of bilirubin glucuronides, a portion is transported into the portal circulation by MRP3 and subjected to reuptake into the hepatocyte by OATP1B1 and OATP1B3. Recent studies indicate that the molecular basis of Rotor syndrome results from simultaneous deficiency of the plasma membrane transporters OATP1B1 and OATP1B3. This results in reduced reuptake of conjugated bilirubin that has been pumped out of the cell into the portal circulation by MRP3.

1281. Which of the following is false about Benign Recurrent Intrahepatic Cholestasis (BRIC)?
Harrison's 20th Ed. Chapter 331 Page 2346

A. Recurrent attacks of pruritus and jaundice
B. Normal serum aminotransferase levels
C. Elevations in alkaline phosphatase
D. Does not lead to cirrhosis

BRIC is characterized by recurrent attacks of pruritus and jaundice. Laboratory findings include elevations in serum conjugated bilirubin, aminotransferase and alkaline phosphatase levels. BRIC is an autosomal recessive benign disorder in that it does not lead to cirrhosis or end-stage liver disease.

1282. Mutation in which of the following genes produce the Benign Recurrent Intrahepatic Cholestasis (BRIC)?
Harrison's 20th Ed. Chapter 331 Page 2346

A. ABCC2
B. NTCP
C. MRP2
D. FIC1

Gene FIC1 is mutated in patients with BRIC.

1283. Gene FIC1 is mainly expressed in?

Harrison's 20th Ed. Chapter 331 Page 2346

- A. Liver
- B. Small intestine
- C. Kidney
- D. Heart

Gene FIC1 is mainly expressed strongly in the small intestine but only weakly in the liver.

1284. Byler disease is also known as?

Harrison's 20th Ed. Chapter 331 Page 2347

- A. Progressive familial intrahepatic cholestasis type 1
- B. Progressive familial intrahepatic cholestasis type 2
- C. Progressive familial intrahepatic cholestasis type 3
- D. Progressive familial intrahepatic cholestasis type 4

Byler disease is also termed as Progressive Familial Intrahepatic Cholestasis (FIC) type 1. This is also a consequence of an FIC1 mutation and may progresses to malnutrition, growth retardation, and end-stage liver disease during childhood.

1285. Mutation of MDR3 gene results in?

Harrison's 20th Ed. Chapter 331 Page 2347

- A. Progressive familial intrahepatic cholestasis type 1
- B. Progressive familial intrahepatic cholestasis type 2
- C. Progressive familial intrahepatic cholestasis type 3
- D. Progressive familial intrahepatic cholestasis type 4

Progressive FIC type 3 has been associated with a mutation of MDR3, a protein that is essential for normal hepatocellular excretion of phospholipids across the bile canaliculus.

Acute Viral Hepatitis

1286. World Hepatitis Day is observed on?

A. October 01
B. December 01
C. February 04
D. July 28

World Hepatitis Day is recognized annually on July 28th, the birthday of Dr. Baruch Blumberg (1925-2011). Dr. Blumberg discovered hepatitis B virus in 1967 and two years later developed the first hepatitis B vaccine and for these achievements won the Nobel Prize. World Hepatitis Awareness Day - October 01, World AIDS Day - December 1, World Cancer Day - February 04.

1287. DANE particle is the name given to?
N Engl J Med. 1973; 288:1409

A. Hepatitis A virion
B. Hepatitis B virion
C. Hepatitis C virion
D. Hepatitis D virion

D.S. Dane and others discovered the HBV virus particle in 1970 by electron microscopy.

1288. Which of the following is not a RNA virus?
Harrison's 20th Ed. Chapter 332 Page 2347

A. Hepatitis A virus
B. Hepatitis B virus
C. Hepatitis C virus
D. Hepatitis D virus

A, C, D, E human hepatitis viruses are RNA viruses.

1289. Which of the following viruses is a DNA virus?
Harrison's 20th Ed. Chapter 332 Page 2347

A. Hepatitis A
B. Hepatitis B
C. Hepatitis C
D. Hepatitis D

Hepatitis B is a DNA virus but replicates like a retrovirus.

1290. Which of the following is not a bloodborne type virus?
Harrison's 20th Ed. Chapter 332 Page 2347

A. Hepatitis A
B. Hepatitis B
C. Hepatitis C
D. Hepatitis D

HBV, HCV, and HDV are bloodborne type viruses.

1291. Which of the following about Hepatitis A virus is false?
Harrison's 20th Ed. Chapter 332 Page 2347

A. Enveloped
B. Heat resistant
C. Acid resistant
D. Ether resistant

Hepatitis A virus is a nonenveloped 27-nm, heat, acid, and ether-resistant RNA virus in the hepatovirus genus of the picornavirus family.

1292. Four capsid polypeptides of Hepatitis A virion are designated as?
Harrison's 20th Ed. Chapter 332 Page 2347

A. SP1 to SP4
B. HP1 to HP4
C. VP1 to VP4
D. WP1 to WP4

Hepatitis A virion contains four capsid polypeptides, designated VP1 to VP4. These are cleaved posttranslationally from the polyprotein product of a 7500-nucleotide genome.

1293. Inactivation of Hepatitis A virus can be achieved by?
Harrison's 20th Ed. Chapter 332 Page 2347

A. Formaldehyde
B. Chlorine
C. Ultraviolet irradiation
D. All of the above

Inactivation of viral activity can be achieved by boiling for 1 minute, by formaldehyde and chlorine, or by ultraviolet irradiation.

1294. Hepatitis A has an incubation period of?
Harrison's 20th Ed. Chapter 332 Page 2347

A. ~ 2 weeks
B. ~ 4 weeks
C. ~ 6 weeks
D. ~ 8 weeks

Hepatitis A has an incubation period of ~4 weeks.

1295. Replication of Hepatitis A virus occurs in?
Harrison's 20th Ed. Chapter 332 Page 2347

A. Liver
B. Bile
C. Blood
D. All of the above

Hepatitis A virus replication is limited to liver. But, the virus is present in liver, bile, stools, and blood during the late incubation period and acute preicteric phase of illness.

1296. Which of the following statements about Hepatitis A virus is false?
Harrison's 20th Ed. Chapter 332 Page 2347

A. HAV can be cultivated reproducibly in vitro
B. Virus is present in liver, bile, stools and blood during late incubation period & acute preicteric phase of illness
C. Viral shedding in feces, viremia and infectivity diminish rapidly once jaundice becomes apparent
D. None of the above

Despite persistence of virus in liver, viral shedding in feces, viremia, and infectivity diminish rapidly once jaundice becomes apparent.

1297. After acute illness, anti-HAV of IgM class remains detectable for?
Harrison's 20th Ed. Chapter 332 Page 2347

A. Up to 3 months
B. Up to 6 months
C. Up to 12 months
D. Up to 18 months

Early antibody response to HAV infection is predominantly of the IgM class and persists for ~3 months, rarely for 6-12 months.

1298. After acute illness, anti-HAV of IgG class remains detectable for?
Harrison's 20th Ed. Chapter 332 Page 2347

A. 3 months
B. 6 months
C. 12 months
D. Indefinitely

After acute illness, anti-HAV of the IgG class remains detectable indefinitely.

1299. Which of the following has the largest virus particle size?
Harrison's 20th Ed. Chapter 332 Page 2348 Figure 332-1

A. Hepatitis A
B. Hepatitis D
C. Hepatitis C
D. Hepatitis E

1300. Which of the following has the smallest virus particle size?
Harrison's 20th Ed. Chapter 332 Page 2348 Figure 332-1

A. Hepatitis A
B. Hepatitis D
C. Hepatitis C
D. Hepatitis E

Hepatitis A virus (27-nm), Hepatitis B virus (42-nm), Hepatitis C virus (55-nm), Hepatitis D virus (35–37 nm) and Hepatitis E virus (32–34 nm)

1301. Which of the following has the largest viral genome size?
Harrison's 20th Ed. Chapter 332 Page 2348 Figure 332-1

A. Hepatitis A
B. Hepatitis B
C. Hepatitis C
D. Hepatitis E

1302. Which of the following has the smallest viral genome size?
Harrison's 20th Ed. Chapter 332 Page 2348 Table 332-1

A. Hepatitis A
B. Hepatitis B
C. Hepatitis C
D. Hepatitis D

1303. Which of the following has the smallest viral genome size?
Harrison's 20th Ed. Chapter 332 Page 2348 Table 332-1

A. Hepatitis A
B. Hepatitis B
C. Hepatitis C
D. Hepatitis E

HAV - 7.5 kb, HBV 3.2 kb, HCV - 9.4 kb, HDV - 1.7 kb, HEV - 7.6 kb.

1304. HBV belongs to which family of viruses?
Harrison's 20th Ed. Chapter 332 Page 2347

A. Hepadnaviruses
B. Hepatovirus
C. Hepacivirus
D. Hepevirus

HBV belongs to hepadnaviruses family of viruses, type 1 ("hepa" from hepatotrophic and "dna" because it is a DNA virus), HAV is a Hepatovirus, HCV is Hepacivirus and HEV is a Hepevirus. HDV resembles viroids and plant satellite viruses.

1305. The four overlapping genes of encoding proteins in Hepatitis B virus are?
Harrison's 20th Ed. Chapter 332 Page 2347

A. S, C, P and X
B. S, T, U and V
C. S, O, M and Z
D. S, Q, C, and Y

In Hepatitis B virus, the four overlapping genes encoded by the genome are S, C, P and X.

1306. Hepadnaviruses also infect which of the following?
Harrison's 20th Ed. Chapter 332 Page 2347

A. Woodchucks
B. Ground and tree squirrels
C. Pekin ducks
D. All of the above

Hepadnavirus type 1 viruses infect species of woodchucks, ground & tree squirrels, and Pekin ducks.

1307. Out of the following, who is related to the discovery of Australia antigen?
N Engl J Med. 1970; 283:349-354

A. Alter MJ
B. Baruch Blumberg
C. Bouchard MJ
D. Zuckerman AJ

In 1965, American physician & geneticist Baruch Blumberg (1925-2011), working at National Institutes of Health (NIH), discovered the Australia antigen (later known to be Hepatitis B surface antigen, or HBsAg) in the blood of Australian aboriginal people. He was the co-recipient of the 1976 Nobel Prize in Physiology or Medicine.

1308. Additional name for Australia antigen is?
N Engl J Med. 1970; 283:349-354

A. Hepatitis antigen
B. SH antigen
C. Hepatitis-associated antigen
D. All of the above

1309. Which of the following is false about HBV genome?
Harrison's 20th Ed. Chapter 332 Page 2348

A. Circular genome
B. Partially double-strand and partially single-strand
C. Replicates through an RNA intermediate form by reverse transcription
D. None of the above

Hepatitis B is a non-retroviral virus which uses reverse transcription for its replication.

1310. Which of the following about Hepatitis B virus is false?
N Engl J Med. 2004;351:2832-8

A. Enveloped, double-stranded DNA virus
B. Smallest dsDNA virus known to infect humans
C. Primary reservoir is chronically infected people
D. Insects can transmit HBV

1311. Which of the following about Hepatitis B virus is false?
N Engl J Med. 2004;351:2832-8

A. Blood contains highest concentrations of virus
B. Not transmitted by fecal-oral route
C. Vertical transmission from mother to child possible
D. Breast milk can cause viral transmission

1312. Which of the following about Hepatitis B virus is false?
N Engl J Med. 2004;350:1118-29

A. Replication of DNA genome by reverse transcription of RNA intermediate
B. Covalently closed circular DNA (cccDNA) is formed in hepatocyte nucleus
C. Most abundant protein in HBV genome is S protein
D. Risk of development of chronicity is directly related to age at time of infection

1313. Entry of HBV into hepatocytes is mediated by binding to?
Harrison's 20th Ed. Chapter 332 Page 2348

A. Sodium taurocholate cotransporting polypeptide receptor
B. Sodium deoxycholate cotransporting polypeptide receptor
C. Sodium lithocholate cotransporting polypeptide receptor
D. All of the above

Entry of HBV into hepatocytes is mediated by binding to the sodium taurocholate cotransporting polypeptide receptor. Hepatitis B virus entry into hepatocytes requires the binding of myristolated N-terminal pre-S1 peptide of large HBsAg to sodium taurocholate co-transporting peptide, the functional receptor for HBV into hepatocytes.

1314. Which is the largest overlapping gene in Hepatitis B virus?
Harrison's 20th Ed. Chapter 332 Page 2348 Figure 332-3

A. S
B. C
C. P
D. X

The P gene of HBV is the largest gene and codes for DNA polymerase.

1315. Which of the following statements about overlapping genes in Hepatitis B virus is false?
Harrison's 20th Ed. Chapter 332 Page 2348 Figure 332-3

A. S gene codes for HBsAg
B. P gene codes for DNA polymerase
C. C gene codes for HBeAg
D. X gene codes for HBcAg

1316. Which of the following may bind to p53?
Harrison's 20th Ed. Chapter 332 Page 2348 Figure 332-3

A. HBsAg
B. HBcAg
C. HBeAg
D. HBxAg

The S gene codes for the "major" envelope protein, HBsAg. The largest gene, P, codes for DNA polymerase. C gene codes for nucleocapsid proteins—HBeAg and HBcAg. X gene codes for HBxAg which can transactivate the transcription of cellular and viral genes and may contribute to carcinogenesis by binding to p53.

1317. Which particulate form of HBV is most numerous in blood?
Harrison's 20th Ed. Chapter 332 Page 2348

A. 22-nm
B. 27-nm
C. 42-nm
D. All of the above

Of the three particulate forms of HBV, the most numerous are the 22-nm particles, which appear as spherical or long filamentous forms. These are antigenically indistinguishable from outer surface or envelope protein of HBV and are thought to represent excess viral envelope protein.

1318. Which of the following represents the intact hepatitis B virion?
Harrison's 20th Ed. Chapter 332 Page 2348

A. 22-nm
B. 27-nm
C. 42-nm
D. All of the above

Large, 42-nm, double-shelled spherical particles represent the intact hepatitis B virion.

1319. Which of the following about hepatitis B surface antigen (HBsAg) is false?
Harrison's 20th Ed. Chapter 332 Page 2348

A. It is the product of the S gene of HBV
B. Envelope protein
C. Expressed on outer surface of virion and on smaller spherical & tubular structures
D. None of the above

1320. Which is the common group-reactive antigen in different HBsAg subdeterminants?
Harrison's 20th Ed. Chapter 332 Page 2348

A. a
B. b
C. c
D. d

In different HBsAg subdeterminants, common group-reactive antigen, "a" is shared by all HBsAg isolates.

1321. Number of genotypes in Hepatitis B isolates is?
Harrison's 20th Ed. Chapter 332 Page 2348

A. 4
B. 10
C. 12
D. 16

In 1988, hepatitis B virus (HBV) was classified into four genotypes by a sequence divergence in the entire genome exceeding 8%, and designated by capital letters of the alphabet from A to D. Later, six more were added from E to J. Genotype H is phylogenetically closely related to genotype F.

1322. Genotypes of HBV were defined by a sequence divergence greater than what percentage in the entire genome?
Harrison's 20th Ed. Chapter 332 Page 2348

A. 2
B. 4
C. 6
D. 8

Genotypes of HBV were defined by a sequence divergence greater than 8% in the entire genome.

1323. Which of the following is not a major serotype of HBV?
Harrison's 20th Ed. Chapter 332 Page 2348

A. add
B. adw
C. ayr
D. ayw

HBV virus is divided into 4 major serotypes (adr, adw, ayr, ayw) based on antigenic epitopes present on its envelope proteins, and into ten genotypes (A-J) according to overall nucleotide sequence variation of the genome. Genotypes of HBV were defined by a sequence divergence > 8% in the entire genome. HBsAg serotypes adw, adr, ayw and ayr are readily determined by immunological methods, and they were regarded the phenotypic expression of HBV genotypes. All HBV isolates of genotype A or B isolates were adw and all genotype D isolates were ayw. Isolates of genotype C were heterogeneous and covered adw, adr and ayr.

1324. The protein product of S region in Hepatitis B virus is?
Harrison's 20th Ed. Chapter 332 Page 2348

A. Major protein
B. Middle protein
C. Large protein
D. All of the above

1325. The protein product of S gene in Hepatitis B virus is?
Harrison's 20th Ed. Chapter 332 Page 2348

A. Major protein
B. Middle protein
C. Large protein
D. All of the above

1326. The protein product of S region plus pre-S2 region in Hepatitis B virus is?
Harrison's 20th Ed. Chapter 332 Page 2348

A. Major protein
B. Middle protein
C. Large protein
D. All of the above

1327. The protein product of pre-S1 plus pre-S2 plus S regions in Hepatitis B virus is?
Harrison's 20th Ed. Chapter 332 Page 2348

A. Major protein
B. Middle protein
C. Large protein
D. All of the above

The envelope protein, HBsAg, is the product of the S gene of HBV. HBsAg gene is one long open reading frame but contains 3 in frame "start" (ATG) codons that divide the gene into 3 sections, pre-S1, pre-S2, and S. S gene codes for the "major" envelope protein - HBsAg. "Large" protein is the product of pre-S1 + pre-S2 + S. "Middle" protein is the product of pre-S2 + S.

1328. HBsAg is also called?
Harrison's 20th Ed. Chapter 332 Page 2348

A. Major protein
B. Middle protein
C. Large protein
D. All of the above

The S gene codes for the "major" envelope protein, HBsAg.

1329. Nucleocapsid proteins are coded for by?
Harrison's 20th Ed. Chapter 332 Page 2348

A. Pre-S1 gene
B. Pre-S2 gene
C. S gene
D. C gene

Nucleocapsid proteins are coded for by the C gene. The C gene codes for two nucleocapsid proteins, HBeAg, a soluble, secreted protein (initiation from the pre-C region of the gene), and HBcAg, the intracellular core protein (initiation after pre-C).

1330. Which of the following is not a nucleocapsid protein?
Harrison's 20th Ed. Chapter 332 Page 2348

A. HBsAg
B. HBeAg
C. HBcAg
D. All of the above

The C gene codes for two nucleocapsid proteins, HBeAg and HBcAg. If translation is initiated at the precore region of C gene, the protein product is HBeAg, while if translation begins with the core region of C gene, HBcAg is the protein product.

1331. Which of the following represents excess virus coat material?
Harrison's 20th Ed. Chapter 332 Page 2348

A. HBsAg
B. HBeAg
C. HBcAg
D. HBxAg

1332. In Hepatitis B virus, which of the following is a 'secreted' nucleocapsid protein?
Harrison's 20th Ed. Chapter 332 Page 2348

A. HBsAg
B. HBeAg
C. HBcAg
D. HBxAg

HBeAg is a soluble, secreted nucleocapsid protein. HBeAg provides a convenient, readily detectable, qualitative marker of HBV replication and relative infectivity. HBeAg has a signal peptide that binds it to the smooth endoplasmic reticulum and leads to its secretion into the circulation.

1333. Which of the following is qualitative marker of HBV replication & relative infectivity?
Harrison's 20th Ed. Chapter 332 Page 2349

A. HBsAg
B. HBeAg
C. HBcAg
D. HBxAg

HBsAg-positive serum containing HBeAg is highly infectious and associated with presence of hepatitis B virions than HBeAg-negative or anti-HBe-positive serum. Anti-HBeAg positivity usually indicates low infectivity and no replication, unless patient is precore mutant.

1334. Persistence of HBeAg in serum beyond how many months of acute infection is predictive of chronic infection?
Harrison's 20th Ed. Chapter 332 Page 2349

A. 1 month
B. 2 month
C. 3 month
D. Any of the above

HBeAg appears transiently and early during acute hepatitis B infection. Persistence of HBeAg in serum beyond the first three months of acute infection may be predictive of the development of chronic infection.

1335. HBsAg-positive mothers rarely infect their offspring, if their serum contains?
Harrison's 20th Ed. Chapter 332 Page 2349

A. HBsAg
B. HBeAg
C. Anti-HBs
D. Anti-HBe

HBsAg-positive mothers who are HBeAg-positive almost invariably (>90%) transmit hepatitis B infection to their offspring, whereas HBsAg-positive mothers with anti-HBe rarely infect their offspring.

1336. Presence of HBeAg during chronic hepatitis B tends to be associated with?
Harrison's 20th Ed. Chapter 332 Page 2349

A. Ongoing viral replication
B. Infectivity
C. Inflammatory liver injury
D. All of the above

1337. Which of the following particles of HBV do not circulate in the serum?
Harrison's 20th Ed. Chapter 332 Page 2349

A. HBsAg
B. HBcAg
C. HBeAg
D. All of the above

HBcAg is intracellular. When in serum, it is within an HBsAg coat. Therefore, naked HBcAg particles do not circulate in serum and are not detectable routinely in serum of patients with HBV infection.

1338. Hepatitis B patients contain which of the following circulating antibodies?
Harrison's 20th Ed. Chapter 332 Page 2349

A. Anti-HBe Ag
B. Anti-HBs Ag
C. Anti HBcAg
D. All of the above

Hepatitis B patients contain circulating antibodies against HBcAg (hepatitis B core antigen), & develop antibodies against HBeAg & HBsAg (anti-HBe & anti-HBs) at later stages.

1339. Which of the following HBV genes codes for DNA polymerase?
Harrison's 20th Ed. Chapter 332 Page 2349

A. S
B. C
C. P
D. X

Gene P of the HBV genes is the largest and codes for DNA polymerase which has both DNA-dependent DNA polymerase and RNA-dependent reverse transcriptase activities.

1340. Which of the following about HBV DNA polymerase is false?
Harrison's 20th Ed. Chapter 332 Page 2349

A. Encoded by P gene
B. Has DNA-dependent DNA polymerase activity
C. Has RNA-dependent reverse transcriptase activity
D. None of the above

1341. Which of the following is a nonparticulate protein of HBV?
Harrison's 20th Ed. Chapter 332 Page 2349

A. HBeAg
B. HBcAg
C. HBxAg
D. All of the above

1342. Which of the following HBV antigens stimulates HBV reverse transcription and HBV DNA replication?
Harrison's 20th Ed. Chapter 332 Page 2349

A. HBsAg
B. HBeAg
C. HBcAg
D. HBxAg

Hepatitis B x antigen (HBxAg) activates signal-transduction pathways that lead to stimulation of HBV reverse transcription and HBV DNA replication.

1343. Clinical association is observed between expression of which of the following & severe chronic hepatitis & hepatocellular carcinoma?
Harrison's 20th Ed. Chapter 332 Page 2349

A. HBsAg
B. HBeAg
C. HBcAg
D. HBxAg

Because HBxAg transactivation enhances replication of HBV, clinical association is observed between its expression with severe chronic hepatitis and hepatocellular carcinoma.

1344. Expression of which of the following HBV antigens induces programmed cell death (apoptosis)?
Harrison's 20th Ed. Chapter 332 Page 2349

A. HBsAg
B. HBeAg
C. HBcAg
D. HBxAg

Expression of HBxAg induces programmed cell death (apoptosis).

1345. Which of the following is transactivated by expression of HBxAg?
Harrison's 20th Ed. Chapter 332 Page 2350

A. Transcription & replication of HIV
B. Transactivation of human interferon gene
C. Transactivation of class I major histocompatibility genes
D. All of the above

1346. After infection with HBV, the first virologic marker detectable in serum is?

Harrison's 20th Ed. Chapter 332 Page 2350

A. HBsAg
B. HBeAg
C. HBcAg
D. HBxAg

Upon HBV infection, the first virologic marker detectable in serum within 1-12 weeks, usually between 8-12 weeks is HBsAg.

1347. Which of the following statements is true?

Harrison's 20th Ed. Chapter 332 Page 2350

A. Circulating HBsAg precedes elevations of SGOT/SGPT
B. Circulating HBsAg follow elevations of SGOT/SGPT
C. Circulating HBsAg coincide with elevations of SGOT/SGPT
D. None of the above

Circulating HBsAg precedes elevations of serum aminotransferase activity and clinical symptoms by 2-6 weeks and remains detectable during the entire icteric or symptomatic phase of acute hepatitis B and beyond.

1348. After the onset of jaundice, HBsAg rarely persists beyond how many months?

Harrison's 20th Ed. Chapter 332 Page 2350

A. 1 month
B. 3 months
C. 6 months
D. 9 months

In typical cases, HBsAg becomes undetectable 1-2 months after the onset of jaundice and rarely persists beyond 6 months.

1349. Of the following antibodies against HBV, which one is first to appear?

Harrison's 20th Ed. Chapter 332 Page 2350

A. Anti-HBc
B. Anti-HBs
C. Anti-HBe
D. None of the above

1350. Of the following antibodies against HBV, which one is detected last?

Harrison's 20th Ed. Chapter 332 Page 2350

A. Anti-HBc
B. Anti-HBs
C. Anti-HBe
D. None of the above

Of the 3 antibodies against HBV, anti-HBc develops first, whereas anti-HBs antibody is detected last. Anti-HBc appears in serum within the first 1-2 weeks after appearance of HBsAg & preceding anti-HBs by weeks to months. Anti-HBs becomes detectable after HBsAg disappears in serum and remains detectable indefinitely thereafter.

1351. Which of the following about HBsAg in acute HBV infection is false?

Harrison's 20th Ed. Chapter 332 Page 2350

A. Precedes rise in ALT
B. Precedes clinical symptoms
C. Detectable during entire icteric or symptomatic phase
D. Rarely persists beyond 3 months

Circulating HBsAg precedes rise in serum aminotransferase levels & clinical symptoms by 2-6 weeks and remains detectable during the entire icteric or symptomatic phase of acute hepatitis B & beyond. HBsAg becomes undetectable 1-2 months after onset of jaundice & rarely persists beyond 6 months.

1352. Which of the following about serology in acute HBV infection is false?

Harrison's 20th Ed. Chapter 332 Page 2350

A. Anti-HBs appears after HBsAg disappears
B. Anti-HBs remains detectable indefinitely
C. Anti-HBs precedes appearance of anti-HBc
D. HBeAg appears almost concurrently with HBsAg

After HBsAg disappears, antibody to HBsAg (anti-HBs) becomes detectable in serum & remains detectable indefinitely. HBcAg naked core particles do not circulate in serum & therefore, HBcAg is not detectable routinely in serum of patients with HBV infection. Anti-HBc is readily demonstrable in serum, beginning within first 1-2 weeks after appearance of HBsAg & preceding detectable levels of anti-HBs by weeks to months. HBeAg appears concurrently with or shortly after HBsAg.

1353. Which of the following is true during "gap" or "window" period in acute HBV infection?

Harrison's 20th Ed. Chapter 332 Page 2350

A. Absence of HBsAg
B. Absence of anti-HBs
C. Presence of IgM anti-HBc
D. All of the above

At times a gap of several weeks or longer may separate disappearance of HBsAg & appearance of anti-HBs. During this "gap" or "window" period, anti-HBc may be the only serologic evidence of current or recent HBV infection & blood containing IgM anti-HBc in the absence of HBsAg & anti-HBs has been implicated in development of transfusion-associated hepatitis B. HBV DNA may be low or undetected.

1354. Presence of which of the following represents hepatitis B infection in remote past?

Harrison's 20th Ed. Chapter 332 Page 2350

A. Anti-HBc
B. Anti-HBs
C. Anti-HBe
D. Any of the above

Isolated anti-HBc represent hepatitis B infection in the remote past. IgM anti-HBc predominates during the first six months after acute infection, whereas IgG anti-HBc persists beyond six months. Generally, in persons who have recovered from hepatitis B, anti-HBs and anti-HBc persist indefinitely.

1355. Isolated presence of which of the following suggests hepatitis B infection in remote past?

Harrison's 20th Ed. Chapter 332 Page 2350

A. HBsAg
B. Anti-HBs
C. IgM anti-HBc
D. IgG anti-HBc

After HBV infection, anti-HBc may persist in circulation longer than anti-HBs. Isolated anti-HBc does not indicate active virus replication but indicates HBV infection in remote past.

1356. Recent and remote HBV infections can be distinguished by determination of?

Harrison's 20th Ed. Chapter 332 Page 2350

A. Anti-HBs
B. IgM anti-HBc

C. IgG anti-HBc

D. All of the above

IgM anti-HBc predominates in first 6 months after acute infection, whereas IgG anti-HBc predominates beyond 6 months. In persons who have recovered from hepatitis B, anti-HBs & anti-HBc persist indefinitely.

1357. Presence of isolated anti-HBc suggests?

Harrison's 20th Ed. Chapter 332 Page 2350

A. Hepatitis B infection in the remote past

B. Low-level hepatitis B viremia (HBsAg below threshold)

C. Cross-reacting or false-positive immunologic specificity

D. Any of the above

Isolated anti-HBc does not necessarily indicate active virus replication.

1358. Which of the following genotype of HBV is frequent in India?

Hepatol Res. 2009;39(2):157-63

A. A

B. B

C. C

D. Any of the above

1359. Which of the following is false about the serology in first stage of HBV patient?

Harrison's 20th Ed. Chapter 332 Page 2350

A. Presence of HBsAg

B. Presence of HBeAg

C. Presence of anti-HBs antibody

D. Presence of IgM anti-HBc antibody

First stage of HBV infection is characterized by presence of HBsAg, HBeAg, and IgM class of anti-HBc antibodies. In intermediate stage, patients lose HBeAg, develop anti-HBe antibodies & enter into clinical remission. Finally, loss of HBsAg & rise of the anti-HBs antibody indicate recovery from infection.

1360. Which of the following about HBV viremia titer is false?

Int. J. Med. Sci. 2005;2(1)

A. Highest during HBeAg phase of infection

B. Declines during the anti-HBe phase

C. Disappears at the anti-HBs phase

D. None of the above

1361. Which of the following is false about expression of core protein and HBeAg?

Int. J. Med. Sci. 2005;2(1)

A. Core protein is translated from pregenomic mRNA, using the ATG codon at 1901 as initiation site

B. HBeAg is translated from precore mRNA, using ATG at 1814

C. G1896A nonsense mutation in precore region specifically prevents translation of HBeAg

D. None of the above

Core protein is translated from pregenomic mRNA, using the ATG codon at 1901 as initiation site. HBeAg is translated from the precore mRNA, using ATG at 1814. G1896A nonsense mutation in the precore region specifically prevents translation of HBeAg.

1362. HBeAg differs from HBcAg by a?

Journal of General Virology. 1995;76(4):1041-5

A. Longer N-terminus and longer C-terminal tail

B. Shorter N-terminus and shorter C-terminal tail

C. Shorter N-terminus and longer C-terminal tail

D. Longer N-terminus and shorter C-terminal tail

HBeAg differs from core protein (HBcAg) by a longer N-terminus and shorter C-terminal tail. HBeAg is a 15 kDa soluble antigen derived from a precursor protein (precore protein) by two processing events, cleavage of the N-terminal signal peptide and cleavage of the C-terminal 34 amino acids.

1363. Which of the following statements about HBV is false?

Harrison's 20th Ed. Chapter 332 Page 2350

A. HBeAg is not part of the virus particle

B. Anti-HBc antibody rises soon after infection

C. HBeAg expression is not essential for virus replication

D. None of the above

1364. HBeAg-negative chronic hepatitis B or e-CHB is characterised by all except?

Harrison's 20th Ed. Chapter 332 Page 2350

A. HBsAg-positive for at least 6 months

B. HBeAg-positive

C. Anti-HBe-positive

D. HBV DNA detectable in serum unamplified assays

e-CHB or HBeAg-negative chronic hepatitis B patients are HBsAg-positive for at least 6 months, HBeAg-negative, anti-HBe-positive, with HBV DNA detectable in serum unamplified assays, and active liver disease (elevated AST or ALT, liver histology showing chronic hepatitis with or without cirrhosis).

1365. Which of the following is expressed during periods of peak replication?

Harrison's 20th Ed. Chapter 332 Page 2350

A. HBeAg

B. Pre-S1 proteins

C. Pre-S2 proteins

D. All of the above

HBeAg, appears concurrently with or shortly after HBsAg and its appearance coincides expression of pre-S1 and pre-S2 proteins marking high levels of virus replication and presence of circulating intact virions and detectable HBV DNA.

1366. Which of the following is the qualitative marker of the replicative stage of HBV infection?

Harrison's 20th Ed. Chapter 332 Page 2351

A. HBsAg

B. HBcAg

C. HBeAg

D. HBxAg

Replicative stage of HBV infection is the time of maximal infectivity & liver injury. HBeAg is a qualitative marker & HBV DNA a quantitative marker of replicative phase, during which all three forms of HBV circulate, including intact virions.

1367. Replicative phase of chronic HBV infection converts to relatively nonreplicative phase at a rate of?

Harrison's 20th Ed. Chapter 332 Page 2351

A. 10% per year

B. 20% per year

C. 30% per year

D. 40% per year

Replicative phase of chronic HBV infection converts to a relatively nonreplicative phase at a rate of 10% per year accompanied by seroconversion from HBeAg-positive to anti-HBe-positive.

1368. Seroconversion from HBeAg-positive to anti-HBe-positive is accompanied by which of the following?
Harrison's 20th Ed. Chapter 332 Page 2351

A. Acute elevation in alanine aminotransferase (ALT) activity
B. Hemoglobinuria
C. Anemia
D. All of the above

Seroconversion from HBeAg-positive to anti-HBe-positive is accompanied by a transient, acute hepatitis-like elevation in aminotransferase activity, believed to reflect cell-mediated immune clearance of virus-infected hepatocytes.

1369. Spontaneous reactivation of replicative HBV infection from nonreplicative phase is marked by which of the following?
Harrison's 20th Ed. Chapter 332 Page 2351

A. Re-expression of HBeAg
B. Re-expression of HBV DNA
C. Reappearance of IgM anti-HBc
D. All of the above

Spontaneous reactivations i.e. nonreplicative HBV infection converting back to replicative infection is accompanied by re-expression of HBeAg and HBV DNA, IgM anti-HBc and exacerbations of liver injury.

1370. HBV infections is self-limited if?
Harrison's 20th Ed. Chapter 332 Page 2351

A. HBeAg becomes undetectable after peak rise in ALT
B. HBeAg becomes undetectable before disappearance of HBsAg
C. Anti-HBe becomes detectable before disappearance of HBsAg
D. All of the above

1371. Which of the following about HBeAg in acute HBV infection is false?
Harrison's 20th Ed. Chapter 332 Page 2351

A. Appears with HBsAg
B. Appearance coincides with high viral replication
C. Undetectable after peak rise in ALT
D. Undetectable after disappearance of HBsAg

HBeAg presence coincides with high levels of virus replication and reflects the presence of circulating intact virions and detectable HBV DNA. In self-limited HBV infections, HBeAg becomes undetectable shortly after peak elevations in aminotransferase activity, before the disappearance of HBsAg, and anti-HBe then becomes detectable, coinciding with a period of relatively lower infectivity.

1372. Which of the following about chronic HBV infection is false?
Harrison's 20th Ed. Chapter 332 Page 2351

A. HBsAg detectable > 6 months
B. IgG anti-HBc present
C. Anti-HBs low to absent
D. None of the above

In chronic HBV infection, HBsAg remains detectable beyond 6 months, anti-HBc is primarily of the IgG class, and anti-HBs is either undetectable or detectable at low levels.

1373. Replicative chronic hepatitis B in the absence of HBeAg occurs in which of the following situations?
Harrison's 20th Ed. Chapter 332 Page 2351

A. Patients with core mutations
B. Patients with precore mutations
C. Patients with pre S1 mutations
D. Patients with pre S2 mutations

Replicative chronic hepatitis B in the absence of HBeAg occurs in patients with precore mutations who cannot synthesize HBeAg.

1374. HBeAg-negative chronic hepatitis with mutations in the precore region is now the most frequently encountered form of hepatitis B in which region of the world?
Harrison's 20th Ed. Chapter 332 Page 2351

A. North America
B. South America
C. Mediterranean countries
D. Southeast Asia

HBeAg-negative chronic hepatitis with mutations in the precore region is now the most frequently encountered form of hepatitis B in Mediterranean countries and in Europe.

1375. Which of the following is false about severe chronic HBV infection due to precore region HBV mutant?
Harrison's 20th Ed. Chapter 332 Page 2351

A. Detectable HBV DNA
B. HBeAg negative
C. Anti-HBe positive
D. None of the above

Molecular variants of HBV may not express typical viral proteins i.e. nucleocapsid proteins, envelope proteins, or both. Severe chronic HBV infection due to precore region HBV mutation have detectable HBV DNA (> 105 copies/ml), and anti-HBe but no HBeAg as the mutant virus is incapable of encoding HBeAg. This is an example of single base substitution, from G to A, which occurs in the second to last codon of pre-C gene at nucleotide 1896 results in the replacement of the TGG tryptophan codon by a stop codon (TAG), which prevents the translation of HBeAg.

1376. HBV escape mutants best relate to which of the following?
Harrison's 20th Ed. Chapter 332 Page 2351

A. Single base substitution
B. Single base addition
C. Single amino acid substitution
D. Single amino acid addition

In escape mutants of HBV there occurs a single amino acid substitution, from glycine to arginine at position 145 of the immunodominant "a" determinant common to all subtypes of HBsAg. This change in HBsAg leads to a loss of neutralizing activity by anti-HBs. This HBV/a mutant is seen in active and passive immunization, and in liver transplant recipients who underwent the procedure for hepatitis B and who were treated with a high-potency human monoclonal anti-HBs preparation.

1377. Extrahepatic site where Hepatitis B antigen and HBV DNA has been identified is?
Harrison's 20th Ed. Chapter 332 Page 2351

A. Bone marrow
B. Spleen
C. Pancreas
D. All of the above

Although not associated with tissue injury, extrahepatic site where Hepatitis B antigens and HBV DNA have been identified include lymph nodes, bone marrow, circulating lymphocytes, spleen, and pancreas.

1378. Which of the following is a member of the genus Deltavirus?
Harrison's 20th Ed. Chapter 332 Page 2351

A. Hepatitis D virus
B. Marburg virus
C. California encephalitis virus
D. All of the above

Delta hepatitis agent (HDV) is the only member of the genus Deltavirus.

1379. Which of the following is false about delta hepatitis virus?
Harrison's 20th Ed. Chapter 332 Page 2351

A. Defective RNA virus
B. 35- to 37-nm in size
C. 1700-nucleotide genome
D. Has antigenic homology with HBV antigens

HDV is a defective RNA virus that coinfects with and requires the helper function of HBV for its replication & expression. It is formalin-sensitive, 35- to 37-nm virus with a hybrid structure. Its genome is a 1700-nucleotide, circular, single-strand RNA. Delta antigen bears no antigenic homology with any of the HBV antigens.

1380. Delta core of HDV is "encapsidated" by an outer envelope of?
Harrison's 20th Ed. Chapter 332 Page 2351

A. HBcAg
B. HBsAg
C. HBeAg
D. None of the above

The delta core of HDV is "encapsidated" by an outer envelope of HBsAg quite like that of HBV.

1381. The single-stranded RNA genome of HDV is homologous to an extent with which gene of HBV?
Harrison's 20th Ed. Chapter 332 Page 2351

A. S
B. C
C. P
D. X

HDV genome is a small, 1700-nucleotide, circular, single-strand RNA of negative polarity that is nonhomologous with HBV DNA, except for a small area of the polymerase gene.

1382. HDV RNA requires which of the following for its replication?
Harrison's 20th Ed. Chapter 332 Page 2351

A. Host RNA polymerase I
B. Viral RNA polymerase I
C. Host RNA polymerase II
D. Viral RNA polymerase II

HDV RNA requires host RNA polymerase II for its replication via RNA-directed RNA synthesis by transcription of genomic RNA to a complementary antigenomic (plus strand) RNA. The antigenomic RNA, in turn, serves as a template for subsequent genomic RNA synthesis.

1383. When HDV infects a person simultaneously with HBV, it is called?
Harrison's 20th Ed. Chapter 332 Page 2352

A. Super-infection
B. Co-infection
C. Multiple infection
D. Sub-infection

Co-infection means HDV infecting a person simultaneously with HBV. Superinfection means HDV infecting a person already infected with HBV.

1384. Which of the following is false about delta hepatitis virus?
Harrison's 20th Ed. Chapter 332 Page 2352

A. HDV relies absolutely on HBV
B. HDV replication tends to suppress HBV replication
C. In chronic HDV infection, anti-HDV circulates in high titer
D. None of the above

1385. Which of the following is false about delta hepatitis virus?
Harrison's 20th Ed. Chapter 332 Page 2352

A. HDV antigen is expressed in hepatocyte nuclei
B. Intracellular replication of HDV RNA can occur without HBV
C. Duration of HDV infection determined by duration of HBV infection
D. In acute HDV infection, anti-HDV detected before symptoms appear

In acute HDV infection, anti-HDV is detected 30–40 days after symptoms appear.

1386. Which of the following is an HDV protein?
Harrison's 20th Ed. Chapter 332 Page 2352

A. HDAg
B. HDsAg
C. HDeAg
D. All of the above

HDV RNA has only one open reading frame, and delta antigen (HDAg), a product of the antigenomic strand is the only known HDV protein. When HDV infection is transmitted from a donor with a particular HBsAg subtype to an HBsAg-positive recipient with a different subtype, HDV assumes the HBsAg subtype of the recipient, rather than the donor.

1387. Which of the following hepatitis was earlier called "non-A, non-B hepatitis"?
Harrison's 20th Ed. Chapter 332 Page 2352

A. Hepatitis A
B. Hepatitis B
C. Hepatitis C
D. Hepatitis E

Before its identification, Hepatitis C virus was labeled as "non-A, non-B hepatitis".

1388. Hepatitis C virus was first identified in which year?
Liver Int. 2009;29(1):82-8

A. 1986
B. 1989
C. 1992
D. 1995

The non-A, non-B hepatitis virus, later known as Hepatitis C virus was first identified in 1989 by scientists at a California biotechnology company called Chiron Corporation who were collaborating with investigators at the Centers for Disease Control and Prevention (CDC).

1389. Which of the following genera belong to the family Flaviviridae?
Harrison's 20th Ed. Chapter 332 Page 2352

A. Pestivirus
B. Hepacivirus
C. Flavivirus
D. All of the above

The genera Pestivirus, Hepacivirus and Flavivirus are grouped together in the family Flaviviridae.

1390. Which of the following is a hepacivirus?
Harrison's 20th Ed. Chapter 332 Page 2352

A. Hepatitis C virus
B. Hepatitis D virus
C. Hepatitis E virus
D. All of the above

HCV is the only member of the genus Hepacivirus in the family Flaviviridae.

1391. **Which of the following is a member of family Flaviviridae?**
   Harrison's 20th Ed. Chapter 332 Page 2352
   A. Yellow fever virus
   B. Dengue virus
   C. Hepatitis C virus
   D. All of the above

   Members of family Flaviviridae are Yellow fever virus, Dengue virus, St. Louis encephalitis virus, West Nile virus, Hepatitis C virus (HCV) and Hepatitis G virus.

1392. **Which of the following is a structural protein in HCV?**
   Harrison's 20th Ed. Chapter 332 Page 2352
   A. C
   B. E1
   C. E2
   D. All of the above

   The three structural genes at the 5' end of hepatitis C virus genome are C - which codes for nucleocapsid, and E1 and E2 - which code for envelope glycoproteins.

1393. **In hepatitis C virus genome, which of the following functions as an ion channel?**
   Harrison's 20th Ed. Chapter 332 Page 2352
   A. C
   B. E1
   C. E2
   D. p7

   Placed adjacent to the structural proteins, p7 is a membrane protein that appears to function as an ion channel.

1394. **Which of the following is present between structural & nonstructural regions of hepatitis C virus genome?**
   Harrison's 20th Ed. Chapter 332 Page 2352 Figure 332-6
   A. NS3
   B. NS4
   C. NS5A
   D. p7

1395. **NS2 codes for which of the following enzymes?**
   Harrison's 20th Ed. Chapter 332 Page 2352 Figure 332-6
   A. Cysteine protease
   B. Serine protease
   C. RNA helicase
   D. All of the above

   NS2 codes for a cysteine protease. NS3 codes for a serine protease and an RNA helicase.

1396. **Which of the following nonstructural regions of hepatitis C virus genome codes for RNA-dependent RNA polymerase?**
   Harrison's 20th Ed. Chapter 332 Page 2352 Figure 332-6
   A. NS3
   B. NS4
   C. NS5A
   D. NS5B

   At 3' end are seven nonstructural (NS) proteins: p7, NS2, NS3, NS4A, NS4B, NS5A, and NS5B. NS5B codes for an RNA-dependent RNA polymerase.

1397. **Which of the following is false about HCV?**
   Harrison's 20th Ed. Chapter 332 Page 2352
   A. 40–60 nm in diameter
   B. 9600-nucleotide RNA virus
   C. Its half-life is 2.7 hours
   D. None of the above

1398. **Which of the following is false about HCV?**
   Harrison's 20th Ed. Chapter 332 Page 2352
   A. HCV enters hepatocyte via CD81 receptor
   B. Does not induce lasting immunity against reinfection
   C. Most sensitive indicator is the presence of HCV RNA
   D. None of the above

   HCV gains entry into the hepatocyte via the nonliver-specific CD81 receptor and the liver-specific tight junction protein claudin-1. Most sensitive indicator of HCV infection is presence of HCV RNA, that requires molecular amplification by PCR or transcription-mediated amplification (TMA).

1399. **Host receptor to which HCV binds on cell entry is?**
   Harrison's 20th Ed. Chapter 332 Page 2352
   A. Occludin
   B. Scavenger receptor B1
   C. Epidermal growth factor receptor
   D. All of the above

   Other host receptors to which HCV binds on cell entry includes occludin, low-density lipoprotein receptors, glycosaminoglycans, scavenger receptor B1 and epidermal growth factor receptor.

1400. **HCV masquerades as which of the following?**
   Harrison's 20th Ed. Chapter 332 Page 2352
   A. Viroid
   B. Nucleocapsid protein
   C. Lipoprotein
   D. CD81 receptor

   HCV is a lipoviroparticle and masquerades as a lipoprotein.

1401. **Internal ribosomal entry site (IRES) is situated at which end of the HCV genome?**
   Harrison's 20th Ed. Chapter 332 Page 2352
   A. 3' end
   B. 5' end
   C. Both 3' end and 5' end
   D. Any of the above

   The 5' end of HCV genome consists of an untranslated region containing an internal ribosomal entry site (IRES) adjacent to the genes for three structural proteins, C, E1 and E2.

1402. **Host cofactor involved in HCV replication is?**
   Harrison's 20th Ed. Chapter 332 Page 2352
   A. Cyclophilin A
   B. Cyclophilin B
   C. Cyclophilin C
   D. Cyclophilin D

1403. **Which of the following is a liver-specific host microRNA?**
   Harrison's 20th Ed. Chapter 332 Page 2352
   A. miR-122
   B. miR-146a

C. miR-155
D. miR-21

Host cofactors involved in HCV replication include cyclophilin A (which binds to NS5A), and liver-specific host microRNA miR-122.

1404. Number of HCV genotypes identified is?
Harrison's 20th Ed. Chapter 332 Page 2352

A. 2
B. 3
C. 4
D. 6

Till date HCV genotypes identified are 6 as well as >50 subtypes within genotypes.

1405. HCV genotypes differ one from another in sequence homology by?
Harrison's 20th Ed. Chapter 332 Page 2352

A. 10%
B. 20%
C. 30%
D. 40%

1406. HCV subtypes differ one from another in sequence homology by?
Harrison's 20th Ed. Chapter 332 Page 2352

A. 10%
B. 20%
C. 30%
D. 40%

Genotypes differ one from another in sequence homology by 30%, subtypes differ by ~ 20%. Those with less differences in sequence homology are referred to as quasispecies.

1407. Which of the following interferes with effective humoral immunity in HCV infection?
Harrison's 20th Ed. Chapter 332 Page 2352

A. High replication rate
B. Large hypervariable region
C. High mutation rate
D. Intragenotypic differences

High mutation rate of HCV virus interferes with effective humoral immunity. Neither heterologous nor homologous immunity develops commonly after acute HCV infection.

1408. In which HCV genotype, hepatic steatosis & clinical progression are more likely?
Harrison's 20th Ed. Chapter 332 Page 2352

A. 1
B. 2
C. 3
D. 4

In HCV genotype 3, hepatic steatosis & clinical progression are more likely.

1409. Differences exist among HCV genotypes in as regards?
Harrison's 20th Ed. Chapter 332 Page 2352

A. Responsiveness to antiviral therapy
B. Pathogenicity
C. Clinical progression
D. All of the above

There are no differences among HCV genotypes in pathogenicity or clinical progression. However, differences exist among HCV genotypes in responsiveness to antiviral therapy.

1410. In acute HCV infection, immunoassays detect anti-HCV antibodies against which of the following proteins?
Harrison's 20th Ed. Chapter 332 Page 2352

A. Core
B. NS3 region
C. NS5 region
D. All of the above

1411. HCV RNA is reported as?
Harrison's 20th Ed. Chapter 332 Page 2353

A. International units (IUs) per milliliter
B. Microgram per milliliter
C. Copies per milliliter
D. Virions per milliliter

HCV RNA is reported as international units (IUs) per milliliter.

1412. Which of the following is useful to detect the presence of HCV RNA?
Harrison's 20th Ed. Chapter 332 Page 2353

A. Transcription-mediated amplification (TMA)
B. Ligase chain reaction (LCR)
C. Enzyme immunoassays (EIAs)
D. Gas liquid chromatography assays

The most sensitive indicator of HCV infection is the presence of HCV RNA, which requires molecular amplification by PCR or transcription-mediated amplification (TMA).

1413. Which of the following is the first detectable event during acute hepatitis C progressing to chronicity?
Harrison's 20th Ed. Chapter 332 Page 2353 Figure 332-7

A. HCV RNA
B. HCV DNA
C. Elevated alanine aminotransferase (ALT)
D. Elevation and appearance of anti-HCV

During acute hepatitis C progressing to chronicity, HCV RNA is the first detectable event, preceding alanine aminotransferase (ALT) elevation and the appearance of anti-HCV.

1414. "Epidemic, non-A, non-B hepatitis" relates to which of the following?
N Engl J Med. 2012;367:1237-44, Harrison's 20th Ed. Chapter 332 Page 2353

A. Hepatitis A
B. Hepatitis B
C. Hepatitis C
D. Hepatitis E

Hepatitis E was initially identified in 1980 as "epidemic or enterically transmitted, non-A, non-B hepatitis", an infectious, waterborne illness similar to hepatitis A.

1415. In India, most common cause of acute hepatitis is?
Harrison's 20th Ed. Chapter 332 Page 2353

A. Hepatitis A
B. Hepatitis B

C. Hepatitis C
D. Hepatitis E

In India, enterically transmitted HEV is the most common cause of acute hepatitis.

1416. Which of the following about HEV is false?
N Engl J Med. 2012;367:1237-44, Harrison's 20th Ed. Chapter 332 Page 2353

A. Enveloped virus
B. Single-stranded, positive-sense RNA genome
C. Genome is 7.2 kb in length
D. Genome contains three open reading frames (ORFs)

HEV is a small (32- to 34-nm), nonenveloped virus with a single-strand, positive-sense RNA genome (7.2 kb in length) which contains three partially overlapping open reading frames (ORFs) bracketed by short 5' and 3' nontranslated regions.

1417. ORF1 encodes which of the following nonstructural proteins?
N Engl J Med. 2012;367:1237-44

A. Methyl transferase (MT)
B. Cysteine protease (Pro)
C. Helicase (Hel)
D. All of the above

ORF1 encodes nonstructural proteins namely methyl transferase (MT), cysteine protease (Pro), helicase (Hel), and RNA polymerase (Pol). ORF1 also encodes three regions of unknown function (Y, H, and X).

1418. Which of the following ORF in Hepatitis E virus genome encodes the nonstructural, enzymatic activities required for viral replication?
N Engl J Med. 2012;367:1237-44, Harrison's 20th Ed. Chapter 332 Page 2353

A. ORF1
B. ORF2
C. ORF3
D. All of the above

Largest of three ORFs, ORF1 encodes the nonstructural, enzymatic activities required for viral replication.

1419. In HEV, which of the following genes encode the nucleocapsid protein?
Harrison's 20th Ed. Chapter 332 Page 2353

A. ORF1
B. ORF2
C. ORF3
D. All of the above

The middle-sized open reading frame 2 (ORF2) gene in HEV encodes the nucleocapsid protein. Largest ORF1 encodes nonstructural proteins involved in virus replication. The smallest ORF3, encodes a structural protein whose function remains undetermined.

1420. ORF gene relates to?
Harrison's 20th Ed. Chapter 332 Page 2353

A. Hepatitis A
B. Hepatitis B
C. Hepatitis C
D. Hepatitis E

HEV has three open reading frames (ORF) genes.

1421. Which of the following acts as an animal reservoir contributing to the perpetuation of HEV?
Harrison's 20th Ed. Chapter 332 Page 2353

A. Swine
B. Bird
C. Fish
D. Dog

Contributing to the perpetuation of HEV are animal reservoirs, most notably in swine. Others include camels, deer, rats, and rabbits.

1422. Which of the following best relates to HEV?
N Engl J Med. 2012;367:1237-44, Harrison's 20th Ed. Chapter 332 Page 2353

A. Flaviviridae
B. Hepeviridae
C. Rhabdoviridae
D. Arenaviridae

HEV was the first member to be identified in the Hepeviridae family.

1423. Which of the following about HEV is false?
N Engl J Med. 2012;367:1237-44

A. HEV replicates in cytoplasm
B. Genotypes 1 and 2 are human viruses
C. Genotypes 3 and 4 are swine viruses
D. None of the above

HEV replicates in cytoplasm. Four genotypes of HEV have been categorized into two major groups. Genotypes 1 and 2 are human viruses that cause epidemic hepatitis with waterborne and fecal-oral transmission. Genotypes 3 and 4 are swine viruses.

1424. Which of the following about HEV infection is false?
N Engl J Med. 2012;367:1237-44

A. HEV RNA is detectable in stool during incubation period
B. HEV RNA is detectable in serum during incubation period
C. IgM antibody is undetectable during recovery
D. None of the above

Both IgM anti-HEV and IgG anti-HEV appear early during acute infection, but both fall rapidly after acute infection, reaching low levels within 9–12 months.

1425. Incubation period of acute hepatitis E infection is?
N Engl J Med. 2012;367:1237-44

A. 1 to 2 weeks
B. 2 to 4 weeks
C. 3 to 8 weeks
D. 6 to 12 weeks

Acute hepatitis E has an incubation period of 3 to 8 weeks.

1426. Average case fatality rate in acute HEV infections is?
N Engl J Med. 2012;367:1237-44

A. 0%
B. 2%
C. 3%
D. 5%

Acute hepatitis E is mostly self-limited without progression to chronic hepatitis. Average case fatality rate is ~ 5%.

1427. Clinical features of autochthonous hepatitis E include all except?
N Engl J Med. 2012;367:1237-44

A. Disease rates highest among older adults
B. Hepatitis E is preventable by vaccination

C. No neurologic complications
D. Ribavirin, peginterferon indicated

In endemic, or autochthonous hepatitis E, the average age was more than 60 years, and men outnumbered women by at least 3 to 1. Hepatitis E is preventable by vaccination. Autochthonous HEV infection is usually subclinical and mild. Autochthonous hepatitis E has frequent serious complications, including "acute-on-chronic" liver failure, neurologic disorders (polyradiculopathy, the GBS, Bell's palsy, peripheral neuropathy, ataxia, and mental confusion), and chronic hepatitis. Chronic hepatitis E is also susceptible to antiviral therapy (peginterferon, ribavirin, or a combination of two).

1428. Chronic infection in Hepatitis E has been identified almost exclusively among?
N Engl J Med. 2012;367:1237-44

A. Pre-existing liver disease
B. Blood transfusion recipients
C. Pork eaters
D. Immunocompromised persons

Chronic HEV infection has been identified almost exclusively among immunocompromised persons (organ transplant recipients, patients receiving cancer chemotherapy, and HIV-infected persons). Blood transfusion is a potential but rare route of HEV transmission. Chronic hepatitis E is characterized by the persistence of HEV RNA in serum & stool, accompanied by fluctuating, mild-to-moderate elevations in serum ALT levels and low or moderate titers of IgG and IgM anti-HEV antibodies.

1429. Which of the following hepatitis viruses is directly cytopathic to hepatocytes?
Harrison's 20th Ed. Chapter 332 Page 2353

A. Hepatitis A
B. Hepatitis B
C. Hepatitis C
D. None of the above

None of the hepatitis viruses is directly cytopathic to hepatocytes.

1430. Which of the following statements is false?
Harrison's 20th Ed. Chapter 332 Page 2353

A. Hepatitis B virus is not directly cytopathic
B. HBcAg invites cytolytic T cells to destroy hepatocytes
C. Inactive hepatitis B carriers can have normal liver histology
D. None of the above

1431. Which of the following nucleocapsid protein of HBV invites cytolytic T cells to destroy HBV-infected hepatocytes?
Harrison's 20th Ed. Chapter 332 Page 2353

A. HBsAg
B. HBcAg
C. HBxAg
D. All of the above

Nucleocapsid proteins (HBcAg and HBeAg) on the cell membrane are the viral target antigens that, with host antigens, invite cytolytic T cells to destroy HBV-infected hepatocytes.

1432. Acute hepatitis B patients who would recover or progress to chronic hepatitis is determined by?
Harrison's 20th Ed. Chapter 332 Page 2353

A. HBV-specific helper CD4+ T cells levels
B. Polyclonality of CD8+ cytolytic T cell responsiveness
C. Antiviral cytokine elaboration by T cells
D. All of the above

Whether or not, acute hepatitis B patient would recover or progress to chronic hepatitis is determined by differences in robustness & broad polyclonality of CD8+ cytolytic T cell responsiveness; in HBV-specific helper CD4+ T cells level; in virus-specific T cells level; in viral T cell epitope escape mutations; and in elaboration of antiviral cytokines by T cells.

1433. Which of the following participate in the early immune response to HBV infection?
Harrison's 20th Ed. Chapter 332 Page 2353

A. Cytopathic antiviral mechanisms
B. Innate immune system
C. Inflammatory cytokines
D. All of the above

Early immune response to HBV infection leads to elimination of HBV replicative intermediates from cytoplasm & covalently closed circular viral DNA from the nucleus of infected hepatocytes.

1434. Which of the following participates in innate immune response to HBV infection?
Harrison's 20th Ed. Chapter 332 Page 2353

A. Natural killer (NK) cell cytotoxicity
B. Interleukin 10 (IL10) & transforming growth factor β (TGFβ)
C. Major histocompatibility complex
D. All of the above

Ultimately, HBV-HLA–specific cytolytic T cell responses of the adaptive immune system are responsible for recovery from HBV infection.

1435. Fibrosing cholestatic hepatitis best relates to?
Harrison's 20th Ed. Chapter 332 Page 2353

A. Gallstones
B. Liver transplantation
C. HIV infection
D. Cholangiocarcinoma

In patients who undergo liver transplantation for end-stage chronic hepatitis B, occasionally, rapidly progressive liver injury appears in the new liver with an unusual histologic pattern - fibrosing cholestatic hepatitis. Ultrastructurally, it represents a choking of the cell with overwhelming quantities of HBsAg.

1436. Which of the following statements is false?
Harrison's 20th Ed. Chapter 332 Page 2353

A. Patients with defects in cellular immune competence are more likely to remain chronically infected with HBV
B. Chronic HBV infection can occur in the absence of serum hepatitis Be antigen (HBeAg)
C. Most characteristic histologic feature of chronic HBV infection is "ground-glass hepatocyte" due to intracellular accumulation of HBsAg
D. None of the above

1437. Which of the following is associated with a more severe outcome of HBV infection?
Harrison's 20th Ed. Chapter 332 Page 2353

A. Infection with precore genetic mutants of HBV
B. Concomitant HDV and HBV infections
C. In liver transplantation for end-stage chronic hepatitis B
D. All of the above

1438. **HBV infection in neonatal period is associated with all except?**
Harrison's 20th Ed. Chapter 332 Page 2354
   A. Acquisition of immunologic tolerance to HBV
   B. Absence of acute-hepatitis illness
   C. Almost invariable establishment of chronic infection
   D. Never go into cirrhosis & hepatocellular carcinoma

Neonatally acquired HBV infection can may culminate into cirrhosis & hepatocellular carcinoma.

1439. **HBV infection acquired during adolescence or early adulthood is associated with all except?**
Harrison's 20th Ed. Chapter 332 Page 2354
   A. Robust host-immune response
   B. Acute hepatitis-like illness
   C. Failure to recover is the exception
   D. Chronicity is common

Chronicity is uncommon and risk of hepatocellular carcinoma is very low.

1440. **Which of the following is a HBV infection phase?**
Harrison's 20th Ed. Chapter 332 Page 2354
   A. "Immunotolerant" phase
   B. "Immunoreactive" phase
   C. "Inactive" phase
   D. All of the above

1441. **In which of the following, there is no period of immunologic tolerance?**
Harrison's 20th Ed. Chapter 332 Page 2354
   A. Babies born to mothers with replicative chronic HBV infection
   B. Adulthood-acquired HBV infection
   C. Elderly-acquired HBV infection
   D. All of the above

A typical adult living in West has self-limited acute hepatitis B. There is no period of immunologic tolerance.

1442. **Which of the following HLA allele has been linked with self-limited hepatitis C?**
Harrison's 20th Ed. Chapter 332 Page 2354
   A. HLA-B*1501
   B. HLA-B*5701
   C. Single nucleotide polymorphism T allele at IL28B locus
   D. C/C haplotype of the IL28B gene

*C/C haplotype of the IL28B gene has been linked with self-limited hepatitis C. It codes for interferon l3, a component of innate immune antiviral defense. The IL28B association is even stronger when combined with HLA class II DQB1*03:01.*

1443. **Which of the following is type II interferon (IFN)?**
Clin Microbiol Infect. 2014;20:1237-1245
   A. IFN-α
   B. IFN-β
   C. IFN-γ
   D. IFN-λ

IFNs are categorized into three different families: type I IFNs (IFN-α and IFN-β, with least 13 subtypes), type II IFN (IFN-γ), and type III IFN (IFN-λ1–4).

1444. **Interleukin (IL)-28B is also known as?**
Clin Microbiol Infect. 2014;20:1237-1245
   A. IFN-λ1
   B. IFN-λ2
   C. IFN-λ3
   D. IFN-λ4

1445. **IL-28B gene resides on the short arm of chromosome?**
Clin Microbiol Infect. 2014;20:1237-1245
   A. 11
   B. 15
   C. 19
   D. 21

IL-28B gene resides on the short arm of chromosome 19 (19q13.13) and encodes IFN-λ3, which, together with IFN-λ1 (IL-29), IFN-λ2 (IL-28A), and IFN-λ4, constitutes the IFN-λ family.

1446. **Which of the following is related to the association between hepatitis C and autoimmune hepatitis?**
Harrison's 20th Ed. Chapter 332 Page 2354
   A. HCV NS3
   B. HCV NS5A
   C. Cytochrome P450 2D6
   D. All of the above

Cross-reactivity between viral antigens (HCV NS3 & NS5A) and host autoantigens (cytochrome P450 2D6) explain the association between hepatitis C & patients with autoimmune hepatitis and antibodies to liver-kidney microsomal (LKM) antigen (anti-LKM).

1447. **Which of the following plays a pathogenetic role in the extrahepatic manifestations of acute hepatitis B?**
Harrison's 20th Ed. Chapter 332 Page 2354
   A. Cytopathic role of virus
   B. Immune complex - mediated tissue damage
   C. Cryoprecipitable immune complexes
   D. All of the above

Immune complex - mediated tissue damage (HBsAg-anti-HBs with activation of complement system) plays a pathogenetic role in the extrahepatic manifestations of acute hepatitis B.

1448. **Which of the following is an extrahepatic manifestation of chronic hepatitis B?**
Harrison's 20th Ed. Chapter 332 Page 2354
   A. Glomerulonephritis with nephrotic syndrome
   B. Polyarteritis nodosa
   C. Essential mixed cryoglobulinemia (EMC)
   D. All of the above

1449. **Deposition of which of the following occurs in glomerular basement membrane in patients of chronic hepatitis B?**
Harrison's 20th Ed. Chapter 332 Page 2354
   A. HBsAg
   B. Immunoglobulin
   C. C3
   D. All of the above

Glomerulonephritis with nephrotic syndrome seen in chronic hepatitis B is due to deposition of HBsAg, immunoglobulin, and C3 in the glomerular basement membrane.

1450. What percentage of patients with polyarteritis nodosa have HBsAg in their serum?
Harrison's 20th Ed. Chapter 332 Page 2354

A. 5–10%
B. 10–20%
C. 20–30%
D. 30–40%

20–30% of patients with polyarteritis nodosa have HBsAg in their serum.

1451. Which of the following is strongly associated with HCV infection?
N Engl J Med. 2011; 364:1479-80

A. Necrolytic acral erythema
B. Porphyria cutanea tarda
C. Leucocytoclastic vasculitis
D. Lichen planus (LP)

1452. Necrolytic acral erythema closely resembles?
N Engl J Med. 2011; 364:1479-80

A. Atopic dermatitis
B. Pemphigus vulgaris
C. Psoriasis
D. Scleroderma

1453. Necrolytic acral erythema is best related to?
N Engl J Med. 2011; 364:1479-80

A. Calcific chronic pancreatitis
B. Penicillamine therapy
C. Myeloproliferative disorders
D. Zinc deficiency

Necrolytic acral erythema, first described in 1996, is strongly associated with hepatitis C, often an early cutaneous marker of HCV infection. It is described as a well-defined, pruritic or burning, hyperkeratotic erythematous eruption that most often affects the acral surfaces. The pathogenesis of necrolytic acral erythema is related to zinc dysregulation due to hepatitis C induced metabolic alteration. Necrolytic acral erythema closely resembles psoriasis.

1454. Mixed cryoglobulinemia (MC) is associated with which of the following?
Harrison's 20th Ed. Chapter 308 Page 2149

A. HAV
B. HCV
C. HDV
D. HEV

Mixed cryoglobulinemia (MC) is unequivocally associated with HCV. Cryoglobulinemia can be seen with multiple myeloma, lymphoproliferative disorders, connective tissue diseases, infection & liver disease, in many instances it is idiopathic. When there is apparent absence of an underlying disease and presence of cryoprecipitate containing oligoclonal / polyclonal immunoglobulins, this entity is called essential mixed cryoglobulinemia (EMC). Vast majority of patients who were considered to have EMC have cryoglobulinemic vasculitis related to hepatitis C infection.

1455. Monoclonal cryoglobulinemia is associated with which of the following?
Harrison's 20th Ed. Chapter 54 Page 354

A. Plasma cell dyscrasias
B. Chronic lymphocytic leukemia
C. Lymphoma
D. All of the above

Monoclonal cryoglobulinemia is associated with plasma cell dyscrasias, chronic lymphocytic leukemia and lymphoma.

1456. Classic triad of cryoglobulinemic syndrome includes all except?
Harrison's 20th Ed. Chapter 356 Page 2586

A. Purpura
B. Arthralgias
C. Weakness
D. Acrocyanosis

Classic triad of cryoglobulinemic syndrome consists of palpable purpura, arthralgias & weakness. Others are glomerulonephritis, peripheral neuropathy, generalized vasculitis, livedo reticularis, ischemic ulcers, acrocyanosis and hemorrhagic bullae.

1457. What percentage of patients with chronic hepatitis C will develop cryoglobulinemic vasculitis?
Harrison's 20th Ed. Chapter 356 Page 2586

A. 5%
B. 10%
C. 20%
D. 40%

5% of patients with chronic hepatitis C will develop cryoglobulinemic vasculitis.

1458. Which of the following glomerulonephritis is responsible for most renal lesions in cryoglobulinemic vasculitis?
Harrison's 20th Ed. Chapter 356 Page 2586

A. Minimal change glomerulonephritis
B. Membranoproliferative glomerulonephritis
C. Membranous glomerulonephritis (MGN)
D. Mesangioproliferative glomerulonephritis

Membranoproliferative glomerulonephritis is responsible for 80% of all renal lesions in cryoglobulinemic vasculitis.

1459. In cryoglobulinemic vasculitis, immune complexes consisting of?
Harrison's 20th Ed. Chapter 356 Page 2586

A. Hepatitis C antigens
B. Polyclonal hepatitis C-specific IgG
C. Monoclonal IgM rheumatoid factor
D. All of the above

Cryoglobulinemic vasculitis occurs when an aberrant immune response to hepatitis C infection leads to the formation of immune complexes consisting of hepatitis C antigens, polyclonal hepatitis C-specific IgG, and monoclonal IgM rheumatoid factor. The deposition of these immune complexes in blood vessel walls triggers an inflammatory cascade that results in cryoglobulinemic vasculitis.

1460. Which of the following is almost always found in cryoglobulinemic vasculitis?
Harrison's 20th Ed. Chapter 356 Page 2586

A. Antinuclear antibodies
B. Anti-smooth muscle antibodies
C. Antiplatelet antibodies
D. Rheumatoid factor

Rheumatoid factor is almost always found in cryoglobulinemic vasculitis and may be a useful clue to the disease when cryoglobulins are not detected. Hypocomplementemia occurs in 90% of patients An elevated ESR and anemia occur frequently. Evidence for hepatitis C infection must be sought in all patients by testing for hepatitis C antibodies and hepatitis C RNA.

1461. Which of the following about cryoglobulins is false?
Harrison's 20th Ed. Chapter 107 Page 802

A. Mixed cryoglobulins are not associated with malignancy
B. 10% of macroglobulins are cryoglobulins
C. For cryoglobulins, blood is drawn into a warm syringe
D. None of the above

Mixed cryoglobulins are composed of IgM or IgA complexed with IgG, for which they are specific.

1462. Morphologic lesions of viral hepatitis are all except?
Harrison's 20th Ed. Chapter 332 Page 2355

A. Panlobular mononuclear cells infiltration
B. Hepatic cell necrosis
C. Cholestasis
D. Atrophy of Kupffer cells

Typical morphologic lesions of all types of viral hepatitis are panlobular infiltration with mononuclear cells, hepatic cell necrosis, Kupffer cells hyperplasia & variable cholestasis. Hepatic cell regeneration is present.

1463. Hepatic cell regeneration is evidenced by?
Harrison's 20th Ed. Chapter 332 Page 2355

A. Numerous mitotic figures
B. Multinucleated cells
C. "Rosette" or "pseudoacinar" formation
D. All of the above

Hepatic cell regeneration is evidenced by numerous mitotic figures, multinucleated cells and "rosette" or "pseudoacinar" formation.

1464. Panlobular mononuclear infiltration in viral hepatitis consists "primarily" of?
Harrison's 20th Ed. Chapter 332 Page 2355

A. Plasma cells
B. Small lymphocytes
C. Large lymphocytes
D. Eosinophils

Panlobular mononuclear infiltration in viral hepatitis consists "primarily" of small lymphocytes. Plasma cells & eosinophils are present occasionally.

1465. William Thomas Councilman (1854-1933) was of which nationality?
Science. 1933;77(2009):613-18

A. British
B. American
C. Ireland
D. Canadian

Councilman bodies are named after American pathologist William Thomas Councilman (1854-1933) who discovered them. His work included study of amebiasis, diphtheria, smallpox, and yellow fever.

1466. Councilman bodies are best related to?
Harrison's 20th Ed. Chapter 332 Page 2355

A. Fibrosis
B. Liver cell regeneration
C. Apoptosis
D. Growth arrest

Liver cell damage leads to acidophilic degeneration of hepatocytes called Councilman or apoptotic bodies.

1467. Liver cell damage in viral hepatitis consists of?
Harrison's 20th Ed. Chapter 332 Page 2355

A. Hepatic cell degeneration and necrosis
B. Cell dropout, ballooning of cells
C. Acidophilic degeneration of hepatocytes
D. All of the above

Liver cell damage in viral hepatitis consists of hepatic cell degeneration and necrosis, cell dropout, ballooning of cells, and acidophilic degeneration of hepatocytes (Councilman or apoptotic bodies).

1468. Which of the following is seen in chronic but not in acute HBV infection?
Harrison's 20th Ed. Chapter 332 Page 2355

A. Acidophilic degeneration of hepatocytes
B. Ballooning of hepatocytes
C. Hepatocyte dropout
D. Large hepatocytes with ground-glass appearance of cytoplasm

Large hepatocytes with a ground-glass appearance of the cytoplasm may be seen in chronic but not in acute HBV infection.

1469. Ground-glass appearance of the cytoplasm in chronic HBV infection is due to?
Harrison's 20th Ed. Chapter 332 Page 2355

A. HBsAg
B. HBeAg
C. HBcAg
D. HBxAg

1470. Hepatocytes containing HBsAg can be identified histochemically with?
Harrison's 20th Ed. Chapter 332 Page 2355

A. Orcein or aldehyde fuchsin
B. Congo red
C. Nitroblue tetrazolium (NBT)
D. Crystal violet

Ground-glass appearance of the cytoplasm in chronic HBV infection is due to HBsAg and can be identified histochemically with orcein or aldehyde fuchsin.

1471. In hepatitis C, the most remarkable histologic feature is?
Harrison's 20th Ed. Chapter 332 Page 2355

A. Marked increase in activation of sinusoidal lining cells
B. Relative paucity of inflammation
C. Lymphoid aggregates
D. Bile duct lesions

In hepatitis C, the histologic lesion is remarkable for a relative paucity of inflammation.

1472. In Hepatitis C, which of the following histologic lesion is linked to increased fibrosis?
Harrison's 20th Ed. Chapter 332 Page 2355

A. Increase in activation of sinusoidal lining cells
B. Lymphoid aggregates
C. Presence of fat
D. Bile duct lesions

In hepatitis C, apart from the most notable histologic lesion i.e. relative paucity of inflammation, there is marked increase in activation of sinusoidal lining cells, lymphoid aggregates, presence of fat (more frequent in genotype 3 & linked to increased fibrosis), and, occasionally, bile duct lesions.

1473. **Marked cholestasis is a feature of?**
Harrison's 20th Ed. Chapter 332 Page 2355

   A. HAV
   B. HCV
   C. HDV
   D. HEV

Marked cholestasis is a common histologic feature of hepatitis E.

1474. **Bridging hepatic necrosis is also called?**
Harrison's 20th Ed. Chapter 332 Page 2355

   A. Subacute necrosis
   B. Confluent necrosis
   C. Interface hepatitis
   D. All of the above

In acute hepatitis, bridging hepatic necrosis, also termed subacute or confluent necrosis or interface hepatitis is observed occasionally.

1475. **What was earlier called piecemeal necrosis is now called?**
Harrison's 20th Ed. Chapter 334 Page 2375

   A. Gradual hepatitis
   B. Interface hepatitis
   C. Coupled hepatitis
   D. Destruction hepatitis

Piecemeal necrosis or limiting plate necrosis is now called "interface hepatitis".

1476. **In bridging hepatic necrosis, the bridge consists of?**
Harrison's 20th Ed. Chapter 332 Page 2355

   A. Condensed reticulum
   B. Inflammatory debris
   C. Degenerating liver cells
   D. All of the above

1477. **The bridge in bridging hepatic necrosis spans?**
Harrison's 20th Ed. Chapter 332 Page 2355

   A. Adjacent portal areas
   B. Portal to central veins
   C. Central vein to central vein
   D. Any of the above

In bridging hepatic necrosis, the bridge consists of condensed reticulum, inflammatory debris, and degenerating liver cells that span adjacent portal areas, portal to central veins, or central vein to central vein. There is collapse of the reticulin framework.

1478. **Postmortem examination finding of a small, shrunken, soft liver is seen in?**
Harrison's 20th Ed. Chapter 332 Page 2355

   A. Massive hepatic necrosis
   B. Fulminant hepatitis
   C. Acute yellow atrophy
   D. All of the above

Massive hepatic necrosis, fulminant hepatitis and acute yellow atrophy are synonymous.

1479. **Which of the following histologic changes occur in liver injury?**
World J Gastroenterol. 2011;17(17):2172-77

   A. Ballooned hepatocytes
   B. Mallory–Denk bodies
   C. Apoptotic hepatocytes
   D. All of the above

In liver disease, histologic examination of biopsied liver tissue may demonstrate steatosis, inflammation, ballooned hepatocytes, Mallory–Denk bodies, apoptotic hepatocytes, and fibrosis or cirrhosis.

1480. **Mallory-Denk Bodies (MDB) are seen in?**
World J Gastroenterol. 2011;17(17):2172-77

   A. Hepatitis C
   B. Primary biliary cirrhosis (PBC)
   C. Nonalcoholic fatty liver disease (NAFLD)
   D. All of the above

1481. **Which of the following is localized to hepatocyte nucleus?**
Harrison's 20th Ed. Chapter 332 Page 2355

   A. HAV antigen
   B. HCV antigen
   C. HDV antigen
   D. HEV antigen

1482. **Which of the following antigens are localized to the cytoplasm?**
Harrison's 20th Ed. Chapter 332 Page 2355

   A. HAV
   B. HCV
   C. HEV
   D. All of the above

HDV antigen is localized to hepatocyte nucleus, while HAV, HCV & HEV antigens are localized to the cytoplasm. HBsAg is localized to the cytoplasm & plasma membrane of infected liver cells.

1483. **Which of the following hepatitis can be transmitted by fecal-oral route?**
Harrison's 20th Ed. Chapter 332 Page 2356 Table 332-2

   A. Hepatitis B
   B. Hepatitis C
   C. Hepatitis D
   D. None of the above

Hepatitis A is transmitted almost exclusively by the fecal-oral route.

1484. **Hepatitis virus with longest incubation period is?**
Harrison's 20th Ed. Chapter 332 Page 2356 Table 332-2

   A. Hepatitis A
   B. Hepatitis B
   C. Hepatitis C
   D. Hepatitis E

1485. **Hepatitis virus with an incubation period of ~2 weeks is?**
Harrison's 20th Ed. Chapter 332 Page 2356 Table 332-2

   A. Hepatitis A
   B. Hepatitis C
   C. Hepatitis E
   D. All of the above

Incubation period in days: HAV - 15–45, mean 30, HBV - 30–180, mean 60–90, HCV - 15–160, mean 50, HDV - 30–180, mean 60–90, HEV - 14–60, mean 40.

1486. Viral hepatitis with an insidious onset only is?
Harrison's 20th Ed. Chapter 332 Page 2356 Table 332-2

A. Hepatitis A
B. Hepatitis B
C. Hepatitis C
D. Hepatitis E

Onset : HAV - acute, HBV - insidious or acute, HCV - insidious, HDV - insidious or acute, HEV - acute

1487. Chronicity is invariable in which of the following infections?
Harrison's 20th Ed. Chapter 332 Page 2356 Table 332-2

A. HBV / HDV coinfection
B. HBV / HDV superinfection
C. HBV / HIV co-infection
D. All of the above

1488. Which of the following hepatitis is not transmitted by sexual route?
Harrison's 20th Ed. Chapter 332 Page 2356 Table 332-2

A. Hepatitis A
B. Hepatitis B
C. Hepatitis D
D. Hepatitis E

1489. Which of the following hepatitis, perinatal transmission is least likely?
Harrison's 20th Ed. Chapter 332 Page 2356 Table 332-2

A. Hepatitis A
B. Hepatitis B
C. Hepatitis C
D. Hepatitis D

1490. Which of the following hepatitis, fulminant progression is most common in?
Harrison's 20th Ed. Chapter 332 Page 2356 Table 332-2

A. Hepatitis A
B. Hepatitis B
C. Hepatitis C
D. Hepatitis D

1491. Which of the following hepatitis, prognosis is excellent?
Harrison's 20th Ed. Chapter 332 Page 2356 Table 332-2

A. Hepatitis A
B. Hepatitis B
C. Hepatitis C
D. Hepatitis E

1492. Food material incriminated in transmission of HAV is?
Harrison's 20th Ed. Chapter 332 Page 2355

A. Frozen raspberries & strawberries
B. Green onions imported from Mexico
C. Shellfish
D. All of the above

HAV large outbreaks as well as sporadic cases have been traced to contaminated food, water, milk, frozen raspberries and strawberries, green onions imported from Mexico and shellfish.

1493. Hepatitis A infections tend to occur in?
Harrison's 20th Ed. Chapter 332 Page 2355

A. Early summer
B. Spring
C. Mid - monsoon
D. Late fall and early winter

Epidemiologic observations point towards the fact that hepatitis A infections tend to occur in late fall and early winter.

1494. Which of the following about HAV infections is false?
Harrison's 20th Ed. Chapter 332 Page 2355

A. Intrafamily & intrainstitutional spread common
B. No HAV carrier state identified after acute hepatitis A
C. Hepatitis A tends to be more symptomatic in adults
D. Hepatis A is never bloodborne

Hepatitis A is rarely bloodborne, several outbreaks have been recognized in recipients of clotting-factor concentrates.

1495. Which of the following body fluid from infected persons is most infectious?
Harrison's 20th Ed. Chapter 332 Page 2355

A. Semen
B. Saliva
C. Serum
D. All are equally infectious

HBsAg is identified in almost every body fluid from infected persons. Semen & saliva are infectious though less than serum.

1496. Which of the following is the mode of HBV transmission?
Harrison's 20th Ed. Chapter 332 Page 2356

A. Percutaneous inoculation
B. Sexual contact
C. Perinatal transmission
D. All of the above

HBV transmission by oral ingestion has been documented as a potential but inefficient route of exposure.

1497. What is not true for Hepatitis B virus infections?
Harrison's 20th Ed. Chapter 332 Page 2356, N Engl J Med. 2004;351:2832-8

A. Can be transmitted through breast milk
B. Incubation period for acute infection is 45 to 160 days
C. Risk of chronicity in infected neonates is 90%
D. No known animal reservoirs

~10% of HBV infections are acquired in utero. Most infections occur at the time of delivery and early postpartum period & are not related to breastfeeding.

1498. Perinatal transmission occurs in infants born to HBsAg carrier mothers during?
Harrison's 20th Ed. Chapter 332 Page 2356

A. First trimester of pregnancy
B. Second trimester of pregnancy
C. Third trimester of pregnancy
D. Any of the above

Perinatal transmission occurs primarily in infants born to HBsAg carrier mothers or mothers with acute hepatitis B during third trimester of pregnancy or during the early postpartum period.

1499. Which of the following mothers almost invariably transmit hepatitis B infection to their offspring?
Harrison's 20th Ed. Chapter 332 Page 2356

A. HBsAg-positive + HBeAg-positive
B. HBsAg-negative + HBeAg-negative
C. HBsAg-positive + HBeAg-negative
D. HBsAg-negative + HBeAg-positive

HBsAg positive mothers who are HBeAg-positive almost invariably (>90%) transmit hepatitis B infection to their offspring, whereas HBsAg carrier mothers with anti-HBe rarely (10-15%) infect their offspring.

1500. Likelihood of perinatal transmission of HBV correlates with the presence of?
Harrison's 20th Ed. Chapter 332 Page 2356

A. HBsAg
B. HBcAg
C. HBeAg
D. HBxAg

Likelihood of perinatal transmission of HBV correlates with presence of HBeAg. 90% of HBeAg-positive mothers but only 10–15% of anti-HBe-positive mothers transmit HBV infection to their offspring.

1501. Hepatitis B virus (HBV) chronically infects how many people worldwide?
Harrison's 20th Ed. Chapter 332 Page 2356

A. ~50 million
B. ~100 million
C. ~250 million
D. ~350 million

Hepatitis B virus (HBV) chronically infects over 350 million people worldwide.

1502. Prevalence of HBV sero-positivity is more in?
Harrison's 20th Ed. Chapter 332 Page 2356

A. Down's syndrome
B. Lepromatous leprosy
C. Hodgkin's disease
D. All of the above

Increased prevalence of serum HBsAg is found in Down's syndrome, lepromatous leprosy, leukemia, Hodgkin's disease, polyarteritis nodosa, CKD patients on dialysis and IDUs.

1503. Risk of acquiring HBV infection from a blood transfusion is?
Harrison's 20th Ed. Chapter 332 Page 2356

A. 1 in 50,000
B. 1 in 140,000
C. 1 in 230,000
D. 1 in 320,000

Because of highly sensitive virologic screening of donor blood, risk of acquiring HBV infection from a blood transfusion is 1 in 230,000 while it is 1 in 2.3 million for transfusion-associated HCV infection.

1504. HDV infection is endemic among those with hepatitis B in?
Harrison's 20th Ed. Chapter 332 Page 2357

A. Northern African countries
B. Southern European countries
C. Middle East countries
D. All of the above

1505. Which of the following is related to hepatitis D?
Harrison's 20th Ed. Chapter 332 Page 2357

A. Haverhill fever
B. Lábrea fever
C. Hibernian fever
D. Lassa fever

1506. Hepatitis C virus (HCV) infects how many people worldwide?
Harrison's 20th Ed. Chapter 332 Page 2357

A. ~80 million
B. ~120 million
C. ~170 million
D. ~250 million

1507. Extraordinarily high prevalences of HCV infection occur in?
Harrison's 20th Ed. Chapter 332 Page 2357

A. Thailand
B. Venezuala
C. Egypt
D. Haiti

Extraordinarily high prevalences of HCV infection occur in Egypt.

1508. Baby boomer generation refers to persons born between?
Harrison's 20th Ed. Chapter 332 Page 2358, N Engl J Med. 2006; 355:758-60

A. 1943 and 1961
B. 1944 and 1962
C. 1945 and 1963
D. 1946 and 1964

The term "baby boomer" refers to individuals born in the United States between mid-1946 and mid-1964.

1509. By 2012, HCV mortality had surpassed deaths from?
Harrison's 20th Ed. Chapter 332 Page 2358

A. HIV
B. Tuberculosis
C. Hepatitis B
D. All of the above

By 2012, HCV mortality had surpassed deaths from HIV, tuberculosis, hepatitis B, and 57 other notifiable infectious diseases (i.e. all infectious diseases)

1510. Which of the following about HCV infection is false?
Harrison's 20th Ed. Chapter 332 Page 2358

A. Accounts for 40% of chronic liver disease
B. Most frequent indication for liver transplantation
C. Worldwide, genotype 1 is the most common
D. Breastfeeding increases risk of HCV vertical infection

Worldwide, genotype 1 is the most common. Genotype 4 predominates in Egypt; genotype 5 is localized to South Africa, and genotype 6 to Hong Kong. Breastfeeding does not increase the risk of HCV infection between an infected mother and her infant.

1511. Which of the following about HEV infection is false?
Harrison's 20th Ed. Chapter 332 Page 2358

A. Enteric mode of spread
B. Secondary person-to-person spread rare

C. Swine is the zoonotic reservoir for HEV
D. None of the above

An epidemiologic feature that distinguishes HEV from other enteric agents is the rarity of secondary person-to-person spread from infected persons to their close contacts.

1512. Which of the following about presentation of acute viral hepatitis is false?
Harrison's 20th Ed. Chapter 332 Page 2359
A. Constitutional symptoms may precede onset of jaundice by 1 - 2 weeks
B. Dark urine & clay-colored stools occur 1 - 5 days before onset of clinical jaundice
C. Alterations in olfaction and taste
D. None of the above

1513. Which of the following is a presentation of acute viral hepatitis?
Harrison's 20th Ed. Chapter 332 Page 2359
A. Splenomegaly
B. Cervical adenopathy
C. Spider angiomas
D. All of the above

1514. Acute hepatitis B is self-limited in what proportion of cases?
Harrison's 20th Ed. Chapter 332 Page 2359
A. 50–69%
B. 69–79%
C. 79–89%
D. 95–99%

Acute hepatitis B is self-limited in 95 - 99% of infections.

1515. Acute hepatitis C is self-limited in what proportion of cases?
Harrison's 20th Ed. Chapter 332 Page 2359
A. 5–9%
B. 15–20%
C. 35–45%
D. 55–75%

Acute hepatitis C is self-limited in 15–20%.

1516. Which of the following is false about infection with HDV?
Harrison's 20th Ed. Chapter 332 Page 2359
A. Can occur in the presence of acute HBV infection
B. Can occur in the presence of chronic HBV infection
C. Duration of HBV infection determines duration of HDV infection
D. None of the above

1517. Acute hepatitis-like clinical events in chronic hepatitis B may be due to?
Harrison's 20th Ed. Chapter 332 Page 2359
A. HDV superinfection
B. Spontaneous HBeAg to anti-HBe seroconversion
C. Reversion from relatively nonreplicative to replicative infection
D. All of the above

Apart from the above conditions, acute clinical exacerbations of chronic hepatitis B may be due to emergence of a precore mutant.

1518. Therapy with which of the following can lead to reactivation of both hepatitis B and C?
Harrison's 20th Ed. Chapter 332 Page 2359
A. Anti-TNF-α therapy
B. Glucocorticoid therapy
C. Extracorporeal liver-assist devices
D. Plasmapheresis

Anti-TNF-α therapy can lead to reactivation of both hepatitis B and C.

1519. The diagnosis of anicteric hepatitis is based on?
Harrison's 20th Ed. Chapter 332 Page 2359
A. S. Aminotransferase levels
B. S. Bilirubin levels
C. S. Alkaline phosphatase levels
D. S. GGT levels

The diagnosis of anicteric hepatitis is based on clinical features & on aminotransferase elevations.

1520. In acute hepatitis, very high serum bilirubin level (20–30 mg/dL) occur in?
Harrison's 20th Ed. Chapter 332 Page 2359
A. Severe disease
B. Glucose-6-phosphate dehydrogenase deficiency
C. Sickle cell anemia
D. All of the above

Bilirubin levels > 20 mg/dL persisting late into the course of viral hepatitis is associated with severe disease. Patients with underlying hemolytic anemia, like glucose-6-phosphate dehydrogenase deficiency and sickle cell anemia, also have high serum bilirubin levels (>30 mg/dL) due to superimposed hemolysis.

1521. Which of the following occur transiently in acute viral hepatitis?
Harrison's 20th Ed. Chapter 332 Page 2359
A. Neutropenia
B. Lymphopenia
C. Steatorrhea
D. All of the above

Neutropenia and lymphopenia are transient and are followed by a relative lymphocytosis. Also, mild and transient steatorrhea, microscopic hematuria and minimal proteinuria have been noted.

1522. Prognostically, which of the following is relevant in acute hepatitis?
Harrison's 20th Ed. Chapter 332 Page 2359
A. Levels of serum bilirubin
B. Levels of aminotransferases
C. Prothrombin time (PT) prolongation
D. All of the above

Prothrombin time (PT) prolongation in acute viral hepatitis reflects a severe hepatic synthetic defect, signify extensive hepatocellular necrosis, and indicates a worse prognosis.

1523. Which of the following is characteristically elevated during acute hepatitis A?
Harrison's 20th Ed. Chapter 332 Page 2359
A. Serum IgG
B. Serum IgM
C. Serum IgA
D. Serum IgE

A diffuse but mild elevation of the gamma globulin fraction is common during acute viral hepatitis. Serum IgM level is elevated more characteristically during acute hepatitis A.

1524. Which of the following antibodies may be present during the acute phase of viral hepatitis?
Harrison's 20th Ed. Chapter 332 Page 2359

A. Rheumatoid factor
B. Nuclear antibody
C. Heterophil antibody
D. All of the above

During the acute phase of viral hepatitis, antibodies to smooth muscle and other cell constituents may be present, and low titers of rheumatoid factor, nuclear antibody, and heterophil antibody can also be found. In hepatitis C and D, antibodies to LKM may be found.

1525. Which of the following can give rise to false-positive results for IgM anti-HAV during acute illness?
Harrison's 20th Ed. Chapter 332 Page 2359

A. Antibodies to LKM
B. Rheumatoid factor
C. Antiphospholipid antibodies
D. Cytoplasmic antineutrophil cytoplasmic antibody (c-ANCA)

1526. If levels of HBsAg are too low to be detected during acute HBV infection, which of the following establishes its diagnosis?
Harrison's 20th Ed. Chapter 332 Page 2359

A. IgM anti-HBc
B. IgG anti-HBc
C. IgM & IgG anti-HBc
D. HBeAg

If levels of HBsAg are too low to be detected during acute HBV infection, presence of IgM anti-HBc establishes its diagnosis. HBeAg is invariably present during early acute hepatitis B, HBeAg testing is indicated primarily during follow-up of chronic infection.

1527. Which of the following about HBsAg is false?
Harrison's 20th Ed. Chapter 332 Page 2359

A. HBsAg titer is not related to severity of clinical disease
B. HBsAg titers are highest in immunosuppressed patients
C. HBsAg titers are very low in acute fulminant hepatitis
D. None of the above

1528. Which of the following about HBeAg is false?
Harrison's 20th Ed. Chapter 332 Page 2360

A. It is an indicator of relative infectivity
B. HBeAg is invariably present during early acute hepatitis B
C. HBeAg testing is indicated primarily in chronic infection
D. None of the above

1529. Which of the following is true in chronic HBV infection?
Harrison's 20th Ed. Chapter 332 Page 2360

A. IgM anti-HBc-positive, IgG anti-HBc-positive
B. IgM anti-HBc-negative, IgG anti-HBc-negative
C. IgM anti-HBc-negative, IgG anti-HBc-positive
D. IgM anti-HBc-positive, IgG anti-HBc-negative

IgM anti-HBc may be useful to distinguish between acute or recent infection (IgM anti-HBc-positive) and chronic HBV infection (IgM anti-HBc-negative, IgG anti-HBc-positive).

1530. A false-positive test for IgM anti-HBc may be found in patients with?
Harrison's 20th Ed. Chapter 332 Page 2360

A. Glucose-6-phosphate dehydrogenase deficiency
B. High-titer rheumatoid factor
C. Sickle cell anemia
D. All of the above

A false-positive test for IgM anti-HBc may be encountered in patients with high-titer rheumatoid factor.

1531. Presence of anti-HBs in the presence of HBsAg in patients with acute hepatitis B indicates which of the following?
Harrison's 20th Ed. Chapter 332 Page 2360

A. Fulminant hepatitis
B. Chronicity
C. Imminent HBsAg clearance
D. None of the above

Anti-HBs is rarely detectable in the presence of HBsAg in patients with acute hepatitis B. When this happens, its of no recognized clinical significance.

1532. After hepatitis B vaccination, which is the only serologic marker to appear?
Harrison's 20th Ed. Chapter 332 Page 2360

A. Anti-HBs
B. Anti-HBe
C. Anti-HBc
D. All of the above

After immunization with hepatitis B vaccine, which consists of HBsAg alone, anti-HBs is the only serologic marker to appear.

1533. In hepatitis B, threshold for infectivity and liver injury is?
Harrison's 20th Ed. Chapter 332 Page 2360

A. $10^1 - 10^2$ IU/mL
B. $10^2 - 10^3$ IU/mL
C. $10^3 - 10^4$ IU/mL
D. $10^5 - 10^6$ IU/mL

1534. Which of the following is related to HBV replication?
Harrison's 20th Ed. Chapter 332 Page 2360

A. Hepatitis D virus
B. HBeAg
C. Serum HBV DNA
D. All of the above

Patients with hepatitis D tend to have lower levels of HBV replication. In hepatitis B is HBeAg. Its principal clinical usefulness is as an indicator of relative infectivity. Serum HBV DNA is an indicator of HBV replication.

1535. In chronic hepatitis B, high levels of HBV DNA indicate increased risk of?
Harrison's 20th Ed. Chapter 332 Page 2360

A. Cirrhosis
B. Hepatic decompensation
C. Hepatocellular carcinoma
D. All of the above

In chronic hepatitis B, high levels of HBV DNA increase the risk of cirrhosis, hepatic decompensation, and hepatocellular carcinoma.

1536. Presence of which of the following confirms that HBV infection is acute?
   Harrison's 20th Ed. Chapter 332 Page 2360
   A. IgM anti-HBcAg
   B. IgM anti-HBsAg
   C. IgM anti-HBeAg
   D. IgM anti-HBxAg

Presence of HBsAg, with or without IgM anti-HBc, represents HBV infection. If IgM anti-HBc is present, the HBV infection is considered acute even in the absence of HBsAg. If IgM anti-HBc is absent, the HBV infection is considered chronic.

1537. HBsAg (+), Anti-HBs (–), IgM Anti-HBc (+), HBeAg (+), Anti-HBe (–) is indicative of?
   Harrison's 20th Ed. Chapter 332 Page 2360 Table 332-5
   A. Acute hepatitis B, high infectivity
   B. Chronic hepatitis B, high infectivity
   C. Low-level hepatitis B carrier
   D. Hepatitis B in remote past

1538. HBsAg (+), Anti-HBs (–), IgG Anti-HBc (+), HBeAg (+), Anti-HBe (–) is indicative of?
   Harrison's 20th Ed. Chapter 332 Page 2360 Table 332-5
   A. Acute hepatitis B, high infectivity
   B. Chronic hepatitis B, high infectivity
   C. Low-level hepatitis B carrier
   D. Hepatitis B in remote past

1539. HBsAg (+), Anti-HBs (–), IgG Anti-HBc (+), HBeAg (–), Anti-HBe (+) is indicative of?
   Harrison's 20th Ed. Chapter 332 Page 2360 Table 332-5
   A. Acute hepatitis B, high infectivity
   B. Late acute or chronic hepatitis B, low infectivity
   C. Anti-HBc "window"
   D. Hepatitis B in remote past

1540. HBsAg (–), Anti-HBs (–), IgM Anti-HBc (+), HBeAg (±), Anti-HBe (±) is indicative of?
   Harrison's 20th Ed. Chapter 332 Page 2360 Table 332-5
   A. Acute hepatitis B, high infectivity
   B. Late acute or chronic hepatitis B, low infectivity
   C. Anti-HBc "window"
   D. Recovery from hepatitis B

1541. HBsAg (–), Anti-HBs (–), IgG Anti-HBc (+), HBeAg (–), Anti-HBe (±) is indicative of?
   Harrison's 20th Ed. Chapter 332 Page 2360 Table 332-5
   A. Recovery from hepatitis B
   B. Immunization with HBsAg
   C. Low-level hepatitis B carrier
   D. Anti-HBc "window"

1542. HBsAg (–), Anti-HBs (+), IgG Anti-HBc (+), HBeAg (–), Anti-HBe (±) is indicative of?
   Harrison's 20th Ed. Chapter 332 Page 2360 Table 332-5
   A. Recovery from hepatitis B
   B. Immunization with HBsAg
   C. Low-level hepatitis B carrier
   D. Anti-HBc "window"

1543. HBsAg (–), Anti-HBs (+), IgG Anti-HBc (–), HBeAg (–), Anti-HBe (–) is indicative of?
   Harrison's 20th Ed. Chapter 332 Page 2360 Table 332-5
   A. Recovery from hepatitis B
   B. Immunization with HBsAg
   C. Low-level hepatitis B carrier
   D. Anti-HBc "window"

1544. HBsAg (–), Anti-HBs (+), IgG Anti-HBc (–), HBeAg (–), Anti-HBe (–) is indicative of?
   Harrison's 20th Ed. Chapter 332 Page 2360 Table 332-5
   A. Hepatitis B in the remote past
   B. Immunization with HBsAg
   C. False-positive
   D. Any of the above

1545. Which of the following may reappear during acute reactivation of chronic hepatitis B?
   Harrison's 20th Ed. Chapter 332 Page 2360 Table 332-5
   A. HBsAg
   B. HBeAg
   C. IgM anti-HBc
   D. IgG anti-HBc

IgM anti-HBc may reappear during acute reactivation of chronic hepatitis B.

1546. Which of the following about anti-HCV is false?
   Harrison's 20th Ed. Chapter 332 Page 2360
   A. Detected in acute hepatitis C
   B. Remains detectable during chronic infection
   C. False positive in persons with circulating rheumatoid factor
   D. None of the above

1547. Which of the following about HCV RNA in HCV infections is false?
   Harrison's 20th Ed. Chapter 332 Page 2360
   A. Most sensitive test for HCV infection - "gold standard"
   B. Can be detected before acute elevation of aminotransferases
   C. Can be detected before appearance of anti-HCV
   D. None of the above

1548. Which of the following about HCV RNA in HCV infections is false?
   Harrison's 20th Ed. Chapter 332 Page 2360
   A. Remains detectable indefinitely in chronic hepatitis C
   B. Values expressed in IU/mL
   C. Reliable marker of disease severity or prognosis
   D. Helps in predicting relative responsiveness to antiviral therapy

Determination of HCV RNA level is not a reliable marker of disease severity or prognosis.

1549. Which of the following is true for "cured" hepatitis C?
Harrison's 20th Ed. Chapter 332 Page 2361

A. Anti-HCV (–), HCV RNA (–)
B. Anti-HCV (+), HCV RNA (–)
C. Anti-HCV (–), HCV RNA (+)
D. Anti-HCV (+), HCV RNA (+)

Detectable anti-HCV in the absence of HCV RNA signifies spontaneous or therapeutically induced recovery from hepatitis C i.e. "cured".

1550. Which of the following is false about HDV infection?
Harrison's 20th Ed. Chapter 332 Page 2361

A. Intrahepatic HDV antigen demonstrable
B. Circulating HDV antigen is detectable only briefly
C. Anti-HDV is undetectable once HBsAg disappears
D. None of the above

Anti-HDV appears after a delay of up to 30–40 days in acute HDV infection.

1551. Which of the following helps to differentiate whether HBV and HDV infections are simultaneous or superimposed?
Harrison's 20th Ed. Chapter 332 Page 2361

A. HBeAg
B. Anti-HDV
C. Anti-HBc
D. Anti-HBe

In simultaneous acute HBV and HDV infections, IgM anti-HBc will be detectable. In acute HDV infection superimposed on chronic HBV infection, anti-HBc will be of IgG class.

1552. HBsAg (+), IgM Anti-HAV (–), IgM Anti-HBc (+), Anti-HCV (–) indicates?
Harrison's 20th Ed. Chapter 332 Page 2361 Table 332-6

A. Acute hepatitis B
B. Chronic hepatitis B
C. Acute hepatitis A superimposed on chronic hepatitis B
D. Acute hepatitis A and B

1553. HBsAg (+), IgM Anti-HAV (–), IgM Anti-HBc (–), Anti-HCV (–) indicates?
Harrison's 20th Ed. Chapter 332 Page 2361 Table 332-6

A. Acute hepatitis B
B. Chronic hepatitis B
C. Acute hepatitis A superimposed on chronic hepatitis B
D. Acute hepatitis A and B

1554. HBsAg (+), IgM Anti-HAV (+), IgM Anti-HBc (–), Anti-HCV (–) indicates?
Harrison's 20th Ed. Chapter 332 Page 2361 Table 332-6

A. Acute hepatitis B
B. Chronic hepatitis B
C. Acute hepatitis A superimposed on chronic hepatitis B
D. Acute hepatitis A and B

1555. HBsAg (+), IgM Anti-HAV (+), IgM Anti-HBc (+), Anti-HCV (–) indicates?
Harrison's 20th Ed. Chapter 332 Page 2361 Table 332-6

A. Acute hepatitis B
B. Chronic hepatitis B
C. Acute hepatitis A superimposed on chronic hepatitis B
D. Acute hepatitis A and B

1556. HBsAg (–), IgM Anti-HAV (+), IgM Anti-HBc (–), Anti-HCV (–) indicates?
Harrison's 20th Ed. Chapter 332 Page 2361 Table 332-6

A. Acute hepatitis A
B. Acute hepatitis A and B (HBsAg below detection threshold)
C. Acute hepatitis B (HBsAg below detection threshold)
D. Acute hepatitis C

1557. HBsAg (–), IgM Anti-HAV (+), IgM Anti-HBc (+), Anti-HCV (–) indicates?
Harrison's 20th Ed. Chapter 332 Page 2361 Table 332-6

A. Acute hepatitis A
B. Acute hepatitis A and B (HBsAg below detection threshold)
C. Acute hepatitis B (HBsAg below detection threshold)
D. Acute hepatitis C

1558. HBsAg (–), IgM Anti-HAV (–), IgM Anti-HBc (+), Anti-HCV (–) indicates?
Harrison's 20th Ed. Chapter 332 Page 2361 Table 332-6

A. Acute hepatitis A
B. Acute hepatitis A and B (HBsAg below detection threshold)
C. Acute hepatitis B (HBsAg below detection threshold)
D. Acute hepatitis C

1559. HBsAg (–), IgM Anti-HAV (–), IgM Anti-HBc (–), Anti-HCV (+) indicates?
Harrison's 20th Ed. Chapter 332 Page 2361 Table 332-6

A. Acute hepatitis A
B. Acute hepatitis A and B (HBsAg below detection threshold)
C. Acute hepatitis B (HBsAg below detection threshold)
D. Acute hepatitis C

1560. Which of the following hepatitis is more likely to be anicteric?
Harrison's 20th Ed. Chapter 332 Page 2361

A. Hepatitis A
B. Hepatitis B
C. Hepatitis C
D. All of the above

1561. Pregnant women with hepatitis E have a case fatality rate of?
Harrison's 20th Ed. Chapter 332 Page 2361

A. 1–2%
B. 5–10%
C. 10–20%
D. 20–30%

In outbreaks of hepatitis E in India, case fatality rate is 1–2% and up to 10–20% in pregnant women.

1562. Relapsing hepatitis is a feature of?
Harrison's 20th Ed. Chapter 332 Page 2361

A. Acute hepatitis A
B. Acute hepatitis B

C. Acute hepatitis C
D. Hepatitis D superinfection

Complications of hepatitis A include relapsing hepatitis appearing weeks to months after apparent recovery from acute hepatitis, cholestatic hepatitis and rarely fulminant hepatitis.

1563. Relapses in relapsing hepatitis are characterized by?
Harrison's 20th Ed. Chapter 332 Page 2362

A. Recurrence of symptoms
B. Aminotransferase elevations
C. Fecal excretion of HAV
D. All of the above

Relapses are characterized by recurrence of symptoms, aminotransferase elevations, occasionally jaundice and fecal excretion of HAV.

1564. Cholestatic hepatitis is unusual variant of?
Harrison's 20th Ed. Chapter 332 Page 2362

A. Acute hepatitis A
B. Acute hepatitis B
C. Acute hepatitis C
D. Hepatitis D superinfection

Cholestatic hepatitis is an unusual variant of acute hepatitis A characterized by protracted cholestatic jaundice and pruritus.

1565. Prodromal phase of acute hepatitis B is often diagnosed erroneously as?
Harrison's 20th Ed. Chapter 332 Page 2362

A. Hematological diseases
B. Sexually transmitted diseases
C. Rheumatologic diseases
D. Malignancy

During prodromal phase of acute hepatitis B, a serum sickness-like syndrome characterized by arthralgia or arthritis, rash, angioedema and rarely hematuria and proteinuria may develop in 5–10% of patients. It occurs before the onset of clinical jaundice and is often diagnosed erroneously as rheumatologic diseases.

1566. Extrahepatic manifestations of HCV include?
Harrison's 20th Ed. Chapter 332 Page 2362

A. Mixed cryoglobulinemia
B. Porphyria cutanea tarda
C. Lichen planus (LP)
D. All of the above

Well-accepted extrahepatic manifestations of HCV include pruritus, mixed cryoglobulinemia & necrolytic acral erythema. Frequently associated conditions include porphyria cutanea tarda, leucocytoclastic vasculitis, lichen planus, sicca syndrome & polyarteritis nodosa.

1567. Which of the following is a complication of HCV infection?
Harrison's 20th Ed. Chapter 332 Page 2362

A. Hepatic steatosis
B. Hypercholesterolemia
C. Insulin resistance
D. All of the above

HCV infection may be complicated by hepatic steatosis, hypercholesterolemia, insulin resistance (and other manifestations of the metabolic syndrome) and type 2 diabetes mellitus.

1568. Which of the following complications of HCV infection blunts responsiveness to antiviral therapy?
Harrison's 20th Ed. Chapter 332 Page 2362

A. Hepatic steatosis
B. Hypercholesterolemia
C. Hepatitis B co-infection
D. All of the above

Hepatic steatosis & insulin resistance accelerate hepatic fibrosis & blunt antiviral therapy response.

1569. Which of the following is false in the original definition of "fulminant hepatic failure"?
N Engl J Med. 2013;369:2525-34

A. Severe liver injury
B. Potentially reversible in nature
C. Hepatic encephalopathy within 2 weeks of first symptoms
D. Absence of pre-existing liver disease

The original term "fulminant hepatic failure" was defined as "a severe liver injury, potentially reversible in nature and with onset of hepatic encephalopathy within 8 weeks of the first symptoms in the absence of pre-existing liver disease."

1570. Which of the following is the most common cause of acute liver failure in United States?
N Engl J Med. 2013;369:2525-34

A. Drug-induced liver injury
B. Hepatitis A, B, and E
C. Autoimmune hepatitis
D. Cocaine use

Drug-induced liver injury is the most common cause of acute liver failure in United States and much of Western Europe.

1571. Which of the following viral infection can cause acute liver failure?
N Engl J Med. 2013;369:2525-34

A. Cytomegalovirus
B. Epstein - Barr virus
C. Parvoviruses
D. All of the above

Rare viral causes of acute liver failure include herpes simplex virus, cytomegalovirus, Epstein–Barr virus, and parvoviruses.

1572. Which of the following is a classification system for acute liver failure?
N Engl J Med. 2013;369:2525-34

A. O'Grady System
B. Bernuau System
C. Japanese System
D. All of the above

1573. Which of the following criteria is used for selection of patients with acute liver failure for transplantation?
N Engl J Med. 2013;369:2525-34

A. King's College criteria
B. Clichy criteria
C. Japanese criteria
D. All of the above

The King's College criteria are from O'Grady et al., the Clichy criteria from Bernuau et al., and Japanese criteria from Mochida et al.

1574. Which of the following is a cause of acute liver failure?
N Engl J Med. 2013;369:2525-34

- A. Heatstroke
- B. Mushroom ingestion
- C. Wilson's disease
- D. All of the above

Causes of acute liver failure also include neoplastic infiltration, acute Budd–Chiari syndrome, heatstroke, mushroom ingestion, Wilson's disease and pregnancy.

1575. Which of the following is decreased in acute liver failure?
N Engl J Med. 2013;369:2525-34

- A. Gluconeogenesis
- B. Lactate clearance
- C. Ammonia clearance
- D. All of the above

1576. In acute liver failure, which of the following is more common particularly in acetaminophen-related disease?
N Engl J Med. 2013;369:2525-34

- A. Acute lung injury
- B. Pancreatitis
- C. Bone marrow suppression
- D. Coagulopathy

Substantial renal dysfunction and pancreatitis more common in patients with acetaminophen-induced acute liver failure.

1577. In acute liver failure and hypotension despite volume repletion, which vasopressor is preferred?
N Engl J Med. 2013;369:2525-34

- A. Norepinephrine
- B. Vasopressin
- C. Vasopressin analogue
- D. Any of the above

In acute liver failure patients who continue to have hypotension despite volume repletion, norepinephrine is the preferred vasopressor, with or without adjunctive use of vasopressin or vasopressin analogues.

1578. Fulminant hepatitis is rare in?
Harrison's 20th Ed. Chapter 332 Page 2362

- A. Hepatitis A
- B. Hepatitis B & D
- C. Hepatitis E
- D. All of the above

Fulminant hepatitis is primarily seen in hepatitis B and D, and hepatitis E. It is rare in hepatitis A.

1579. Which of the following predispose to fulminant cases of hepatitis A?
Harrison's 20th Ed. Chapter 332 Page 2362

- A. Older adults
- B. Chronic hepatitis B
- C. Chronic hepatitis C
- D. All of the above

1580. Out of the following, fulminant hepatitis is most common in?
Harrison's 20th Ed. Chapter 332 Page 2362

- A. Hepatitis A
- B. Hepatitis B
- C. Hepatitis C
- D. Hepatitis E

Hepatitis B accounts for >50% of fulminant cases of viral hepatitis.

1581. Fulminant hepatitis is hardly ever seen in?
Harrison's 20th Ed. Chapter 332 Page 2362

- A. Hepatitis A
- B. Hepatitis B
- C. Hepatitis C
- D. Hepatitis E

Fulminant hepatitis is hardly ever seen in hepatitis C.

1582. Which of the following variables does not indicate impending hepatic failure with encephalopathy?
Harrison's 20th Ed. Chapter 332 Page 2362

- A. Shrunken liver
- B. Excessively prolonged PT
- C. Rapidly rising bilirubin level
- D. Rapidly rising aminotransferase levels

Aminotransferase levels may register a fall due to reduced hepatocyte mass in massive hepatic necrosis.

1583. Likelihood of remaining chronically infected after acute HBV infection is high in all except?
Harrison's 20th Ed. Chapter 332 Page 2362

- A. Old
- B. Down's syndrome
- C. Chronically hemodialyzed patients
- D. HIV infection

Likelihood of remaining chronically infected after acute HBV infection is high among neonates, Down's syndrome, chronically hemodialyzed patients & immunosuppressed patients, including those with HIV infection.

1584. Progression of acute to chronic hepatitis B is likely if?
Harrison's 20th Ed. Chapter 332 Page 2362

- A. HBeAg persists for >3 months
- B. HBsAg persists for >6 months
- C. AST/ALT do not normalise within 6–12 months
- D. All of the above

Progression of acute hepatitis to chronic hepatitis is likely if clinical symptoms do not resolve, AST/ALT, bilirubin and globulin levels fail to normalise within 6–12 months, HBeAg persists for >3 months and HBsAg persists for >6 months.

1585. Which of the following is false about hepatitis D superinfection?
Harrison's 20th Ed. Chapter 332 Page 2362

- A. Can transform inactive chronic hepatitis B into severe, progressive chronic hepatitis and cirrhosis
- B. Can accelerate course of chronic hepatitis B
- C. Can potentiate chronic hepatitis B to fulminant hepatitis
- D. Can increase likelihood of chronicity of acute hepatitis B

Acute hepatitis D infection does not increase likelihood of chronicity of simultaneous acute hepatitis B.

1586. The annual rate of cirrhosis in patients with chronic hepatitis D is?
Harrison's 20th Ed. Chapter 332 Page 2362

A. 1%
B. 2%
C. 3%
D. 4%

The annual rate of cirrhosis in patients with chronic hepatitis D is 4%.

1587. Likelihood of remaining chronically infected after acute HCV infection is?
Harrison's 20th Ed. Chapter 332 Page 2362

A. 25–40%
B. 40–60%
C. 65–75%
D. 85–90%

After acute HCV infection, the likelihood of remaining chronically infected approaches 85–90%.

1588. Progression of chronic hepatitis C is be influenced by?
Harrison's 20th Ed. Chapter 332 Page 2362

A. Advanced age of acquisition
B. Coexisting excessive alcohol use
C. HIV coinfection
D. All of the above

Progression of chronic hepatitis C may be influenced by advanced age of acquisition, long duration of infection, immunosuppression, coexisting excessive alcohol use, concomitant hepatic steatosis, other hepatitis virus infection or HIV coinfection.

1589. Condition leading to chronicity in hepatitis E is?
Harrison's 20th Ed. Chapter 332 Page 2362

A. Immunosuppressed organ-transplant recipients
B. Persons receiving cytotoxic chemotherapy
C. Persons with HIV infection
D. All of the above

1590. Enhanced risk of hepatocellular carcinoma in chronic hepatitis B is more in?
Harrison's 20th Ed. Chapter 332 Page 2362

A. Those infected in infancy or early childhood
B. Those with HBeAg
C. Those with high-level HBV DNA
D. All of the above

1591. The annual rate of hepatocellular carcinoma in patients with chronic hepatitis D and cirrhosis is?
Harrison's 20th Ed. Chapter 332 Page 2362

A. ~ 1%
B. ~ 2%
C. ~ 3%
D. ~ 4%

1592. Annual risk of hepatocellular carcinoma in cirrhotic patients with chronic hepatitis C is?
Harrison's 20th Ed. Chapter 332 Page 2362

A. ~ 1–4%
B. ~ 4–8%
C. ~ 8–12%
D. ~ 12–14%

1593. Gianotti-Crosti syndrome is best related to?
Harrison's 20th Ed. Chapter 332 Page 2363

A. Hepatitis A
B. Hepatitis B
C. Hepatitis C
D. Hepatitis E

Gianotti-Crosti syndrome or papular acrodermatitis of childhood refers to hepatitis B that presents with anicteric hepatitis, nonpruritic papular rash of face, buttocks & limbs & lymphadenopathy.

1594. Autoimmune hepatitis can be triggered by?
Harrison's 20th Ed. Chapter 332 Page 2363

A. Hepatitis A
B. Hepatitis B
C. Hepatitis C
D. All of the above

1595. Which of the following is a heterophile test?
Harrison's 20th Ed. Chapter 332 Page 2363

A. Weil Felix test
B. Paul Bunnel test or mononuclear spot test
C. Cold agglutination test
D. All of the above

Similar antigens present on dissimilar organisms are heterophile antigens. Antibodies thus produced are called hererophile antibodies or an antibody that reacts with antigens other than the antigen that stimulated it, i.e. an antibody that cross reacts.

1596. Clinical condition that may mimic acute hepatitis is?
Harrison's 20th Ed. Chapter 332 Page 2363

A. Right ventricular failure
B. Hypoperfusion syndromes
C. Budd-Chiari syndrome
D. All of the above

1597. Clinical condition that may mimic acute hepatitis is?
Harrison's 20th Ed. Chapter 332 Page 2363

A. Constrictive pericarditis
B. Right atrial myxoma
C. Venoocclusive disease
D. All of the above

Clinical constellation that may mimic acute hepatitis is right ventricular failure with passive hepatic congestion or hypoperfusion syndromes (shock, severe hypotension and severe left ventricular failure), right atrial myxoma, constrictive pericarditis, hepatic vein occlusion (Budd-Chiari syndrome) or venoocclusive disease. Others include acute fatty liver of pregnancy, cholestasis of pregnancy, eclampsia, and HELLP syndrome. Very rarely, malignancies metastatic to liver can mimic acute or even fulminant viral hepatitis. Genetic or metabolic liver disorders (Wilson's disease, α1 antitrypsin deficiency) and nonalcoholic fatty liver disease are confused with acute viral hepatitis.

1598. For severe acute hepatitis B, which of the following drugs is useful?
Harrison's 20th Ed. Chapter 332 Page 2363

A. Tenofovir
B. Ribavirin
C. Telaprevir
D. Boceprevir

1599. Which of the following is false about antiviral therapy for severe acute hepatitis B?
Harrison's 20th Ed. Chapter 332 Page 2363

- A. Nucleoside analogue tenofovir is potent & least resistance prone agent
- B. To be continued till 3 months after HBsAg seroconversion
- C. To be continued till 6 months after HBeAg seroconversion
- D. None of the above

Recovery occurs in ~99% of patients with acute hepatitis B. Rarely, for severe, not mild-moderate, acute hepatitis B, treatment has been attempted successfully with nucleoside analogue (entecavir or tenofovir). Treatment should continue until 3 months after HBsAg seroconversion or 6 months after HBeAg seroconversion. Other drugs used are Interferon, Lamivudine, Adefovir, Pegylated interferon, Telbivudine.

1600. Which of the following drugs provides high efficacy in treatment of acute hepatitis C?
Harrison's 20th Ed. Chapter 332 Page 2363

- A. Ribavirin
- B. Pegylated interferon
- C. Telaprevir
- D. Boceprevir

In typical cases of acute hepatitis C, recovery is rare and progression to chronic hepatitis is the rule. Pegylated interferon-based therapy for acute hepatitis C is efficacious.

1601. Sofosbuvir is best related to which of the following?
Cleveland Clinic Journal of Medicine. 2014;81(3):159

- A. NS3 protease inhibitor
- B. NS5A inhibitor
- C. NS5B nucleoside inhibitor
- D. NS5B non-nucleoside inhibitor

Sofosbuvir is a uridine nucleotide analogue that selectively inhibits HCV NS5B RNA-dependent RNA polymerase. It targets the highly conserved nucleotide binding pocket of this enzyme and functions as a chain terminator.

1602. Simeprevir is best related to which of the following?
Cleveland Clinic Journal of Medicine. 2014;81(3):159

- A. NS3 protease inhibitor
- B. NS5A inhibitor
- C. NS5B nucleoside inhibitor
- D. NS5B non-nucleoside inhibitor

Simeprevir belongs to the macrocyclic class with FDA approval only for HCV genotype 1 and in combination with interferon alfa and ribavirin. It is a weak inhibitor of the CYP3A4 enzyme and hence has less drug-drug interactions. Patients infected with HCV genotype 1a should be screened for the NS3 Q80K polymorphism at baseline, as it has been associated with substantially reduced response to simeprevir.

1603. Complications of Ribavirin treatment include which of the following?
Cleveland Clinic Journal of Medicine. 2014;81(3):159

- A. Hemolysis
- B. Skin complications
- C. Teratogenicity
- D. All of the above

Ribavirin causes hemolysis and skin complications and is teratogenic.

1604. Complications of Interferon treatment include which of the following?
Cleveland Clinic Journal of Medicine. 2014;81(3):159

- A. Seizures
- B. Peripheral neuropathy
- C. Bone marrow suppression
- D. All of the above

Interferon causes fatigue, flu-like symptoms, psychiatric symptoms (including depression or psychosis), weight loss, seizures, peripheral neuropathy, and bone marrow suppression.

1605. Patients with which of the following *IL28B* HCV genotype have a better chance of sustained virologic response with interferon?
Cleveland Clinic Journal of Medicine. 2014;81(3):159

- A. IL28B CC
- B. IL28B CT
- C. IL28B TT
- D. All of the above

When using interferon for HCV infected patient, information of IL28B genotype is essential i.e. single-nucleotide polymorphism (C or T) on chromosome 19q13 (rs12979860) upstream of the IL28B gene encoding for interferon lambda-3. Patients with the IL28B CC genotype have a much better chance of a sustained virologic response with interferon than do patients with CT or TT.

1606. Boceprevir and telaprevir are best related to which of the following?
Cleveland Clinic Journal of Medicine. 2014;81(3):159

- A. NS3/4 protease inhibitor
- B. NS5A inhibitor
- C. NS5B nucleoside inhibitor
- D. NS5B non-nucleoside inhibitor

Telaprevir & boceprevir are NS3/4A protease inhibitors that belong to the alfa-ketoamid derivative class. In May 2011, the FDA approved NS3/4A protease inhibitors boceprevir & telaprevir for treating HCV genotype 1 being highly specific for the amino acid target sequence of the NS3 region. These direct-acting antiviral agents had to be used in combination with interferon alfa and ribavirin.

1607. Dysgeusia is a adverse effect of which of the following drugs used to treat HCV infection?
Cleveland Clinic Journal of Medicine. 2014;81(3):159

- A. Boceprevir
- B. Telaprevir
- C. Sofosbuvir
- D. Simeprevir

Dysgeusia is seen with boceprevir, rash with telaprevir, and anemia with both.

1608. Principal enzyme responsible for boceprevir & telaprevir metabolism is?
Cleveland Clinic Journal of Medicine. 2014;81(3):159

- A. CYP2C9
- B. CYP2D6
- C. CYP3A4
- D. CYP2C19

Serious drug-drug interactions occur with the use of boceprevir & telaprevir with other medications that interact with CYP3A4, the principal enzyme responsible for their metabolism.

1609. Which of the following improves survival in patients of fulminant hepatitis?
Harrison's 20th Ed. Chapter 332 Page 2364

- A. Protein intake restriction
- B. Glucocorticoid therapy
- C. Prophylactic antibiotic coverage
- D. Plasmapheresis

Orthotopic liver transplantation provides excellent results in patients with fulminant hepatitis.

1610. Active immunization with vaccines is the preferable approach for prevention of?
Harrison's 20th Ed. Chapter 332 Page 2364

A. Hepatitis A
B. Hepatitis B
C. Hepatitis E
D. All of the above

1611. Hepatitis A vaccination is recommended for?
Harrison's 20th Ed. Chapter 332 Page 2364

A. Patients with chronic hepatitis B
B. Patients with chronic hepatitis C
C. Patients receiving clotting-factor concentrates
D. All of the above

1612. Hepatitis A vaccines provide adequate protection how many weeks after a primary inoculation?
Harrison's 20th Ed. Chapter 332 Page 2364

A. 1 week
B. 2 weeks
C. 3 weeks
D. 4 weeks

Formalin-inactivated vaccines made from strains of HAV attenuated in tissue culture are safe, immunogenic, and effectively prevent hepatitis A. Hepatitis A vaccines provide adequate protection beginning 4 weeks after a primary inoculation.

1613. Hepatitis A vaccine is administered by which route?
Harrison's 20th Ed. Chapter 332 Page 2364

A. Intradermal
B. Subcutenuous
C. Intramuscular
D. Intravenous

Hepatitis A vaccine is administered intramuscularly.

1614. The first vaccine for hepatitis B active immunization was prepared from?
Harrison's 20th Ed. Chapter 332 Page 2365

A. 22-nm spherical forms of HBsAg
B. 27-nm spherical forms of HBsAg
C. 42-nm spherical forms of HBsAg
D. All of the above

First vaccine for active immunization (1982) was prepared from purified, noninfectious 22-nm spherical forms of HBsAg derived from plasma of healthy HBsAg carriers.

1615. Which of the following is the difference between plasma-derived vaccine and genetically engineered Hepatitis B vaccine?
Harrison's 20th Ed. Chapter 332 Page 2365

A. Nonglycosylated
B. Hydrolyzed
C. Oxidized
D. Heat attenuated

Plasma-derived Hepatitis B vaccine is prepared from purified, noninfectious 22-nm spherical forms of HBsAg derived from plasma of healthy HBsAg carriers, while genetically engineered Hepatitis B vaccine is derived from recombinant yeast and consists of HBsAg particles that are nonglycosylated but are otherwise indistinguishable from natural HBsAg;

1616. Hepatitis B vaccine is administered?
Harrison's 20th Ed. Chapter 332 Page 2365

A. Intradermally
B. Subcuteneously
C. Intramuscularly
D. Intravenously

1617. In adults, recommended site of Hepatitis B vaccine is?
Harrison's 20th Ed. Chapter 332 Page 2365

A. Thigh muscle
B. Triceps muscle
C. Deltoid muscle
D. Gluteal muscle

1618. After the first dose of Hepatitis B vaccine, the third dose is given after?
Harrison's 20th Ed. Chapter 332 Page 2365

A. One month
B. Three months
C. Six months
D. Twelve months

For preexposure prophylaxis against hepatitis B, three IM injections of hepatitis B vaccine in deltoid, not gluteal muscle are recommended at 0, 1, and 6 months.

1619. Engerix-B for adults contains what amount of HBsAg in 1 mL?
Harrison's 20th Ed. Chapter 332 Page 2365

A. 5 µg
B. 10 µg
C. 15 µg
D. 20 µg

1620. For postexposure HBV prophylaxis, dose of HbIg is?
Harrison's 20th Ed. Chapter 332 Page 2365

A. 0.02 mL/kg
B. 0.04 mL/kg
C. 0.06 mL/kg
D. 0.08 mL/kg

For postexposure HBV prophylaxis, dose of HbIg is a single intramuscular dose of HbIg, 0.06 mL/kg, administered as soon after exposure as possible and followed by a complete course of hepatitis B vaccine to begin within the first week.

1621. Which of the following statements about Hepatitis B vaccination is false?
Harrison's 20th Ed. Chapter 332 Page 2365

A. Pregnancy is not a contraindication to vaccination
B. Booster immunizations are not recommended routinely
C. Booster recommended if anti-HBs levels are <10 mIU/mL
D. None of the above

1622. True nonresponse after proper HBV vaccination means antibody level of less than?
Harrison's 20th Ed. Chapter 332 Page 2365, N Engl J Med. 2004;351:2832-8

A. 10 mIU/mL
B. 15 mIU/mL

C. 20 mIU/mL
D. 50 mIU/mL

Booster immunizations are not recommended routinely in immunocompetent persons. Booster doses are recommended when anti-HBs levels fall to <10 mIU/mL.

1623. HBV inactive carriers have serum HBV DNA level below?
N Engl J Med. 2008;359:1486-500

A. 1000 IU per milliliter
B. 10000 IU per milliliter
C. 100000 IU per milliliter
D. 1000000 IU per milliliter

Persons with a serum HBV DNA level below 1000 IU per milliliter and a normal ALT level consistently are considered to be inactive carriers.

1624. Hepatitis B immune globulin (HbIg) is used in?
N Engl J Med. 2004;351:2832-8

A. Infants born to HBsAg + mothers
B. Contact with HBsAg + blood / bodily fluid
C. Sexual contact with person who is HBsAg +
D. All of the above

1625. Groups for whom Hepatitis B vaccine is recommended include all except?
N Engl J Med. 2004;351:2832-8

A. All infants
B. Patients on peritoneal dialysis
C. Persons at occupational risk
D. Clients & staff of institutions for developmentally disabled

1626. Groups for whom Hepatitis B vaccine is recommended include all except?
N Engl J Med. 2004;351:2832-8

A. Recipients of clotting-factor concentrates
B. Household members & sexual partners of HBV carriers
C. Adoptees from countries where HBV infection is endemic
D. Travelers spending > 6 weeks in HBV endemic areas

1627. Which of the following is false about hepatitis C vaccination?
Harrison's 20th Ed. Chapter 332 Page 2366

A. IG is ineffective in preventing hepatitis C
B. Hepatitis C vaccination is not feasible practically
C. No special precautions are recommended for babies born to mothers with hepatitis C
D. Breastfeeding to be restricted

Breastfeeding does not have to be restricted.

1628. Leser-Trelat sign mostly points towards which pathology?
Harrison's 20th Ed. Chapter 54 Page 346

A. Infection
B. Neoplasm
C. Nutritional deficiency
D. Environmental toxin

Leser-Trelat sign refers to multiple pruritic seborrheic keratoses of sudden onset. Mostly associated with gastrointestinal adenocarcinomas, breast, lung, urinary tract cancers & lymphoid malignancies.

1629. Which drug should be included in ART regimen when Hepatitis B and HIV occur together?
Harrison's 20th Ed. Chapter 334 Page 2379

A. Interferon alpha
B. Entecavir
C. Tenofovir
D. None of the above

1630. Wickman's striae are best related to?
N Engl J Med. 2018;379:567

A. Necrolytic acral erythema
B. Porphyria cutanea tarda
C. Leucocytoclastic vasculitis
D. Lichen planus (LP)

LP is an inflammatory disease of skin & mucous membranes, characterized by pruritic, purple, polygonal, papules with an overlying fine reticulate pattern of dots and lines called Wickman's striae. Lichen planus has a known association with HCV infection.

Toxic and Drug-induced Hepatitis

1631. Drugs affect a normal hepatocyte by?
Harrison's 20th Ed. Chapter 333 Page 2368 Figure 333-1
A. Disruption of intracellular calcium homeostasis
B. Disruption of actin filaments next to the canaliculus
C. Covalent binding of cytochrome P450 enzyme
D. All of the above

1632. Drugs affect a normal hepatocyte by?
Harrison's 20th Ed. Chapter 333 Page 2368 Figure 333-1
A. Stimulating immune response by cytolytic T cells & cytokines
B. Activation of apoptotic pathways by TNF-α receptor or Fas
C. Inhibition of mitochondrial function
D. All of the above

1633. Phase I reaction in drug metabolism include which of the following chemical process?
N Engl J Med. 2005;352:2211-21
A. Oxidation
B. Reduction
C. Hydrolysis
D. All of the above

1634. Phase II reaction in drug metabolism include which of the following chemical process?
N Engl J Med. 2005;352:2211-21
A. Glucuronidation
B. Sulfation
C. Acetylation
D. All of the above

1635. Phase II reactions in drug metabolism include all except?
N Engl J Med. 2005;352:2211-21
A. Sulfation
B. Glucuronidation
C. Acetylation
D. Hydrolysis

Drugs may be metabolized by sequential or competitive chemical processes involving oxidation, reduction & hydrolysis (phase I reactions) or glucuronidation, sulfation, acetylation & methylation (phase II reactions). CYP is important for phase I metabolism and are located primarily in endoplasmic reticulum, while phase 2 conjugation enzymes are cytosolic.

1636. Which of the following is not a feature of direct toxic hepatitis?
Harrison's 20th Ed. Chapter 333 Page 2367
A. Predictable regularity
B. Dose-dependent
C. Latent period usually long
D. Morphologic abnormalities reproducible for each toxin

In direct toxic hepatitis, latent period between exposure and liver injury is usually short (often several hours), although clinical manifestations may be delayed for 24–48 hours.

1637. Which of the following is not a feature of idiosyncratic drug hepatotoxicity?
Harrison's 20th Ed. Chapter 333 Page 2367
A. Unpredictability
B. Not dose-dependent
C. Extrahepatic manifestations of hypersensitivity
D. None of the above

1638. Which of the following is involved in the pathogenesis of drug-induced cholestasis?
Harrison's 20th Ed. Chapter 333 Page 2367, J Clin Exp Hepatol. 2012;2(3):247-259
A. Farnesoid X receptor (FXR)
B. Pregnane X receptor (PXR)
C. Constitutive androstane receptor (CXR)
D. All of the above

1639. Hepatocellular injury produced by idiosyncratic reactions resembles that observed in?
Harrison's 20th Ed. Chapter 333 Page 2367
A. Acute viral hepatitis A
B. Acute viral hepatitis B
C. Acute viral hepatitis C
D. All of the above

1640. Antibody to liver-kidney microsomes associated with drug induced hepatitis is?
Harrison's 20th Ed. Chapter 333 Page 2367
A. Anti LKM 1
B. Anti LKM 2
C. Anti LKM 3
D. All of the above

Drug hepatotoxicity may be associated with the appearance of autoantibodies, including a class of antibodies to liver-kidney microsomes, anti-LKM2, directed against a cytochrome P450 enzyme.

1641. Amoxicillin-clavulanic acid produces which type of drug-induced cholestasis?
Harrison's 20th Ed. Chapter 333 Page 2367
A. Bland cholestasis
B. Inflammatory cholestasis
C. Sclerosing cholangitis
D. Ductopenic cholestasis

1642. Distinction between hepatocellular and cholestatic reaction is indicated by?
Harrison's 20th Ed. Chapter 333 Page 2367
A. Q value
B. R value
C. S value
D. T value

Distinction between hepatocellular and cholestatic reaction is indicated by R value which is the ratio of alanine aminotransferase (ALT) to alkaline phosphatase values, both expressed as multiples of the upper limit of normal. An R value of >5.0 is indicative of hepatocellular injury, R <2.0 of cholestatic injury, and R between 2.0 and 5.0 of mixed hepatocellular-cholestatic injury. R value was established by the Council for International Organizations of Medical Sciences. R = (ALT value ÷ ALT ULN) ÷ (Alk P value ÷ Alk P ULN).

1643. Which of the following is a causality assessment method for assessing causality in drug-induced liver injury (DILI)?
Harrison's 20th Ed. Chapter 333 Page 2367

- A. Benichou Causality Assessment Method
- B. Roussel Uclaf Causality Assessment Method
- C. Lachin Danan Causality Assessment Method
- D. Watkins Navarro Causality Assessment Method

The Roussel Uclaf Causality Assessment Method (RUCAM) was developed to quantify the strength of association between a liver injury and the medication implicated as causing the injury. RUCAM is composed of seven different criteria including time to onset, clinical course, risk factors, concomitant drugs, non-drug-causes, published information on hepatotoxicity, and the response to any re-administration. RUCAM score ranges from −8 to + 14, with higher values signifying a greater degree of association.

1644. Which of the following is a causality assessment method for assessing causality in drug-induced liver injury (DILI)?
J Clin Exp Hepatol. 2012;2(3):247-59

- A. Roussel Uclaf Causality Assessment Method (RUCAM)
- B. Maria and Victorino (M and V) method
- C. DILIN (Drug-Induced Liver Injury Network) expert opinion
- D. All of the above

1645. Name of the prognostic law stating that a pure drug-induced liver injury (DILI) leading to jaundice, without a hepatic transplant, has a case fatality rate of 10% to 50% is?
Harrison's 20th Ed. Chapter 333 Page 2367

- A. Zy's law
- B. Ky's law
- C. Hy's law
- D. Wy's law

Hy's Law criteria: >3x ULN AST or ALT + >2x ULN TBL, no initial cholestasis (normal AP), no other prior or concomitant reason for liver function abnormality. Rezulin Rule is also a prognostic rule of DILI. Rezulin is the trade name of banned drug troglitazone.

1646. Portal hypertension in the absence of cirrhosis may result from the use of?
Harrison's 20th Ed. Chapter 333 Page 2369

- A. Vitamin A
- B. Arsenic intoxication
- C. Exposure to vinyl chloride
- D. All of the above

1647. Which of the following are associated with angiosarcoma of the liver?
Harrison's 20th Ed. Chapter 333 Page 2369

- A. Arsenic intoxication
- B. Vinyl chloride
- C. Thorium dioxide
- D. All of the above

Arsenic intoxication, industrial exposure to vinyl chloride, or administration of thorium dioxide have been associated with angiosarcoma of the liver.

1648. Peliosis hepatis refers to?
Harrison's 20th Ed. Chapter 333 Page 2369

- A. Trauma of liver
- B. Blood cysts of liver
- C. Ectopic liver
- D. Unilobular liver

Peliosis hepatis refers to blood cysts of the liver.

1649. Peliosis hepatis is seen in patients treated with?
Harrison's 20th Ed. Chapter 333 Page 2369

- A. Halothane
- B. Anabolic steroids
- C. Chlorpromazine
- D. Methotrexate

Peliosis hepatis has been observed in some patients treated with anabolic steroids.

1650. Which of the following about acetaminophen metabolism is false?
N Engl J Med. 2008;359:285-92

- A. >90% is metabolized by glucuronidation or sulfation
- B. ~5% is metabolized by cytochrome P450 2E1 to NAPQI
- C. NAPQI is detoxified by glutathione to cysteine & mercapturic acid
- D. None of the above

As long as sufficient glutathione is present, the liver is protected from injury. N-acetylcysteine prevents hepatic injury primarily by restoring hepatic glutathione, improving hemodynamics and oxygen use, increasing clearance of indocyanine green and decreasing cerebral edema.

1651. Which of the following histopathologic changes occur after toxic quantity of acetaminophen ingestion?
Harrison's 20th Ed. Chapter 333 Page 2371

- A. Periportal hepatic necrosis
- B. Centrilobular hepatic necrosis
- C. Massive hepatic necrosis
- D. Bridging hepatic necrosis

Acetaminophen causes dose-related centrilobular hepatic necrosis after single time-point ingestions.

1652. Fatal fulminant liver disease is usually associated with ingestion of what amount of acetaminophen?
Harrison's 20th Ed. Chapter 333 Page 2371

- A. 5 grams
- B. 10 grams
- C. 20 grams
- D. 25 grams

A single dose of 10–15 grams may produce clinical evidence of liver injury. Fatal fulminant liver disease is usually associated with ingestion of over 25 grams of acetaminophen.

1653. What level of acetaminophen in blood is predictive of severe liver damage?
Harrison's 20th Ed. Chapter 333 Page 2371

- A. > 100 µg/mL
- B. > 150 µg/mL
- C. > 200 µg/mL
- D. > 300 µg/mL

Blood levels of acetaminophen of >300 µg/mL, 4 hours after ingestion are predictive severe liver damage. Levels <150 µg/mL suggest that hepatic injury is highly unlikely.

1654. Maximal hepatic injury and hepatic failure occurs after how many days of acetaminophen ingestion?
Harrison's 20th Ed. Chapter 333 Page 2371

A. 1–2 days
B. 2–3 days
C. 3–5 days
D. 7–9 days

Maximal hepatic injury & hepatic failure appear 3–5 days after acetaminophen ingestion. Extremely high aminotransferase levels in association with low bilirubin levels are characteristic.

1655. Which of the following is "hepatoprotective"?
Harrison's 20th Ed. Chapter 333 Page 2371

A. Activated charcoal
B. Cholestyramine
C. Glutathione
D. All of the above

Alcohol suppresses hepatic glutathione production.

1656. Glutathione is synthesized from which of the following amino acids?
N Engl J Med. 2008;359:285-92

A. Cysteine
B. Glutamate
C. Glycine
D. All of the above

Glutamate & glycine are present in abundance in hepatocytes. Availability of cysteine is the rate-limiting factor in glutathione synthesis. Cysteine itself is not well absorbed after oral administration. Acetylcysteine, in contrast, is readily absorbed & rapidly enters cells, where it is hydrolyzed to cysteine, thus providing the limiting substrate for glutathione synthesis.

1657. Nomogram to define risk of acetaminophen hepatotoxicity is called?
N Engl J Med. 2008;359:285-92

A. Makin-Mitchell nomogram
B. Rumack-Matthew nomogram
C. Jollow-Devlin nomogram
D. Trey-Daly nomogram

The Rumack–Matthew nomogram was first published in 1975. It estimates the likelihood of hepatic injury due to acetaminophen toxicity for patients with a single ingestion at a known time.

1658. Which of the following is the hepatotoxic metabolite formed from acetaminophen?
Harrison's 20th Ed. Chapter 333 Page 2371

A. 4-pentenoic acid
B. Electrophilic arene oxides
C. NAPQI
D. Betaine

N-acetyl-p-benzoquinone imine (NAPQI) is the hepatotoxic metabolite formed from acetaminophen by cytochrome P450 CYP2E1 by a phase 1 reaction. When excessive amounts of NAPQI are formed or when glutathione levels are low, glutathione levels are depleted and overwhelmed, permitting covalent binding to nucleophilic hepatocyte macromolecules forming acetaminophen-protein "adducts" which can be measured in serum by high performance liquid chromatography.

1659. N-acetyl-benzoquinone-imine (NAPQI) is best related to which of the following?
Harrison's 20th Ed. Chapter 333 Page 2371

A. Acetaminophen
B. Quinidine
C. Azathioprine
D. Carbamazine

1660. Which of the following is the end product of acetaminophen metabolism?
Harrison's 20th Ed. Chapter 333 Page 2371

A. Gamma-aminobutyric acid
B. Mercapturic acid
C. Boric acid
D. Butyric acid

Most of acetaminophen is metabolized by phase II reaction to sulfate & glucuronide metabolites. Phase I reaction by CYP2E1 metabolizes a small amount of acetaminophen to N-acetyl-benzoquinone-imine (NAPQI) which is hepatotoxic. However, "hepatoprotective" glutathione binds NAPQI to form harmless mercapturic acid that is excreted through kidneys. Alcohol induces cytochrome P450 CYP2E1.

1661. With acetaminophen, hepatic injury may be potentiated by?
Harrison's 20th Ed. Chapter 333 Page 2371

A. Alcohol
B. Phenobarbital
C. INH
D. All of the above

Hepatic injury may be potentiated by prior administration of alcohol, phenobarbital, INH, & starvation.

1662. Which of the following about alcohol is false?
Harrison's 20th Ed. Chapter 333 Page 2371

A. Direct hepatotoxin
B. Induces cytochrome P450 CYP2E1
C. Suppresses hepatic glutathione production
D. None of the above

1663. Oral activated charcoal or cholestyramine is useless how much time after acetaminophen ingestion?
Harrison's 20th Ed. Chapter 333 Page 2371

A. > 30 minutes
B. > 60 minutes
C. > 90 minutes
D. > 120 minutes

Oral activated charcoal or cholestyramine to prevent absorption of residual drug is useless if given >30 minutes after acetaminophen ingestion.

1664. Which of the following has a role in the management of acetaminophen hepatotoxicity?
Harrison's 20th Ed. Chapter 333 Page 2371

A. Cysteamine
B. Cysteine
C. N-acetylcysteine
D. All of the above

If given within 8 hours of ingestion of acetaminophen, administration of sulfhydryl compounds (cysteamine, cysteine, or N-acetylcysteine) reduces the severity of hepatic necrosis. These agents act by providing a reservoir of sulfhydryl groups to bind toxic metabolites or by stimulating synthesis and repletion of hepatic glutathione. If these fail, liver transplantation may be the only option.

1665. Patients of acetaminophen hepatotoxicity who present with hepatic failure have a mortality rate of?
N Engl J Med. 2008;359:285-92

   A. 5 to 20%
   B. 20 to 40%
   C. 40 to 60%
   D. 60 to 80%

Acetaminophen hepatotoxicity patients presenting with hepatic failure have a mortality rate of 20 to 40%.

1666. In acute acetaminophen ingestion, oral acetylcysteine is given as a loading dose of?
N Engl J Med. 2008;359:285-92

   A. 40 mg per kilogram of body weight
   B. 140 mg per kilogram of body weight
   C. 240 mg per kilogram of body weight
   D. 340 mg per kilogram of body weight

1667. In acute acetaminophen ingestion, maintenance dose of oral acetylcysteine is?
N Engl J Med. 2008;359:285-92

   A. 40 mg per kilogram of body weight
   B. 50 mg per kilogram of body weight
   C. 60 mg per kilogram of body weight
   D. 70 mg per kilogram of body weight

Oral acetylcysteine is given as a loading dose of 140 mg per kilogram of body weight, with maintenance doses of 70 mg per kilogram that are repeated every 4 hours for a total of 17 doses. Rechecking the alanine aminotransferase & serum acetaminophen concentrations is particularly important to increase the duration of treatment.

1668. In acute acetaminophen ingestion, intravenous loading dose of acetylcysteine is?
N Engl J Med. 2008;359:285-92

   A. 120 mg per kilogram of body weight
   B. 150 mg per kilogram of body weight
   C. 200 mg per kilogram of body weight
   D. 220 mg per kilogram of body weight

The intravenous loading dose of acetylcysteine in acute acetaminophen ingestion is 150 mg per kilogram, followed by an infusion of 12.5 mg per kilogram per hour over a 4-hour period, and finally an infusion of 6.25 mg per kilogram per hour over a 16-hour period.

1669. Which of the following is an adverse effect of intravenous acetylcysteine?
N Engl J Med. 2008;359:285-92

   A. Pruritus
   B. Angioedema, bronchospasm
   C. Tachycardia, hypotension
   D. All of the above

The most commonly reported adverse effects of intravenous acetylcysteine are anaphylactoid reactions, including rash, pruritus, angioedema, bronchospasm, tachycardia, and hypotension.

1670. In acetaminophen hepatotoxicity, which of the following may identify patients highly likely to require liver transplantation?
Harrison's 20th Ed. Chapter 333 Page 2372

   A. Arterial blood ammonia levels
   B. Arterial blood mercaptan levels
   C. Arterial blood lactate levels
   D. All of the above

Early arterial blood lactate levels of >3.5 mmol/L in patients with acute liver failure due to acetaminophen hepatotoxicity may distinguish patients highly likely to require liver transplantation from those likely to survive without liver replacement.

1671. Which of the following about isoniazid is false?
Clin Infect Dis. 2016;63:e147

   A. Also called isonicotinylhydrazide or isonicotinic acid hydrazine
   B. Synthetic antibiotic
   C. Bactericidal against replicating Mycobacterium tuberculosis
   D. None of the above

1672. In USA, which of the following is the commonest cause of drug-induced acute liver failure (ALF)?
J Clin Exp Hepatol. 2012;2(3):247-259

   A. Paracetamol
   B. Antituberculosis drugs
   C. Antiepileptic drugs
   D. Herbal drugs

1673. In India, which of the following is the commonest cause of drug-induced acute liver failure (ALF) in adults and children?
J Clin Exp Hepatol. 2012;2(3):247-259

   A. Paracetamol
   B. Antituberculosis drugs
   C. Antiepileptic drugs
   D. Herbal drugs

In India antituberculosis drugs are the commonest cause of drug-induced ALF in adults and children.

1674. Isoniazid hepatotoxicity is enhanced by?
Harrison's 20th Ed. Chapter 333 Page 2372

   A. Alcohol
   B. Rifampin
   C. Pyrazinamide
   D. All of the above

Isoniazid hepatotoxicity is enhanced by alcohol, barbiturates, rifampin & pyrazinamide.

1675. Highest frequency of substantial liver injury due to INH use is in patients over the age of?
Harrison's 20th Ed. Chapter 333 Page 2372

   A. 20 years
   B. 30 years
   C. 40 years
   D. 50 years

Substantial liver injury appears to be age-related, increasing substantially after age 35. Highest frequency is in patients over age 50 years and the lowest is in patients under the age of 20.

1676. Which of the following drugs produce toxic and idiosyncratic reactions?
Harrison's 20th Ed. Chapter 333 Page 2372

   A. Isoniazid
   B. Sodium valproate

C. Amiodarone
D. All of the above

1677. Which of the following drugs act as a direct toxin in liver?
Harrison's 20th Ed. Chapter 333 Page 2372

A. Acetaminophen
B. Nitrofurantoin
C. Amoxicillin-clavulanate
D. Simvastatin

Acetaminophen causes dose-related centrilobular hepatic necrosis after single-time-point ingestions.

1678. IV administration of carnitine may be ameliorate hepatotoxicity due to?
Harrison's 20th Ed. Chapter 333 Page 2372

A. Valproate
B. Isoniazid
C. Halothane
D. Acetaminophen

Valproate hepatotoxicity may be ameliorated by IV administration of carnitine. Valproate inhibits biosynthesis of carnitine, by affecting the beta-oxidation of fatty acids. Carnitine supplementation circumvents the defect by increasing the beta-oxidation of valproate.

1679. Which metabolite of sodium valproate may be responsible for hepatic injury?
Harrison's 20th Ed. Chapter 333 Page 2372

A. 1-pentenoic acid
B. 2-pentenoic acid
C. 3-pentenoic acid
D. 4-pentenoic acid

Sodium valproate is not directly hepatotoxic, but its metabolite 4-pentenoic acid may be responsible for hepatic injury.

1680. Which of the following drugs is associated with moderate to severe chronic hepatitis with autoimmune features?
Harrison's 20th Ed. Chapter 333 Page 2372

A. Nitrofurantoin
B. Hydralazine
C. Methyldopa
D. All of the above

Nitrofurantoin, minocycline, hydralazine and methyldopa have been associated with moderate to severe chronic hepatitis with autoimmune features.

1681. "Vanishing bile duct syndrome" best relates to?
Harrison's 20th Ed. Chapter 333 Page 2372

A. Amoxicillin-clavulanate hepatotoxicity
B. Oral contraceptive hepatotoxicity
C. Anabolic steroid hepatotoxicity
D. All of the above

1682. "Vanishing bile duct syndrome" best relates to?
Harrison's 20th Ed. Chapter 45 Page 280, Chapter 338 Page 2420

A. Chronic liver transplant rejection
B. Graft-versus-host disease after bone marrow transplantation
C. Sarcoidosis
D. All of the above

1683. Pure cholestasis is due to which of the following drug toxicity?
Harrison's 20th Ed. Chapter 45 Page 280 Table 45-3

A. Chlorpromazine
B. Erythromycin estolate
C. Anabolic and contraceptive steroids
D. Prochlorperazine

1684. Cholestatic hepatitis is due to which of the following drug toxicity?
Harrison's 20th Ed. Chapter 45 Page 280 Table 45-3

A. Anabolic steroids
B. Erythromycin estolate
C. Contraceptive steroids
D. Prochlorperazine

1685. Chronic cholestasis is due to which of the following drug toxicity?
Harrison's 20th Ed. Chapter 45 Page 280 Table 45-3

A. Anabolic steroids
B. Erythromycin estolate
C. Contraceptive steroids
D. Chlorpromazine

1686. Which of the following about halothane hepatotoxicity is false?
Hepat Mon. 2011;11(1):3-6

A. Idiosyncratic reaction
B. Halothane is not a direct hepatotoxin
C. Cause severe centrilobular hepatic necrosis
D. Cross-reactions between halothane & methoxyflurane

The pathologic changes produced by halothane hepatotoxicity are indistinguishable from massive hepatic necrosis resulting from viral hepatitis. Severe centrilobular hepatic necrosis is typical of acetaminophen toxicity.

1687. Which of the following is false about methyldopa hepatotoxicity?
The American Journal of Medicine. 1976;60(7):941-948

A. Toxic reaction
B. Idiosyncratic reaction
C. Resolves with discontinuation of drug
D. None of the above

1688. A defect in epoxide hydrolase activity could cause hepatotoxicity due to which drug?
Harrison's 20th Ed. Chapter 333 Page 2372

A. Valproate
B. Phenytoin
C. Halothane
D. Acetaminophen

A defect in epoxide hydrolase activity could cause hepatotoxicity due to Phenytoin.

1689. Stevens-Johnson syndrome may be a presentation of toxicity due to?
Harrison's 20th Ed. Chapter 333 Page 2372

A. Valproate
B. Phenytoin

C. Halothane
D. Acetaminophen

Apart from drug induced hepatitis, fever, lymphadenopathy, rash (Stevens-Johnson syndrome or exfoliative dermatitis), leukocytosis & eosinophilia may manifest in hepatotoxicity due to Phenytoin.

1690. Histopathologically, abundance of eosinophils in liver points towards the toxicity with which of the following drug?
Harrison's 20th Ed. Chapter 333 Page 2372

A. Valproate
B. Phenytoin
C. Halothane
D. Acetaminophen

1691. Hepatic injury manifests within what period after beginning phenytoin therapy?
Harrison's 20th Ed. Chapter 333 Page 2372

A. First day
B. First week
C. First month
D. Two months

Hepatic injury manifests within the first 2 months after beginning phenytoin therapy.

1692. Which of the following is a major metabolite of Amiodarone?
Harrison's 20th Ed. Chapter 333 Page 2373

A. Desmethylamiodarone
B. Desethylamiodarone
C. Levomethylamiodarone
D. Levoethylamiodarone

1693. Amiodarone metabolite desethylamiodarone accumulate in which of the following?
Harrison's 20th Ed. Chapter 333 Page 2373

A. Hepatocyte lysosomes
B. Hepatocyte mitochondria
C. Bile duct epithelium
D. All of the above

1694. Pseudoalcoholic liver injury best relates to toxicity with?
Harrison's 20th Ed. Chapter 333 Page 2373

A. Valproate
B. Phenytoin
C. Halothane
D. Amiodarone

In amiodarone toxicity, pseudoalcoholic liver injury can range from steatosis, to alcoholic hepatitis like neutrophilic infiltration and Mallory's hyaline, to cirrhosis.

1695. Phospholipidosis is best related to which of the following drug toxicity?
Harrison's 20th Ed. Chapter 333 Page 2373

A. Valproate
B. Phenytoin
C. Halothane
D. Amiodarone

Electron-microscopic demonstration of phospholipid-laden lysosomal lamellar bodies (ultrastructural phospholipidosis) can help to distinguish amiodarone hepatotoxicity from typical alcoholic hepatitis.

1696. Toxicity with which of the following produces cholestatic idiosyncratic reaction?
Harrison's 20th Ed. Chapter 333 Page 2373

A. Acetaminophen
B. Erythromycin
C. Azathioprine
D. Carbamazine

1697. Drugs producing cholestatic reaction and portal inflammation is?
Harrison's 20th Ed. Chapter 333 Page 2373

A. Erythromycin
B. Oral contraceptive
C. Amiodarone
D. 17, α-Alkyl-Substituted Anabolic Steroids

1698. Which of the following rises most in liver injury due to anabolic steroids?
Harrison's 20th Ed. Chapter 333 Page 2373

A. Serum aminotransferases
B. Serum alkaline phosphatase
C. Serum bilirubin
D. Serum globulin

In liver injury due to anabolic steroids, serum aminotransferase levels are usually <100 IU/L, serum alkaline phosphatase levels are generally moderately elevated with bilirubin levels frequently exceeding 20 mg/dL.

1699. In Trimethoprim-Sulfamethoxazole toxicity, hepatotoxicity is attributable to which component of the drug?
Harrison's 20th Ed. Chapter 333 Page 2373

A. Sulfamethoxazole
B. Trimethoprim
C. Sulfamethoxazole + Trimethoprim
D. None of the above

The hepatotoxicity with the use of Trimethoprim-Sulfamethoxazole is attributable to the sulfamethoxazole component of the drug.

1700. The risk of trimethoprim-sulfamethoxazole hepatotoxicity is increased in persons with?
Harrison's 20th Ed. Chapter 333 Page 2373

A. HIV infection
B. Severe anemia
C. Chronic renal failure
D. Congestive heart failure

Risk of trimethoprim-sulfamethoxazole hepatotoxicity is increased in persons with HIV infection.

1701. Statin hepatotoxicity is increased in which of the following patients?
Harrison's 20th Ed. Chapter 333 Page 2374

A. Chronic hepatitis C
B. Hepatic steatosis
C. Other underlying liver diseases
D. None of the above

Statin hepatotoxicity is "not" increased in patients with chronic hepatitis C, hepatic steatosis, or other underlying liver diseases, and statins can be used safely in these patients.

1702. In Total Parenteral Nutrition (TPN), steatosis or steatohepatitis may result due to an excess of?
Harrison's 20th Ed. Chapter 333 Page 2374

A. Carbohydrate calories
B. Protein calories
C. Fat calories
D. Deficiency of minerals

In Total Parenteral Nutrition (TPN), steatosis or steatohepatitis may result due to an excess of carbohydrate calories. This complication has reduced substantially by introduction of balanced TPN formulas that rely on lipid as an alternative caloric source.

1703. Herbal remedies associated with toxic hepatitis is?
Harrison's 20th Ed. Chapter 333 Page 2374

A. Jin Bu Huan
B. Xiao-chai-hutang
C. Ma huang
D. All of the above

Jin Bu Huan, xiao-chai-hutang, germander, chaparral, senna, mistletoe, skullcap, gentian, comfrey (containing pyrrolizidine alkaloids), ma huang, bee pollen, valerian root, pennyroyal oil, kava, celandine, Impila (Callilepis laureola), LipoKinetix, Hydroxycut, herbal nutritional supplements and herbal teas containing Camellia sinensis (green tea extract).

1704. Which of the following drugs is implicated in the development of cirrhosis?
Harrison's 20th Ed. Chapter 333 Page 2369

A. Oxyphenisatin
B. Methyldopa
C. Isoniazid
D. Methotrexate

Methotrexate, tamoxifen and amiodarone have been implicated in the development of cirrhosis.

1705. Most common cause of liver enzyme elevation is?
Cleveland Clinic Journal of Medicine. 2018;85(8):612

A. Alcohol toxicity
B. Medication overdose
C. Fatty liver disease
D. All of the above

Most common causes of liver enzyme elevation are alcohol toxicity, medication overdose, & fatty liver disease.

1706. Cytochrome P450 (CYP) was first discovered in 1954 by?
J Adv Pract Oncol. 2013;4(4):263-268

A. Wilhelm Kuhnz & Hille Gieschen
B. Bernhardt
C. Martin Klingenberg & David Garfinkel
D. Akio Suzuki

1707. Cytochrome P-450 enzymes (CYPs) are important in the biosynthesis and degradation of?
N Engl J Med. 2005;352:2211-21

A. Steroids
B. Lipids
C. Vitamins
D. All of the above

Cytochrome P-450 enzymes (CYPs) are important in biosynthesis & degradation of endogenous compounds like steroids, lipids, and vitamins.

1708. Cytochrome P-450 enzymes (CYPs) are important in the biosynthesis & degradation of endogenous compounds like?
N Engl J Med. 2005;352:2211-21

A. Steroids
B. Lipids
C. Vitamins
D. All of the above

1709. The P in P450 stands for?
Am Fam Phys 1998;57:107-16

A. Particle
B. Pigment
C. Pattern
D. Protein

The P in P450 stands for "pigment".

1710. "450" in Cytochrome P450 isoenzymes is related to?
J Adv Pract Oncol. 2013;4(4):263-268

A. Number of isoenzymes in liver
B. Number of chemical reactions
C. Number of electron needed for its activity
D. Spectrophotometric absorption peak

Name cytochrome P450 is derived from the fact that these are colored ('chrome') cellular ('cyto') proteins, with a "pigment at 450 nm", so named for the characteristic spectrophotometric absorption peak formed by absorbance of light at wavelengths near 450 nm when the heme iron is reduced and complexed to carbon monoxide.

1711. In CYP2E1, letter '2' indicates?
J Adv Pract Oncol. 2013;4(4):263-268

A. Gene family
B. Gene subfamily
C. Individual gene
D. None of the above

"CYP" stands for cytochrome P450, followed by a numeral indicating gene family, a capital letter indicating subfamily and another numeral for the individual gene.

1712. Which of the following about cytochrome P450 is false?
J Adv Pract Oncol. 2013;4(4):263-268

A. Hemoprotein
B. Monooxygenases
C. Pigment at 450 nm
D. None of the above

Cytochrome P450 belongs to a superfamily of hemoproteins. Most common reaction catalysed by cytochrome P450 is a monooxygenase reaction, i.e. insertion of one atom of oxygen into an organic substrate (RH) while the other oxygen atom is reduced to water: $RH + O_2 + 2H^+ + 2e^- = ROH + H_2O$

1713. The catalytic activity of CYP2D6 in humans is best assessed by using which of the following drug?
Pharmacogenomics. 2009;10(1):17-28

A. Debrisoquine
B. Fluoxetine
C. Perphenazine
D. Dextromethorphan

CYP2D6 or Debrisoquine hydroxylase is second to CYP3A4 in the number of commonly used drugs that it metabolizes. Debrisoquine is a derivative of guanidine. It is an antihypertensive drug similar to guanethidine. Debrisoquine is frequently used for phenotyping the CYP2D6 enzyme.

1714. Which of the following cytochrome P-450 is present in enterocytes?
N Engl J Med. 2005;352:2211-21

A. CYP1A2
B. CYP2D6
C. CYP2C9
D. CYP3A

CYP3A is present in the enterocytes.

1715. Which of the following CYP is found mainly in the glomerulosa zone of adrenal gland?
Harrison's 20th Ed. Chapter 379 Page 2723

A. CYP11B2
B. CYP3A5
C. CYP2D6
D. CYP2C19

CYP11B2 is found mainly if not exclusively in the glomerulosa zone of the adrenal gland.

1716. Which of the following is the primary isoenzyme expressed during the prenatal period?
J Pediatr Pharmacol Ther. 2014;19(4):262-276

A. CYP1A2
B. CYP3A7
C. CYP2D6
D. CYP2C19

CYP3A7 is the primary isoenzyme expressed during the prenatal period. It declines rapidly after birth and is barely measurable in adults.

1717. Which of the following CYP is not expressed in neonates?
J Pediatr Pharmacol Ther. 2014;19(4):262-276

A. CYP1A2
B. CYP3A5
C. CYP2D6
D. CYP2C19

CYP1A2 is not expressed in neonates, making them susceptible to toxicity from drugs such as caffeine.

1718. Drugs having a narrow range between the plasma levels yielding therapeutic and adverse effects include all except?

A. Digoxin
B. Theophylline
C. Lidocaine
D. Amiodarone

1719. Which of the following anti-HIV agent is not a CYP3A inhibitor?
N Engl J Med. 2005;352:2211-21

A. Indinavir
B. Ritonavir
C. Saquinavir
D. Nevirapine

1720. Which of the following macrolide antibiotics is not a CYP3A inhibitor?
N Engl J Med. 2005;352:2211-21

A. Clarithromycin
B. Erythromycin
C. Troleandomycin
D. Azithromycin

1721. Which of the following anticonvulsant agent is not a CYP3A inducer?
N Engl J Med. 2005;352:2211-21

A. Carbamazepine
B. Phenobarbital
C. Phenytoin
D. Lamotrigine

1722. Which of the following enzyme is responsible for metabolism of most of the drugs used?
Harrison's 20th Ed. Chapter 64 Page 430

A. CYP3A4
B. CYP3A5
C. CYP2D6
D. CYP2C19

CYP3A4 is the most abundant hepatic and intestinal CYP and is also the enzyme responsible for metabolism of the greatest number of drugs in therapeutic use. CYP2D6 is second to CYP3A4 in the number of commonly used drugs that it metabolizes. Families or enzymes that are of greatest importance in metabolism of drugs are CYP3A4, 2D6, 2C9, 2C19, 1A2, 2E1, and 2B6.

1723. In liver, the family of cytochrome P450 (CYP) isoforms is present in?
J Adv Pract Oncol. 2013;4(4):263-268

A. Endoplasmic reticulum
B. Cell membrane
C. Golgi bodies
D. Nucleus

1724. Which of the following does not inhibit CYP3A4?
Harrison's 20th Ed. Chapter 139 Page 1053

A. Azithromycin
B. Erythromycin
C. Clarithromycin
D. Telithromycin

Erythromycin, clarithromycin and telithromycin inhibit CYP3A4 hepatic drug metabolizing enzyme and can result in increased levels of coadministered drugs, including benzodiazepines, statins, warfarin, cyclosporine and tacrolimus. Azithromycin does not inhibit CYP3A4 and lacks these drug-drug interactions.

1725. Major hepatic isoenzyme involved in warfarin metabolism is?
Harrison's 20th Ed. Chapter 63 Page 421 Table 63-1

A. CYP 2C9
B. CYP 2C19
C. CYP 2D6
D. CYP 3A

1726. Major hepatic isoenzyme involved in phenytoin metabolism is?
Harrison's 20th Ed. Chapter 63 Page 421 Table 63-1

A. CYP 2C9
B. CYP 2C19

C. CYP 2D6
D. CYP 3A

1727. Major hepatic isoenzyme in omeprazole metabolism is?
Harrison's 20th Ed. Chapter 63 Page 421 Table 63-1
A. CYP 2C9
B. CYP 2C19
C. CYP 2D6
D. CYP 3A

1728. Major hepatic isoenzyme in metoprolol metabolism is?
Harrison's 20th Ed. Chapter 63 Page 421 Table 63-1
A. CYP 2C9
B. CYP 2C19
C. CYP 2D6
D. CYP 3A

1729. Major hepatic isoenzyme in tricyclic antidepressants metabolism is?
Harrison's 20th Ed. Chapter 63 Page 421 Table 63-1
A. CYP 2C9
B. CYP 2C19
C. CYP 2D6
D. CYP 3A

1730. Major hepatic isoenzyme involved in selective serotonin reuptake inhibitors metabolism is?
Harrison's 20th Ed. Chapter 63 Page 421 Table 63-1
A. CYP 2C9
B. CYP 2C19
C. CYP 2D6
D. CYP 3A

1731. Major hepatic isoenzyme involved in codeine metabolism is?
Harrison's 20th Ed. Chapter 63 Page 421 Table 63-1
A. CYP 2C9
B. CYP 2C19
C. CYP 2D6
D. CYP 3A

1732. Major hepatic isoenzyme in cyclosporine metabolism is?
Harrison's 20th Ed. Chapter 63 Page 421 Table 63-1
A. CYP 2C9
B. CYP 2C19
C. CYP 2D6
D. CYP 3A

1733. Major hepatic isoenzyme in statin metabolism is?
Harrison's 20th Ed. Chapter 63 Page 421 Table 63-1
A. CYP 2C9
B. CYP 2C19
C. CYP 2D6
D. CYP 3A

1734. Major hepatic isoenzyme in lidocaine metabolism is?
Harrison's 20th Ed. Chapter 63 Page 421 Table 63-1
A. CYP 2C9
B. CYP 2C19
C. CYP 2D6
D. CYP 3A

1735. Major hepatic isoenzyme in quinidine metabolism is?
Harrison's 20th Ed. Chapter 63 Page 421 Table 63-1
A. CYP 2C9
B. CYP 2C19
C. CYP 2D6
D. CYP 3A

1736. Which of the following has been used in mushroom (Amanita phalloides) toxicity?
J Clin Exp Hepatol. 2012;2(3):247-259
A. N-acetylcysteine (NAC)
B. Silymarin
C. S-adenosine methionine
D. Ursodeoxycholic acid

Silymarin alone or silymarin combination with benzylpenicillin has been used in mushroom (Amanita phalloides) toxicity

Chronic Hepatitis

1737. In chronic hepatitis, hepatic inflammation and necrosis continue for at least?
Harrison's 20th Ed. Chapter 334 Page 2375

A. 3 months
B. 6 months
C. 9 months
D. 12 months

In chronic hepatitis, hepatic inflammation & necrosis continue for at least 6 months.

1738. Chronic hepatitis is due to?
Harrison's 20th Ed. Chapter 334 Page 2375

A. Virus
B. Drug-induced
C. Autoimmune
D. All of the above

Chronic viral hepatitis, drug-induced chronic hepatitis & autoimmune chronic hepatitis can cause chronicity.

1739. Chronic hepatitis is due to?
Harrison's 20th Ed. Chapter 334 Page 2375

A. Wilson's disease
B. α1 antitrypsin deficiency
C. Nonalcoholic fatty liver disease
D. All of the above

1740. Which of the following is the more severe form of chronic hepatitis?
Harrison's 20th Ed. Chapter 334 Page 2375

A. Chronic persistent hepatitis
B. Chronic lobular hepatitis
C. Chronic active hepatitis
D. All of the above

Earlier, chronic hepatitis was defined histopathologically as Chronic persistent hepatitis, chronic lobular hepatitis and chronic active hepatitis. Out of these chronic active hepatitis was considered as the more sever form.

1741. Classification of chronic hepatitis is based on?
Harrison's 20th Ed. Chapter 334 Page 2375

A. Cause
B. Histologic activity, or grade
C. Degree of progression, or stage
D. All of the above

Classification of chronic hepatitis is based on its cause, its histologic assessment of necroinflammatory activity, or grade and its degree of progression, or stage.

1742. Which of the following histologic features is accounted for in grading chronic hepatitis?
Harrison's 20th Ed. Chapter 334 Page 2375

A. Periportal necrosis
B. Bridging necrosis
C. Portal inflammation
D. All of the above

1743. Staging of chronic hepatitis is based on?
Harrison's 20th Ed. Chapter 334 Page 2375

A. Hepatic necrosis
B. Hepatic fibrosis
C. Hepatic inflammation
D. All of the above

The stage of chronic hepatitis is based on the degree of hepatic fibrosis.

1744. Histologic activity index (HAI) scoring for necroinflammatory activity (grade) is done out of?
Harrison's 20th Ed. Chapter 334 Page 2376 Table 334-2

A. 10
B. 14
C. 18
D. 20

Out of a maximum of 18, individual scoring is degree of periportal necrosis (max. 4), degree of intralobular confluent necrosis (max. 6), degree of intralobular focal necrosis (max. 4) & degree of portal inflammation (max. 4).

1745. Histologic activity index (HAI) scoring for fibrosis (stage) is done out of?
Harrison's 20th Ed. Chapter 334 Page 2376 Table 334-2

A. 3
B. 4
C. 6
D. 8

Staging is based on the degree of fibrosis as categorized on a numerical scale from 0-6 (HAI) or 0-4 (METAVIR).

1746. Histologic activity index (HAI) scoring for necroinflammatory activity (grade) includes all except?
Harrison's 20th Ed. Chapter 334 Page 2376 Table 334-2

A. Degree of periportal necrosis
B. Portal fibrosis
C. Intralobular necrosis
D. Degree of portal inflammation

Grade, a histologic assessment of necroinflammatory activity, is done by examination of liver biopsy. It includes assessment of degree of periportal necrosis, degree of hepatocyte degeneration and focal necrosis within lobule and degree of portal inflammation.

1747. In Europe, scoring system for assessment of necroinflammatory activity in liver is?
Harrison's 20th Ed. Chapter 334 Page 2375

A. Child-Pugh
B. Ishak
C. METAVIR
D. All of the above

1748. The likelihood of chronicity after acute hepatitis B depends on?
Harrison's 20th Ed. Chapter 334 Page 2375

A. Mode of transmission
B. Quantum of viral infection
C. Associated medical conditions
D. Age at the time of infection

The likelihood of chronicity after acute hepatitis B varies as a function of age at the time of acquisition. Perinatal transmission can be dramatically reduced by the administration of hepatitis B immunoglobulin at childbirth and the hepatitis B vaccine.

1749. What percentage of HBV infection acquired at birth will become chronic?
Harrison's 20th Ed. Chapter 334 Page 2376

A. 10%
B. 40%
C. 75%
D. 90%

HBV infection at birth is associated with clinically silent acute infection but a 90% chance of chronic infection.

1750. What percentage of HBV infection acquired in immunocompetent young adulthood will become chronic?
Harrison's 20th Ed. Chapter 334 Page 2376

A. ~ 1%
B. ~ 4%
C. ~ 7%
D. ~ 9%

HBV infection in immunocompetent young adulthood carry a risk of chronicity of ~ 1%.

1751. Which of the following has prognostic importance among adults with chronic hepatitis B?
Harrison's 20th Ed. Chapter 334 Page 2376

A. HBV serology
B. HLA DR3 or DR4 markers
C. AST and ALT
D. Liver histology

Among adults with chronic hepatitis B, histologic features are of prognostic importance. Distinctions in HBV replication and in histologic category do not always coincide.

1752. Replicative phase of chronic HBV infection is characterized by?
Harrison's 20th Ed. Chapter 334 Page 2376

A. Presence of HBeAg in serum
B. HBV DNA levels > 10^5–10^6 virions/mL
C. Presence of intrahepatocyte HBcAg in liver
D. All of the above

Replicative phase is characterized by presence of HBeAg & HBV DNA levels over 10^5–10^6 virions/mL in serum, by presence of HBcAg in liver, by high infectivity & by accompanying liver injury.

1753. Nonreplicative phase of chronic HBV infection is characterized by all except?
Harrison's 20th Ed. Chapter 334 Page 2376

A. Absence of HBeAg in serum
B. HBV DNA levels < 10^3 virions/mL
C. Presence of anti-HBe
D. Presence of intrahepatocyte HBcAg in liver

Nonreplicative phase is characterized by the absence of the conventional serum marker of HBV replication (HBeAg), the appearance of anti-HBe, levels of HBV DNA below a threshold of ~10^3 virions/mL, the absence of intrahepatocytic HBcAg, limited infectivity, and minimal liver injury.

1754. What percentage of HBeAg-reactive chronic hepatitis B convert spontaneously from replicative to nonreplicative infection per year?
Harrison's 20th Ed. Chapter 334 Page 2376

A. ~ 5%
B. ~ 10%
C. ~ 15%
D. ~ 20%

~10% patients of HBeAg-reactive chronic hepatitis B convert spontaneously from relatively replicative to nonreplicative infection per year.

1755. Most important risk factor for development of cirrhosis & HCC in chronic HBV infection is?
Harrison's 20th Ed. Chapter 334 Page 2376

A. Levels of HBV DNA
B. Level of HBV replication
C. Levels of aminotransferase activity
D. All of the above

Level of HBV replication is the most important risk factor for the ultimate development of cirrhosis & HCC in both HBeAg-reactive and HBeAg-negative patients.

1756. HBV inactive carriers is characterized by all except?
Harrison's 20th Ed. Chapter 334 Page 2377

A. Circulating HBsAg
B. Raised serum aminotransferase levels
C. Undetectable HBeAg
D. Almost undetectable levels of HBV DNA

Inactive HBV carriers have circulating HBsAg, normal serum aminotransferase levels, undetectable HBeAg, and almost undetectable levels of HBV DNA. This serologic profile occurs also in patients with HBeAg-negative chronic hepatitis B during periods of relative inactivity.

1757. Which of the following is not a complication of chronic hepatitis B?
Harrison's 20th Ed. Chapter 334 Page 2377

A. Hyperglobulinemia
B. Immune-complex glomerulonephritis
C. Generalized vasculitis
D. Leukocytoclastic vasculitis

Hyperglobulinemia & detectable circulating autoantibodies are distinctly absent in chronic hepatitis B in contrast to autoimmune hepatitis.

1758. HBV DNA can be detected in serum at levels as low as?
N Engl J Med. 2008;359:1486-500

A. 20 IU/mL
B. 40 IU/mL
C. 60 IU/mL
D. 80 IU/mL

HBV DNA can be detected in the serum at levels as low as 60 IU/mL.

1759. Histologic improvement is defined as a reduction of 2 or more points in the histologic activity index at?
N Engl J Med. 2008;359:1486-500

A. Month 3
B. Month 6
C. Year 1
D. Year 2

1760. Serum HBV DNA undetectable by PCR is defined as?
N Engl J Med. 2008;359:1486-500

A. < 100 to 200 copies per milliliter
B. < 300 to 400 copies per milliliter
C. < 500 to 1000 copies per milliliter
D. < 1000 to 2000 copies per milliliter

Serum HBV DNA undetectable by PCR is defined as <300 to 400 copies per milliliter (<1000 copies / mL for adefovir) at the end of year 1.

1761. Immunity to HBV infection is characterized by all except?
N Engl J Med. 2008;359:1486-500

A. Loss of HBV surface antigen
B. Loss of HBV e antigen
C. Loss of anti-core antigen IgM
D. Loss of anti-core antigen IgG

Immunity to HBV infection is characterized by loss of HBV surface antigen, DNA, e antigen, & anti-core antigen IgM with development of anti-surface antigen antibody & anti-core antigen IgG (total anti-core antigen antibody).

1762. Which of the following differentiates natural immunity by resolved HBV infection from that which is acquired through vaccination?
N Engl J Med. 2008;359:1486-500

A. Presence of Anti HBs + IgM anti HBc
B. Presence of Anti HBs + IgG anti HBc
C. Presence of Anti HBs + anti HBe
D. All of the above

Presence of anti HBs & IgG anti Hbc together differentiates natural immunity through resolved infection from that which is acquired through vaccination, which is denoted by isolated anti-surface antigen antibody.

1763. Which of the following phase is seen almost exclusively in those who acquired HBV infection vertically or during early childhood?
N Engl J Med. 2008;359:1486-500

A. Immune tolerance phase
B. Immune clearance phase
C. Inactive carrier phase
D. Reactivation phase

Immune tolerance phase, the initial phase of chronic HBV infection, is seen almost exclusively in those who acquired HBV infection vertically or during early childhood.

1764. Predictor of spontaneous e antigen seroconversion is?
N Engl J Med. 2008;359:1486-500

A. Old age
B. Elevated ALT level
C. Acute exacerbation
D. All of the above

The strongest predictors of spontaneous e antigen seroconversion are old age, an elevated ALT level, and an acute exacerbation.

1765. Which of the following phase is also called HBV e antigen negative chronic hepatitis?
N Engl J Med. 2008;359:1486-500

A. Immune tolerance phase
B. Immune clearance phase
C. Inactive carrier phase
D. Reactivation phase

Reactivation phase is also termed as HBV e antigen negative chronic hepatitis.

1766. Liver biopsy findings are normal or nonspecific in which of the following phase of HBV infection?
N Engl J Med. 2008;359:1486-500

A. Immune tolerance phase
B. Immune clearance phase
C. Inactive carrier phase
D. Reactivation phase

Liver biopsy shows findings of chronic hepatitis in immune clearance and reactivation phase. Nonsignificant hepatitis is observed in inactive carrier phase.

1767. e antibody is positive in which of the following phase of HBV infection?
N Engl J Med. 2008;359:1486-500

A. Immune tolerance phase
B. Immune clearance phase
C. Inactive carrier phase
D. All of the above

e antibody is negative in immune tolerance and immune clearance phase.

1768. HBV DNA is high in which of the following phase of HBV infection?
N Engl J Med. 2008;359:1486-500

A. Immune tolerance phase
B. Immune clearance phase
C. Inactive carrier phase
D. Reactivation phase

1769. Inactive HBV carriers with a low risk of clinical progression are those with a serum HBV DNA level below?
N Engl J Med. 2008;359:1486-500

A. 1000 IU per milliliter
B. 5000 IU per milliliter
C. 10000 IU per milliliter
D. 10000 IU per milliliter

Persons with a serum HBV DNA level below 1000 IU per milliliter and a normal ALT level consistently are considered to be inactive carriers with a low risk of clinical progression.

1770. Which of the following drug is beneficial in severe acute hepatitis B?
Harrison's 20th Ed. Chapter 334 Page 2377

A. Lamivudine
B. Interferon monotherapy
C. Ribavirin
D. Glucocorticoid

Oral drugs that have been approved for treatment of chronic hepatitis B include lamivudine, adefovir dipivoxil, entecavir, telbivudine and tenofovir.

1771. Which of the following is approved for treatment of chronic HBV infection?
Harrison's 20th Ed. Chapter 334 Page 2377, Lancet Infect Dis 2005;5:374–82

A. PEG IFN
B. Adefovir dipivoxil
C. Entecavir
D. All of the above

Drugs approved for treatment of chronic hepatitis B are injectable interferon (IFN) α and pegylated interferon (PEG IFN), lamivudine, adefovir dipivoxil, entecavir, telbivudine and tenofovir disoproxil fumarate (TDF).

1772. Which of the following drugs was the first to be approved for treatment of chronic HBV infection?
Harrison's 20th Ed. Chapter 334 Page 2377, Lancet Infect Dis 2005;5:374–82

A. Interferon α
B. Lamivudine
C. Adefovir
D. Entecavir

IFN-α was the first approved therapy for chronic hepatitis B in 1992, Lamivudine in 1998, Adefovir dipivoxil in 2002.

1773. Which of the following is the standard therapy for Interferon α?
Harrison's 20th Ed. Chapter 334 Page 2377

A. 5 million units subcutaneously per day for 12 weeks
B. 5 million units subcutaneously per day for 14 weeks
C. 5 million units subcutaneously per day for 16 weeks
D. 5 million units subcutaneously per day for 18 weeks

Standard therapy by immunomodulator Interferon α in chronic hepatitis B is 16-week course of IFN, subcutaneously at a daily dose of 5 million units, or three times a week at a dose of 10 million units.

1774. IFN-α therapy is not effective in which of the following groups of CHB patients?
Harrison's 20th Ed. Chapter 334 Page 2378

A. Very young children infected at birth
B. Immunosuppressed persons
C. Decompensated chronic hepatitis B
D. All of the above

IFN therapy has not been effective in very young children infected at birth, in immunosuppressed persons, Asian patients with minimal-to-mild ALT elevations, or patients with decompensated chronic hepatitis B.

1775. Which of the following side effects of IFN-α therapy is not reversible upon dose lowering or cessation of therapy?
Harrison's 20th Ed. Chapter 334 Page 2378

A. Autoimmune thyroiditis
B. Bone marrow suppression
C. Alopecia
D. Numbness & tingling of extremities

Except autoimmune thyroiditis, all side effects are reversible upon dose lowering / cessation of IFN-α.

1776. Which of the following is a 'Nucleoside analogue'?
Harrison's 20th Ed. Chapter 334 Page 2378, Lancet Infect Dis 2005;5:374–82

A. Lamivudine
B. Adefovir
C. Entecavir
D. Emtricitabine

Adefovir dipivoxil and Tenofovir are nucleotide analogues. Lamivudine - nucleoside analogue, Entecavir - guanosine analogue polymerase inhibitor, Telbivudine - cytosine analogue, Emtricitabine - fluorinated cytosine analogue, Clevudine - pyrimidine nucleoside analogue.

1777. Lamivudine was approved for hepatitis B treatment in?
Harrison's 20th Ed. Chapter 334 Page 2378

A. 1994
B. 1996
C. 1998
D. 2000

1778. Which of the following about Lamivudine is false?
Harrison's 20th Ed. Chapter 334 Page 2378

A. Dideoxynucleoside
B. Inhibits reverse transcriptase activity of HBV
C. Inhibits reverse transcriptase activity of HIV
D. None of the above

1779. HBV DNA level of ~10^3 IU/mL is equivalent to?
Harrison's 20th Ed. Chapter 334 Page 2378

A. <10^2 copies/mL
B. <10^3 copies/mL
C. <10^4 copies/mL
D. <10^5 copies/mL

HBV DNA level of ~10^3 IU/mL is equivalent to <10^4 copies/mL.

1780. Which of the following statements about lamivudine is false?
Harrison's 20th Ed. Chapter 334 Page 2378, Lancet Infect Dis 2005;5:374–82

A. Anti-HIV & anti-HBV activity
B. Dose lower for blocking HIV replication than HBV replication
C. Not be used as monotherapy in HBV/HIV co-infected patients
D. Anti-HBe seroconversion occurs in minority of patients

1781. The inhibitory dose of Lamivudine for treating HBV/HIV co-infected patients is?
Harrison's 20th Ed. Chapter 334 Page 2379, Lancet Infect Dis 2005;5:374–82

A. 100 mg/day
B. 200 mg/day
C. 300 mg/day
D. 400 mg/day

The inhibitory dose of Lamivudine for blocking HBV replication is 100 mg/day. 300 mg/day should be given when treating HBV/HIV co-infected patients, and should always be combined with at least two other anti-HIV agents.

1782. YMDD mutation best relates to?
Harrison's 20th Ed. Chapter 334 Page 2378

A. Lamivudine-resistant virus
B. IFN nonresponders
C. Lamivudine and IFN nonresponders
D. Any of the above

The term YMDD mutant is applied to patients taking lamivudine who initially become hepatitis B DNA negative and subsequently manifest hepatitis DNA in their serum while on therapy. YMDD mutation can be thought of as lamivudine-resistant virus.

1783. Long-term monotherapy with lamivudine is associated with mutation in which motif of HBV DNA polymerase?
Harrison's 20th Ed. Chapter 334 Page 2378

A. Chemokine (C-C motif) receptor 6
B. RNA-binding motif (RBM)

C. YMDD
D. All of the above

Long-term monotherapy with lamivudine is associated with methionine-to-valine (M204V) or methionine-to-isoleucine (M204I) mutations, primarily at amino acid 204 in the tyrosine-methionine-aspartate-aspartate (YMDD) motif (codons 203~206 of the reverse transcriptase) of HBV DNA polymerase.

1784. YMDD mutation after lamivudine therapy best relates to?
Harrison's 20th Ed. Chapter 334 Page 2379

A. Tyrosine-methionine-aspartate-aspartate
B. Tyrosine-aspartate-methionine-aspartate
C. Tyrosine-aspartate-aspartate-methionine
D. All of the above

The greatest drawback with lamivudine treatment is the emergence of drug-resistant HBV mutants with concomitant rise in ALT, DNA and worsening histology in some patients. This mutation of tyrosine-methionine-aspartate-aspartate (YMDD) motif in the C domain of the HBV DNA polymerase gene is also associated with flares of liver disease.

1785. Which of the following about Lamivudine is false?
Harrison's 20th Ed. Chapter 334 Page 2379

A. Effective in patients with decompensated hepatitis B
B. Not teratogenic
C. Reduces the likelihood of perinatal transmission of hepatitis B
D. None of the above

1786. Which of the following about adefovir dipivoxil is false?
Harrison's 20th Ed. Chapter 334 Page 2379

A. Acyclic nucleotide analogue
B. Prodrug of adefovir
C. Oral formulation, daily dose of 10 mg. for 48-week course
D. None of the above

1787. Adefovir dipivoxil is effective in?
Harrison's 20th Ed. Chapter 334 Page 2379

A. IFN nonresponders
B. Lamivudine-resistant, YMDD mutant HBV
C. Among patients co-infected with HBV and HIV
D. All of the above

1788. Which of the following drugs is least likely to result in HBeAg seroconversion?
Harrison's 20th Ed. Chapter 334 Page 2379

A. Lamivudine
B. Adefovir
C. Tenofovir
D. Entecavir

1789. Which of the following is false for HBV treatment in HIV positive patient?
Lancet Infect Dis 2005;5:374–82

A. Response to Interferon α is lower
B. Indefinite treatment with nucleoside/nucleotide analogues
C. Co-infection with hepatitis C rare
D. Frequent "Flares" while on HAART

1790. Which of the following has the highest rates of co-infection with HBV & HIV?
Lancet Infect Dis 2005;5:374–82

A. Men who have sex with men
B. Intravenous drug users
C. Infection through heterosexual contacts
D. Blood transfusion

1791. Markers of successful anti HBV therapy include?
N Engl J Med. 2004;350:1118-29

A. Loss of HBeAg
B. Seroconversion to anti-HBe antibodies
C. Reduction of circulating viral load
D. All of the above

1792. In CHB, factor that is not predictive of a response to antiviral therapy is?
N Engl J Med. 2008;359:1492

A. Low ALT level
B. Low HBV DNA level
C. Mild-to-moderate histologic activity and stage
D. HBV genotype A>B>C>D

Factors that are most predictive of a response include a high ALT level, a low HBV DNA level, and mild-to-moderate histologic activity & stage. Likelihood of HBeAg loss in PEG IFN alfa-2b treated HBeAg-reactive patients is associated with HBV genotype A > B > C > D.

1793. Which hepatitis virus infection leads to the most severe form of chronic viral hepatitis?
J Viral Hepat. 2010;17(11):749-56

A. Hepatitis A virus (HAV)
B. Hepatitis B virus (HBV)
C. Hepatitis C virus (HCV)
D. Hepatitis D virus (HDV)

Hepatitis D virus (HDV) infection leads to the most severe form of chronic viral hepatitis

1794. For HBeAg-reactive chronic HBV infection, antiviral therapy is indicated for patients with?
N Engl J Med. 2008;359:1492

A. ALT level more than two times upper limit of normal
B. HBV DNA > 20,000 IU per milliliter
C. Risk factors for progression
D. All of the above

For HBeAg-reactive chronic HBV, antiviral therapy is indicated if ALT levels are more than twice the upper limit of normal and HBV DNA >20,000 IU/mL. Risk factors for progression (older than 40 years, family history of HCC, or ALT level in high normal range (up to twice the upper limit of normal).

1795. For HBeAg-negative chronic HBV infection, antiviral therapy is indicated for patients with?
N Engl J Med. 2008;359:1492

A. ALT level more than two times upper limit of normal
B. HBV DNA > 20,000 IU per milliliter
C. Moderate-to-severe necroinflammatory activity or fibrosis
D. All of the above

For HBeAg-negative chronic HBV, antiviral therapy is indicated if ALT levels are more than twice the upper limit of normal and HBV DNA >20,000 IU/mL. If ALT is <2X with HBV DNA >20,000 IU/mL, liver biopsy is indicated. Moderate-to-severe necroinflammatory activity or fibrosis favours antiviral therapy.

1796. Conversion factor for HBV DNA between international units (IU) per milliliter and copies per milliliter is about?
N Engl J Med. 2008;359:1492

A. 2.6
B. 3.6
C. 4.6
D. 5.6

Conversion factor HBV DNA between international units /mL & copies/mL is ~ 5.6 (1 IU/mL is ~ 5.6 copies/mL). Treatment thresholds in copies/mL are 5 times higher than international units/mL.

1797. Nephrotoxicity of adefovir is best related to?
Therapeutic Advances in Gastroenterology 2008; 1; 61-75

A. Acute glomerulonephritis
B. Goodpasteur's syndrome
C. Fanconi-like syndrome
D. All of the above

Adefovir at 30 mg has higher antiviral potency. It's potential nephrotoxicity manifests as a Fanconi-like syndrome with phosphaturia and proteinuria.

1798. PEG stands for?
Harrison's 20th Ed. Chapter 334 Page 2379

A. Polyethylene glycerol
B. Perethylene glycerol
C. Polyethylene glycol
D. Perethylene glycol

Pegylated interferon (PEG IFN) is a long-acting IFN bound to polyethylene glycol (PEG).

1799. Pegylated IFN-α was approved by FDA for chronic hepatitis B in which year?
Harrison's 20th Ed. Chapter 334 Page 2380

A. 2000
B. 2002
C. 2003
D. 2005

1992 - Interferon alfa (IFN-α), 1998 - Lamivudine (LAM), 2002 - Adefovir (ADV), 2005 - Entecavir (ETV), Pegylated IFN-α, 2006 - Telbivudine (LDT), 2008 - Tenofovir (TDF).

1800. The recommended regimen of peg IFNa-2a for CHB is?
Harrison's 20th Ed. Chapter 334 Page 2380

A. 180 μg subcutaneously weekly for 24 weeks
B. 180 μg subcutaneously weekly for 36 weeks
C. 180 μg subcutaneously weekly for 48 weeks
D. 180 μg subcutaneously weekly for 51 weeks

Recommended regimen for peg IFNa-2a in CHB is 180 μg subcutaneously weekly for one year.

1801. Which of the following HBV genotype has the highest rate of IFN-induced HBeAg loss?
Harrison's 20th Ed. Chapter 334 Page 2380

A. Genotype A
B. Genotype B
C. Genotype C
D. Genotype D

Patients with HBV genotype A have the highest rate of IFN-induced HBeAg loss. Genotype A is most common in North America & Europe. HBeAg clearance associated with nucleos(t)ide analogues is independent of HBV genotype (HBV genotype A > B > C > D).

1802. PEG IFN therapy should be discontinued if HBsAg levels fail to reach <20,000 IU/mL by?
Harrison's 20th Ed. Chapter 334 Page 2380

A. Week 12
B. Week 24
C. Week 36
D. Week 48

If HBsAg levels fail to fall within first 12–24 weeks or to reach levels <20,000 IU/mL by week 24, PEG IFN therapy is unlikely to be effective and should be discontinued.

1803. The most potent of the HBV antiviral is?
Harrison's 20th Ed. Chapter 334 Page 2380

A. Entecavir
B. Telbivudine
C. Tenofovir
D. Adefovir Dipivoxil

1804. Which of the following is false about Entecavir?
Harrison's 20th Ed. Chapter 334 Page 2380

A. Oral cyclopentyl guanosine analogue polymerase inhibitor
B. Oral dose 0.5 mg daily
C. Effective against lamivudine-resistant HBV infection
D. Entecavir does not have antiviral activity against HIV

Entecavir is an oral cyclopentyl guanosine analogue polymerase inhibitor and is the most potent of the HBV antivirals. Its high barrier to resistance coupled with its high potency and an excellent safety profile renders entecavir a first-line drug for patients with chronic hepatitis B. Entecavir has low-level antiviral activity against HIV and cannot be used as monotherapy to treat HBV infection in HIV/HBV co-infected persons.

1805. Which of the following is false about Tenofovir?
Harrison's 20th Ed. Chapter 334 Page 2381

A. Acyclic nucleotide analogue
B. Antiretroviral agent
C. Oral once-daily dose of 300 mg
D. None of the above

1806. Tenofovir (TDF) is similar to which of the following?
Harrison's 20th Ed. Chapter 334 Page 2381

A. Entecavir
B. Telbivudine
C. Tenofovir
D. Adefovir Dipivoxil

Tenofovir disoproxil fumarate, an acyclic nucleotide analogue similar to adefovir.

1807. Very high HBV DNA levels refers to?
Harrison's 20th Ed. Chapter 334 Page 2381

A. $\geq 10^4$ IU/mL
B. $\geq 10^6$ IU/mL
C. $\geq 10^8$ IU/mL
D. $\geq 10^{10}$ IU/mL

1808. Which of the following is very similar to lamivudine in structure, efficacy, and resistance profile?
Harrison's 20th Ed. Chapter 334 Page 2381

A. Tenofovir
B. Emtricitabine

C. Clevudine
D. Telbivudine

1809. Which of the following is a prodrug of tenofovir?
Harrison's 20th Ed. Chapter 334 Page 2381

A. Tenofovir rufinamide
B. Tenofovir thionamide
C. Tenofovir alafenamide
D. Tenofovir prolinamide

Tenofovir alafenamide (TAF) is a prodrug of tenofovir that is metabolized to the active agent in its target organ (liver for HBV infection), thus permitting higher dose delivery to liver with reduced systemic exposure.

1810. Inactive "nonreplicative" hepatitis B carriers have?
Harrison's 20th Ed. Chapter 334 Page 2382

A. Undetectable HBeAg
B. Normal ALT
C. HBV DNA ≤10^3 IU/mL
D. All of the above

Inactive "nonreplicative" hepatitis B carriers have undetectable HBeAg with normal ALT and HBV DNA ≤10^3 IU/mL documented serially over time.

1811. Treatment for chronic hepatitis B is recommended by the AASLD for those with?
Harrison's 20th Ed. Chapter 334 Page 2383

A. Detectable HBeAg
B. HBV DNA levels >2 × 10^4 IU/mL
C. ALT levels above 2 × the upper limit of normal
D. All of the above

Antiviral therapy is not recommended currently by American association for the study of the liver diseases (AASLD) for HBeAg-positive patients with ALT ≤2 × the upper limit of normal, in whom sustained responses are not likely.

1812. Which of the following is recommended as first-line therapy in Chronic Hepatitis B?
Harrison's 20th Ed. Chapter 334 Page 2384

A. PEG IFN
B. Entecavir
C. Tenofovir
D. All of the above

Among the drugs for hepatitis B, PEG IFN has supplanted standard IFN, entecavir has supplanted lamivudine, and tenofovir has supplanted adefovir. PEG IFN, entecavir, or tenofovir are recommended as first-line therapy.

1813. Therapy with which of the following is least likely to foster emergence of viral mutations?
Harrison's 20th Ed. Chapter 334 Page 2384

A. Lamivudine
B. Tenofovir
C. Telbivudine
D. Adefovir

Lamivudine and telbivudine foster the emergence of viral mutations, adefovir somewhat less so, and entecavir (except in lamivudine-experienced patients) and tenofovir rarely at all.

1814. For treatment of chronic hepatitis B, which of the following can be used safely during pregnancy?
Harrison's 20th Ed. Chapter 334 Page 2384

A. Tenofovir
B. Entecavir
C. Emtricitabine
D. All of the above

Telbivudine and tenofovir are both pregnancy category B drugs and can be used safely during pregnancy. Despite its Class C designation, lamivudine has an extensive pregnancy safety record in women with HIV/AIDS.

1815. Which of the following should be avoided or used with extreme caution during pregnancy?
Harrison's 20th Ed. Chapter 334 Page 2384

A. PEG IFN
B. Adefovir
C. Entecavir
D. All of the above

Except for lamivudine, other antivirals for hepatitis B should be avoided or used with extreme caution during pregnancy.

1816. Which of the following should not be used in patients with compensated or decompensated cirrhosis?
Harrison's 20th Ed. Chapter 334 Page 2384

A. PEG IFN
B. Entecavir
C. Tenofovir
D. All of the above

PEG IFN should not be used in patients with compensated or decompensated cirrhosis due to unfavorable resistance profile.

1817. In patients with HBV-HIV infection, which of the should never be used as monotherapy?
Harrison's 20th Ed. Chapter 334 Page 2385

A. Lamivudine
B. Adefovir
C. Entecavir
D. Tenofovir

Lamivudine should never be used as monotherapy in HBV-HIV infection, because HIV resistance emerges rapidly to both viruses. Adefovir, entecavir, Tenofovir and tenofovir + emtricitabine can be used for treating HBV infection in HBV-HIV co-infected patients.

1818. Which of the following antiviral drugs has dual antiviral activity against HBV & HIV?
Harrison's 20th Ed. Chapter 334 Page 2385, Lancet Infect Dis 2005;5:374–82

A. Emtricitabine
B. Adefovir
C. Entecavir
D. All of the above

1819. Which of the following antiviral drugs has dual antiviral activity against HBV & HIV?
Harrison's 20th Ed. Chapter 334 Page 2385, Lancet Infect Dis 2005;5:374–82

A. Tenofovir
B. Emtricitabine
C. Lamivudine
D. All of the above

Besides lamivudine, tenofovir and emtricitabine have antiviral activity against HBV & HIV.

1820. **Which combination of antiviral drugs is recommended for HBV-HIV co-infected patients?**

Harrison's 20th Ed. Chapter 334 Page 2385

A. Lamivudine and Adefovir
B. Tenofovir and Emtricitabine
C. Entecavir and Emtricitabine
D. Lamivudine and Entecavir

Combination of tenofovir and emtricitabine is an excellent choice for treating HBV infection in HBV-HIV co-infected patients.

1821. **Which of the following drugs is used for chemotherapy-associated reactivation of hepatitis B?**

Harrison's 20th Ed. Chapter 334 Page 2385

A. Lamivudine
B. Entecavir
C. Tenofovir
D. All of the above

1822. **Variables that favour the treatment of HBV/HIV co-infected patients with pegylated interferon are all except?**

Lancet Infect Dis 2005;5:374–82

A. HBeAg-positive
B. Elevated aminotransferases
C. High CD4 counts
D. Psychiatric disorders

1823. **Which of the following about chronic hepatitis D virus (HDV) is false?**

Harrison's 20th Ed. Chapter 334 Page 2385

A. HDV co-infection can increase severity of acute hepatitis B
B. Does not increase progression of acute to chronic hepatitis B
C. Long-term HDV infection is the rule if HDV infects chronically infected with HBV patients
D. None of the above

1824. **Chronic hepatitis B plus D is similar to chronic hepatitis B alone in all respects except?**

Harrison's 20th Ed. Chapter 334 Page 2385

A. Severity
B. Clinical features
C. Laboratory features
D. Route of infection

1825. **Anti-LKM antibodies are seen in patients with?**

Harrison's 20th Ed. Chapter 334 Page 2385

A. Hepatitis D
B. Autoimmune hepatitis
C. Chronic hepatitis C
D. All of the above

1826. **Which of the following antibody is seen in chronic hepatitis D?**

Harrison's 20th Ed. Chapter 334 Page 2385

A. Anti-LKM1
B. Anti-LKM2
C. Anti-LKM3
D. Anti-LKM4

A distinguishing serologic feature of chronic hepatitis D is the presence in the circulation of anti-LKM3 directed against uridine diphosphate glucuronosyltransferase.

1827. **Which of the following drugs has a role in the treatment of chronic hepatitis D?**

Harrison's 20th Ed. Chapter 334 Page 2385

A. IFN-α & PEG IFN
B. Lonafarnib
C. Myrcludex B
D. All of the above

1828. **Which of the following is a nucleoside analogue antiviral agent for hepatitis B?**

Harrison's 20th Ed. Chapter 334 Page 2385

A. Lamivudine
B. Entecavir
C. Telbivudine
D. All of the above

1829. **Which of the following drugs has a role in the treatment of chronic hepatitis D?**

Harrison's 20th Ed. Chapter 334 Page 2385

A. Glucocorticoids
B. Lamivudine
C. Entecavir
D. None of the above

None of the nucleoside analogue antiviral agents for hepatitis B is effective in hepatitis D.

1830. **Dose of IFN-α in the treatment of chronic hepatitis D is?**

Harrison's 20th Ed. Chapter 334 Page 2385

A. 3 million units three times a week for 12 months
B. 6 million units three times a week for 12 months
C. 9 million units three times a week for 12 months
D. 12 million units three times a week for 12 months

High-dose IFN-α i.e. 9 million units three times a week for 12 months is associated with a sustained loss of HDV replication and clinical improvement.

1831. **Which of the following is an oral prenylation inhibitor?**

Harrison's 20th Ed. Chapter 334 Page 2385

A. Tipifarnib
B. Lonafarnib
C. Sorafenib
D. Sunitinib

Lonafarnib (LNF) is an oral prenylation inhibitor.

1832. **Which of the following about prenylation is false?**

Harrison's 20th Ed. Chapter 334 Page 2385

A. Posttranslational
B. Irreversible covalent addition of prenyl lipid farnesyl to HDV antigen
C. Required for HDV protein to interact & form secreted viral particles with HBsAg
D. None of the above

Prenylation is the posttranslational covalent addition of prenyl lipid farnesyl to large HDV antigen. It is required for HDV protein to interact & form secreted viral particles with HBsAg.

1833. Which of the following prenyltransferase enzymes catalyze prenylation?
ACS Chem. Biol. 2015;10(1):51-62

A. Farnesyltransferase (FTase)
B. Geranylgeranyltransferase type 1 (GGTase-I)
C. Geranylgeranyltransferase type 2 (GGTase-II or Rab geranylgeranyltransferase
D. All of the above

Protein prenylation modification is necessary to maintain malignant activity of oncogenic Ras proteins. Inhibition of prenylation has provided an attractive strategy to inhibit oncogenic activity of Ras and achieve antitumor effects.

1834. Which of the following is the structure of myristic acid?
Immunology. 2016;149(2):139-145

A. 12-carbon saturated fatty acid
B. 13-carbon saturated fatty acid
C. 14-carbon saturated fatty acid
D. 15-carbon saturated fatty acid

1835. Which of the following plays a central role in the interaction between viruses and the receptors?
Immunology. 2016;149(2):139-145

A. Pre-S1 domain
B. Pre-S2 domain
C. Post-S1 domain
D. Post-S2 domain

Unlike bacteria, viruses do not produce their own lipids. However, some viral proteins are lipid modified by using the host cellular machinery through a protein lipidation modification process, referred to as N-myristoylation. Hepatitis B virus entry into hepatocytes requires the binding of myristoylated N-terminal pre-S1 peptide of large HBsAg to sodium taurocholate co-transporting peptide, the functional receptor for HBV into hepatocytes.

1836. Sodium taurocholate cotransporting polypeptide is also named as?
Immunology. 2016;149(2):139-145

A. STCP
B. NTCP
C. MTCP
D. PTCP

Sodium taurocholate co-transporting peptide is the functional receptor for HBV into hepatocytes. This HBV receptor has been identified to be sodium taurocholate cotransporting polypeptide, also known as NTCP. When the gene that codes for NTCP is silenced, HBV infection is greatly reduced.

1837. Which of the following about sodium taurocholate cotransporting polypeptide (NTCP) is false?
Harrison's 20th Ed. Chapter 334 Page 2385

A. Multiple transmembrane transporter mainly expressed in liver
B. Interacts specifically with the L proteins of HBV & HDV
C. Functions as a common receptor for both viruses
D. None of the above

1838. Which of the following about NTCP (Slc10a1) is false?
Immunology. 2016;149(2):139-145

A. Solute carrier protein
B. Hepatic Na+ bile acid symporter
C. Localizes to sinusoidal (basolateral) plasma membrane of hepatocytes
D. None of the above

Interaction between NTCP and L protein of HBV is highly specific, and NTCP is crucial for productive viral entry of hepatocytes.

1839. Which of the following has the capacity to mediate lipopeptide antigen presentation?
Immunology. 2016;149(2):139-145

A. MHC class I
B. MHC class II
C. MHC class III
D. MHC class IV

'Classical' MHC class I molecules have the capacity to mediate lipopeptide antigen presentation.

1840. Which of the following is known to be susceptible to infection by human HBV & HDV?
Immunology. 2016;149(2):139-145

A. Chimpanzees
B. Treeshrew
C. Humans
D. All of the above

In addition to humans, only two species are known to be susceptible to infection by human HBV and HDV - chimpanzees and a small mammal known as the treeshrew.

1841. Which of the following processes is related to post-translational modification (PTM) of proteins?
Immunology. 2016;149(2):139-145

A. Phosphorylation
B. O-linked glycosylation
C. Acetylation
D. All of the above

Phosphorylation, O-linked glycosylation, Acetylation, Formylation, N-myristoylation, Citrullination, Methylation, Deamidation and Cysteinylation are involved in post-translational modification (PTM) of proteins.

1842. Which of the following is a synthetic homologous myristolated lipopeptide?
Harrison's 20th Ed. Chapter 334 Page 2385

A. Myrcludex A
B. Myrcludex B
C. Myrcludex C
D. Myrcludex D

Myrcludex B is a synthetic homologous myristolated lipopeptide that competes for binding with HBsAg. Myrcludex B acts as a hepatitis B and D virus entry inhibitor blocking sodium taurocholate cotransporting polypeptide (SLC10A1).

1843. What is the likelihood of patients having chronic HCV infection after acute hepatitis C?
Harrison's 20th Ed. Chapter 334 Page 2386

A. ~ 15%
B. ~ 35%
C. ~ 55%
D. ~ 85%

From 70% to 80% of acute hepatitis C virus infections persist and become chronic, while 20% to 30% spontaneously resolve.

1844. Which of the following distinguishes between responders & nonresponders to IFN-based antiviral therapy for HCV?
Harrison's 20th Ed. Chapter 334 Page 2386

A. IL25B
B. IL27B
C. IL28B
D. IL29B

Located on chromosome 19, IL28B, which codes for IFN-λ3, distinguishes between responders and nonresponders to IFN-based antiviral therapy for HCV.

1845. The human genome contains how many base pairs?
Cleveland Clinic Journal of Medicine. 2015;82(2):97

A. > 1 billion
B. > 2 billion
C. > 3 billion
D. > 4 billion

The human genome contains more than 3 billion base pairs of nucleotides. Of theses, fewer than 1% differ between individuals, but this 1% is responsible for the diversity of human beings. Differences in genetic sequences among individuals are called genetic polymorphisms. A single-nucleotide polymorphism is a DNA sequence variation that occurs in a single nucleotide in the genome.

1846. Which genotype of hepatitis C virus is more likely to clear the virus spontaneously?
Cleveland Clinic Journal of Medicine. 2015;82(2):97

A. IL28B CC
B. IL28B CT
C. IL28B TT
D. All of the above

In hepatitis C virus infection, people born with nucleotide cytosine (C) at location rs12979860 in both alleles of the gene that codes for interleukin 28B (IL28B CC genotype) are luckier than those born with thymine (T) in this location in one of their alleles (CT genotype) or both of their alleles (TT genotype). Those with CC genotype are more likely to clear the virus spontaneously, and even if infection persists, it is less likely to progress to liver cancer and more likely to respond to treatment with interferon. People who have the IL28B CC genotype are three times more likely to spontaneously clear the virus than those with the CT or TT genotype.

1847. Interferon lambda family consists of which of the following cytokines?
Cleveland Clinic Journal of Medicine 2015;82(2):97

A. Interleukin 29 (interferon lambda 1)
B. Interleukin 28A (interferon lambda 2)
C. Interleukin 28B (interferon lambda 3)
D. All of the above

1848. Which of the following statements about HCV is false?
Harrison's 20th Ed. Chapter 334 Page 2386

A. Most frequent indication for liver transplantation
B. HCV infection always recurs after liver transplantation
C. Tends to be very slowly and insidiously progressive
D. None of the above

1849. Which of the following antibody is prevalent in patients with chronic hepatitis C virus (HCV) infection?
Harrison's 20th Ed. Chapter 334 Page 2386

A. Smooth muscle antibodies (SMA)
B. Antinuclear (ANA) antibodies
C. Anti-liver kidney microsomal type 1 (LKM1) antibody
D. All of the above

Non-organ specific autoantibodies (NOSA), particularly smooth muscle antibodies (SMA) and antinuclear (ANA) antibodies are highly prevalent in patients with chronic hepatitis C virus (HCV) infection. Occasionally, Anti-liver kidney microsomal type 1 (LKM1) antibody, Anti-liver cytosol type 1 (LC1) are found.

1850. Out of the following, which one is the most important as regards progression of liver disease in chronic hepatitis C?
Harrison's 20th Ed. Chapter 334 Page 2386

A. Older age
B. Longer duration of infection
C. HIV infection
D. Obesity

Progression of liver disease in chronic hepatitis C is more likely in older age, longer duration of infection, advanced histologic stage and grade, genotype 1, more complex quasispecies diversity, increased hepatic iron, concomitant other liver disorders (alcoholic liver disease, chronic hepatitis B, hemochromatosis, α_1-antitrypsin deficiency, and steatohepatitis), HIV infection, and obesity. Out of these, duration of infection is the most important.

1851. Which of the following features of chronic hepatitis C is predictive of eventual outcome?
Harrison's 20th Ed. Chapter 334 Page 2386

A. Level of aminotransferase activity
B. Level of HCV RNA
C. Presence or absence of jaundice during acute hepatitis
D. None of the above

No other epidemiologic or clinical features of chronic hepatitis C like severity of acute hepatitis, level of aminotransferase activity, level of HCV RNA, presence or absence of jaundice during acute hepatitis, is predictive of eventual outcome.

1852. Annual rate of HCC in cirrhotic patients with hepatitis C is?
Harrison's 20th Ed. Chapter 334 Page 2386

A. 0.2–0.4%
B. 0.4–1%
C. 1–4%
D. 2.3–5.8%

Annual rate of HCC in cirrhotic patients with hepatitis C is 1–4% in those patients who have had HCV infection for 30 years or more.

1853. Best prognostic indicator in chronic hepatitis C is?
Harrison's 20th Ed. Chapter 334 Page 2386

A. Liver histology
B. Severity of jaundice
C. Levels of aminotransferases
D. HIV status

Best prognostic indicator in chronic hepatitis C is liver histology.

1854. The pace of fibrosis progression in chronic HCV may be accelerated by?
Harrison's 20th Ed. Chapter 334 Page 2386

A. Concomitant HIV infection
B. Excessive alcohol use
C. Hepatic steatosis
D. All of the above

Pace of fibrosis progression may be accelerated by such factors as concomitant HIV infection, excessive alcohol use and hepatic steatosis.

1855. Among HCV patients with compensated cirrhosis associated, which of the following is false?
Harrison's 20th Ed. Chapter 334 Page 2386

A. 10-year survival rate is ~80%
B. Mortality occurs at a rate of 2–6% per year
C. Decompensation occurs at a rate of 4–5% per year
D. None of the above

Among hepatitis C patients with compensated cirrhosis, 10-year survival rate is close to 80%, mortality occurs at a rate of 2–6% per year, decompensation occurs at a rate of 4–5% per year and HCC at a rate of 1–4% per year.

1856. The peak prevalence of chronic HCV was estimated to have occurred in?
Harrison's 20th Ed. Chapter 334 Page 2386

A. 2013
B. 2014
C. 2015
D. 2016

1857. Estimated peak mortality due to chronic HCV has been predicted to occur in?
Harrison's 20th Ed. Chapter 334 Page 2386

A. 2026
B. 2028
C. 2032
D. 2035

1858. Which of the following is the most common symptom in chronic hepatitis C?
Harrison's 20th Ed. Chapter 334 Page 2386

A. Fatigue
B. Jaundice
C. Fever
D. Weight loss

Fatigue is the most common symptom of chronic hepatitis C. Jaundice is rare.

1859. Extrahepatic complications unrelated to immune-complex injury in chronic hepatitis C are all except?
Harrison's 20th Ed. Chapter 334 Page 2387

A. Sjögren's syndrome
B. Porphyria cutanea tarda
C. Essential mixed cryoglobulinemia
D. Lichen planus

Essential mixed cryoglobulinemia is an immune complex–mediated extrahepatic complications of chronic hepatitis C. While those unrelated to immune-complex injury are Sjögren's syndrome, lichen planus, porphyria cutanea tarda, type-2 diabetes mellitus and metabolic syndrome (including insulin resistance & steatohepatitis).

1860. Which of the following in a laboratory feature of chronic hepatitis C?
Harrison's 20th Ed. Chapter 334 Page 2387

A. Fluctuating aminotransferase levels
B. Jaundice is rare
C. Circulating anti-LKM1 antibodies
D. All of the above

1861. Anti-LKM1 are directed against which of the following?
Harrison's 20th Ed. Chapter 334 Page 2387

A. Cytochrome P450 2D6
B. Cytochrome P450 3A4
C. Cytochrome P450 2C9
D. Cytochrome P450 2B6

1862. Which of the following enhances the efficacy of IFN?
Harrison's 20th Ed. Chapter 334 Page 2387

A. Ribavirin
B. Adefovir
C. Entecavir
D. Tenofovir

Oral guanosine nucleoside ribavirin is ineffective when used alone. But, ribavirin enhances the efficacy of IFN by reducing the likelihood of sustained virologic response (SVR) after the achievement of an end-treatment response (ETR) i.e. response measured during, and maintained to the end of treatment.

1863. Which of the following statements is false?
Harrison's 20th Ed. Chapter 334 Page 2387

A. Hepatitis C proteins inhibit JAK-STAT signaling
B. JAK-STAT regulates interferon-stimulated genes
C. Interferon lambda signal through IL10R-IL28R receptor
D. None of the above

1864. Which of the following sustained virologic response (SVR) is now the new standard?
Harrison's 20th Ed. Chapter 334 Page 2387

A. SVR_{12}
B. SVR_{24}
C. SVR_{36}
D. SVR_{48}

SVR_{12} has now become the new standard for therapy responses.

1865. Interferon therapy results in activation of?
Harrison's 20th Ed. Chapter 334 Page 2387

A. Cytokines
B. Chemokines
C. JAK-STAT signal transduction pathway
D. All of the above

Interferon therapy results in activation of the JAK-STAT signal transduction pathway, which results in the intracellular elaboration of genes & their protein products with antiviral properties. Hepatitis C proteins inhibit JAK-STAT signaling pathway, and exogenous interferon restores expression of interferon-stimulated genes and their antiviral effects.

1866. Which of the following is a nucleoside analogue?
Harrison's 20th Ed. Chapter 334 Page 2387

A. Telaprevir
B. Boceprevir
C. Sofosbuvir
D. Ribavirin

Sofosbuvir was the first nucleoside analogue approved in 2013 for the treatment of chronic hepatitis C.

1867. Which of the following variable does not correlate favourably in the IFN-based treatment of chronic hepatitis C?
Harrison's 20th Ed. Chapter 334 Page 2387

A. Genotypes 2 and 3
B. Genotypes 1 and 4
C. Low baseline HCV RNA level
D. Histologically mild hepatitis

Patient variables that tend to correlate with sustained virologic responsiveness to IFN-based therapy include favorable genotype (genotypes 2 and 3 as opposed to genotypes 1 and 4), low baseline HCV RNA level (<2 million copies/mL, which is equivalent to 800,000 IU/ml), histologically mild hepatitis and minimal fibrosis, age <40, absence of obesity as well as insulin resistance and type-II diabetes mellitus, and female gender. Patients with cirrhosis respond less favourably.

1868. Duration of IFN-ribavirin therapy have in patients with genotype 1 should last for?
Harrison's 20th Ed. Chapter 334 Page 2388

A. 12 weeks
B. 24 weeks
C. 48 weeks
D. 72 weeks

1869. Duration of IFN-ribavirin therapy have in patients with genotype 2 and 3 should last for?
Harrison's 20th Ed. Chapter 334 Page 2388

A. 12 weeks
B. 24 weeks
C. 48 weeks
D. 72 weeks

Combination IFN-ribavirin therapy in chronic hepatitis C with genotype 1 should for 48 weeks, while in those with genotypes 2 and 3, a 24-week course of therapy suffices.

1870. Which of the following is relevant for patients treated with PEG IFN and ribavirin?
Harrison's 20th Ed. Chapter 334 Page 2388

A. SLCO1B1
B. HLA-B*1501
C. IL15
D. IL28B

In studies of patients treated with PEG IFN and ribavirin, variants of the IL28B SNP that code for IFN-λ3 correlate significantly with responsiveness. Patients homozygous for the C allele at this locus have the highest frequency of achieving an SVR (80%), those homozygous for the T allele at this locus are least likely to achieve an SVR (25%), and those heterozygous at this locus (C/T) have an intermediate level of responsiveness (SVRs in 35%).

1871. The most pronounced side effect of ribavirin therapy is?
Harrison's 20th Ed. Chapter 334 Page 2388

A. Seizure
B. Agranulocytosis
C. Hemolysis
D. All of the above

The most pronounced side effect of ribavirin therapy is hemolysis.

1872. Which of the following is a side effect of ribavirin therapy?
Harrison's 20th Ed. Chapter 334 Page 2388

A. Pruritus
B. Gout
C. Anemia
D. All of the above

1873. Half-life in serum of Hepatitis C virion is?
Harrison's 20th Ed. Chapter 334 Page 2388

A. 2–3 hours
B. 2–3 days
C. 2–3 monhs
D. 2–3 years

Despite a Hepatitis C virion half life in serum of only 2–3 hours, the level of HCV is maintained by a high replication rate of 10^{12} hepatitis C virions per day.

1874. Null responders are the ones who after therapy have HCV RNA reduction of?
Harrison's 20th Ed. Chapter 334 Page 2387, Figure 334-2

A. $< 1 \log_{10}$ IU/mL
B. $< 2 \log_{10}$ IU/mL
C. $< 3 \log_{10}$ IU/mL
D. $< 4 \log_{10}$ IU/mL

Null responders are the ones who after therapy have HCV RNA reduction of $< 2 \log_{10}$ IU/mL by week 24 of therapy.

1875. Rapid virologic response (RVR) is estimated at what time after institution of therapy in Hepatitis C?
Harrison's 20th Ed. Chapter 334 Page 2387, Figure 334-2

A. 2 weeks
B. 4 weeks
C. 8 weeks
D. 12 weeks

RVR (Rapid virologic response) refers to undetectable HCV RNA at week 4 in responders as shown with sensitive amplification assays.

1876. Early virologic response (EVR) is estimated at what time after institution of therapy in Hepatitis C?
Harrison's 20th Ed. Chapter 334 Page 2387, Figure 334-2

A. 2 weeks
B. 4 weeks
C. 8 weeks
D. 12 weeks

EVR refers to ≥2 $\log_{10}$ IU/mL HCV RNA reduction by week 12. If HCV RNA is undetectable at 12 weeks, the designation is "complete" EVR; or at the end of therapy, 48 weeks (ETR, end-treatment response).

1877. Responder status is estimated at what time after institution of therapy in Hepatitis C?
Harrison's 20th Ed. Chapter 334 Page 2387, Figure 334-2

A. 12 weeks
B. 24 weeks
C. 48 weeks
D. 72 weeks

1878. Sustained virologic response (SVR) is estimated at what time after institution of therapy in Hepatitis C?
Harrison's 20th Ed. Chapter 334 Page 2387, Figure 334-2

A. 12 weeks
B. 24 weeks
C. 48 weeks
D. 72 weeks

In responders, if HCV RNA remains undetectable for 24 weeks after ETR, week 72, the patient has a sustained virologic response (SVR).

1879. Elimination time of PEG IFN is how many times longer than standard IFN?
Harrison's 20th Ed. Chapter 334 Page 2388

A. Three times
B. Five times
C. Seven times
D. Nine times

For the treatment of chronic hepatitis C, standard IFNs have now been supplanted by PEG IFNs and these have elimination times up to seven fold longer than standard IFNs, permitting once a week dosage.

1880. The standard treatment of chronic hepatitis C before 2011 was?
Harrison's 20th Ed. Chapter 334 Page 2388

A. PEG IFN
B. Ribavirin
C. PEG IFN + Ribavirin
D. All of the above

The standard treatment of chronic hepatitis C before 2011 was the combination of long acting pegylated IFN (PEG IFN) and ribavirin for all HCV genotypes.

1881. Dose of PEG IFN α-2a is?
Harrison's 20th Ed. Chapter 334 Page 2388

A. 180 μg daily subcutaneously
B. 180 μg weekly subcutaneously
C. 180 μg daily intramuscularly
D. 180 μg weekly intramuscularly

Two PEG IFNs are available: PEG IFN α-2b and α-2a. PEG IFN α-2a is given 180 μg weekly subcutaneously.

1882. Dose of PEG IFN α-2b is?
Harrison's 20th Ed. Chapter 334 Page 2388

A. 0.5 μg / kg weekly subcutaneously
B. 1.5 μg / kg weekly subcutaneously
C. 2.5 μg / kg weekly subcutaneously
D. 3.5 μg / kg weekly subcutaneously

PEG IFN α-2b is given 1.5 μg / kg weekly subcutaneously.

1883. Duration of PEG IFN / ribavirin therapy in chronic hepatitis C of genotypes 1 and 4 is?
Harrison's 20th Ed. Chapter 334 Page 2388

A. 12 weeks
B. 24 weeks
C. 48 weeks
D. 72 weeks

1884. Duration of PEG IFN / ribavirin therapy in chronic hepatitis C of genotypes 2 and 3 is?
Harrison's 20th Ed. Chapter 334 Page 2388

A. 12 weeks
B. 24 weeks
C. 48 weeks
D. 72 weeks

1885. Telaprevir and boceprevir best relate to?
Harrison's 20th Ed. Chapter 334 Page 2389

A. NS3/4A
B. NS4B
C. NS5A
D. NS5B

Telaprevir and boceprevir are serine protease inhibitors that target NS3/4A.

1886. Triple therapy for chronic HCV includes all except?
Harrison's 20th Ed. Chapter 334 Page 2389

A. PEG IFN
B. Ribavirin
C. Telaprevir
D. Tenofovir

Because resistance developed rapidly during monotherapy with telaprevir & boceprevir, these drugs had to be used in combination with PEG IFN and ribavirin.

1887. Dual therapy for chronic HCV refers to?
Harrison's 20th Ed. Chapter 334 Page 2389

A. PEG IFN plus ribavirin
B. PEG IFN plus telaprevir
C. PEG IFN plus boceprevir
D. Any of the above

Telaprevir and boceprevir regimens consisted of periods of triple therapy and periods of dual therapy based on HCV RNA status at weeks 4 and 12 ("response-guided therapy").

1888. Which of the following is a NS5A inhibitor?
Harrison's 20th Ed. Chapter 334 Page 2390

A. Ledipasvir
B. Velpatasvir
C. Daclatasvir
D. All of the above

NS5A inhibitors include Ledipasvir, velpatasvir, daclatasvir, elbasvir, & ombitasvir. NS5A is a membrane-associated phosphoprotein that is part of the HCV RNA replication complex and is essential for viral replication & assembly.

1889. Which of the following is a NS3/4 protease inhibitor?
Harrison's 20th Ed. Chapter 334 Page 2393

A. Ombitasvir
B. Grazoprevir
C. Dasabuvir
D. Ribavirin

Grazoprevir and Paritaprevir are NS3/4 protease inhibitors.

1890. Sofosbuvir-containing combinations are contraindicated with which of the following drugs?
Harrison's 20th Ed. Chapter 334 Page 2390

A. Cyclosporine
B. Ramipril
C. Amiodarone
D. All of the above

sofosbuvir containing regimens can be associated with severe bradycardia in patients taking the antiarrhythmic agent amiodarone and therefore contraindicated.

1891. **Sofosbuvir / ledipasvir fixed-dose regimen for chronic HCV is not effective for which genotype?**
Harrison's 20th Ed. Chapter 334 Page 2396
- A. 3
- B. 4
- C. 5
- D. 6

The most popular of the regimens for chronic HCV is sofosbuvir / ledipasvir, which is effective for all genotypes except 2 and 3.

1892. **For HCV genotypes 2 and 3, which of the following is the combination of choice?**
Harrison's 20th Ed. Chapter 334 Page 2396
- A. Paritaprevir / ritonavir
- B. Elbasvir / grazoprevir
- C. Sofosbuvir / velpatasvir
- D. All of the above

For HCV genotypes 2 and 3, fixed dose, single-pill sofosbuvir / velpatasvir is the combination of choice.

1893. **Standard indication for antiviral therapy of chronic hepatitis C is?**
Harrison's 20th Ed. Chapter 334 Page 2391 Table 334-6
- A. Detectable HCV RNA (with or without elevated ALT)
- B. Portal/bridging fibrosis on liver biopsy
- C. Moderate to severe hepatitis on liver biopsy
- D. All of the above

1894. **Antiviral therapy is not recommended in which of the following patients of chronic hepatitis C?**
Harrison's 20th Ed. Chapter 334 Page 2391 Table 334-6
- A. Age > 70 years
- B. Mild hepatitis on liver biopsy
- C. Persons with severe renal insufficiency
- D. All of the above

1895. **Which of the following patients of chronic hepatitis C are not candidates for IFN-based antiviral therapy?**
Harrison's 20th Ed. Chapter 334 Page 2391 Table 334-6
- A. Decompensated cirrhosis
- B. Pregnancy
- C. Contraindications to use of interferon or ribavirin
- D. All of the above

Patients with decompensated cirrhosis are not candidates for IFN-based antiviral therapy but should be referred for liver transplantation. Interferons are antiproliferative and ribavirin is teratogenic.

1896. **Which of the following is recommended for the success of therapy with PEG IFN / ribavirin in chronic hepatitis C?**
Harrison's 20th Ed. Chapter 334 Page 2395
- A. HCV genotype should be determined prior to therapy
- B. Measure HCV RNA at 12 weeks
- C. Pretreatment liver biopsy
- D. All of the above

1897. **Which of the following is advocated in those who have not responded to treatment with PEG IFN/ribavirin in chronic hepatitis C?**
Harrison's 20th Ed. Chapter 334 Page 2395
- A. Longer duration of treatment
- B. Higher doses of either PEG IFN, ribavirin, or both
- C. Switching to a different IFN preparation
- D. All of the above

For those who have not responded to treatment with PEG IFN / ribavirin in chronicn hepatitis C, following may be tried : longer duration of treatment; higher doses of either PEG IFN, ribavirin, or both and switching to a different IFN preparation. However, none of these approaches achieves more than a marginal benefit.

1898. **Which of the following associated with hepatitis C may respond to antiviral therapy?**
Harrison's 20th Ed. Chapter 334 Page 2395
- A. Essential mixed cryoglobulinemia
- B. Porphyria cutanea tarda
- C. Lichen planus
- D. All of the above

1899. **Which of the following drug is beneficial in acute hepatitis C?**
Harrison's 20th Ed. Chapter 334 Page 2395
- A. Lamivudine
- B. Interferon monotherapy
- C. Ribavirin
- D. Glucocorticoid

In acute hepatitis C, interferon monotherapy (3 million units SC three times a week) is beneficial. Long-acting pegylated interferon plus ribavirin is superior to interferon monotherapy.

1900. **Drugs that have been recommended in acute liver failure are all except?**
Harrison's 20th Ed. Chapter 334 Page 2395
- A. Lamivudine
- B. Telbivudine
- C. Adefovir
- D. Entecavir

Nucleoside/nucleotide analogues recommended in acute liver failure are lamivudine, telbivudine and entecavir. Adefovir has a slow action & potential nephrotoxicity. Interferon drugs are contraindicated because they can worsen hepatitis.

Autoimmune Hepatitis

1901. Autoimmune hepatitis is a kind of?
Harrison's 20th Ed. Chapter 334 Page 2396

A. Acute hepatitis
B. Subacute hepatitis
C. Chronic hepatitis
D. Any of the above

Autoimmune hepatitis is a chronic disorder characterized by continuing hepatocellular necrosis & inflammation, usually with fibrosis, which can progress to cirrhosis & liver failure.

1902. Which of the following is prominent in cases of autoimmune hepatitis?
Harrison's 20th Ed. Chapter 334 Page 2396

A. Extrahepatic features of autoimmunity
B. Serologic abnormalities
C. Immunologic abnormalities
D. All of the above

In autoimmune hepatitis, extrahepatic features of autoimmunity & seroimmunologic abnormalities are prominent & supports an autoimmune process in its pathogenesis, though autoantibodies do not occur in all cases.

1903. Which class of serum globulins is elevated in autoimmune hepatitis?
Harrison's 20th Ed. Chapter 334 Page 2396, N Engl J Med. 2006;354:54-66

A. Alpha globulin
B. Beta globulin
C. Gamma globulin
D. Delta globulin

One characteristic laboratory feature of autoimmune hepatitis is a generalized elevation of serum globulins, particularly gamma globulin and IgG, which are generally 1.2 to 3.0 times normal.

1904. Which of the following virus has been implicated in pathogenesis of autoimmune hepatitis?
N Engl J Med. 2006;354:54-66, Harrison's 20th Ed. Chapter 334 Page 2396

A. Hepatitis viruses
B. Measles virus
C. Epstein–Barr virus
D. All of the above

Measles virus, hepatitis viruses, cytomegalovirus, and Epstein–Barr virus have been implicated as initiators of autoimmune hepatitis in genetically predisposed. Most evidence is related to hepatitis viruses - A, B, or C.

1905. Which of the following drug has been implicated in pathogenesis of autoimmune hepatitis?
N Engl J Med. 2006;354:54-66, Harrison's 20th Ed. Chapter 334 Page 2396

A. Minocycline
B. Atorvastatin
C. Interferon
D. All of the above

Oxyphenisatin, methyldopa, nitrofurantoin, diclofenac, interferon, pemoline, minocycline & atorvastatin can induce hepatocellular injury that mimics autoimmune hepatitis.

1906. Autoimmune disorder that occur with increased frequency in autoimmune hepatitis patients is?
Harrison's 20th Ed. Chapter 334 Page 2396

A. Thyroiditis
B. Rheumatoid arthritis
C. Autoimmune hemolytic anemia
D. All of the above

Autoimmune disorders that occur with increased frequency in autoimmune hepatitis patients are thyroiditis, rheumatoid arthritis, autoimmune hemolytic anemia, ulcerative colitis, membranoproliferative glomerulonephritis, type 1 diabetes mellitus, celiac disease & Sjögren's syndrome.

1907. Which of the following autoantibody is present in patients of autoimmune hepatitis?
Harrison's 20th Ed. Chapter 334 Page 2396

A. Antinuclear antibodies (ANAs)
B. Anti-LKM
C. Antibodies to soluble liver antigen
D. All of the above

Autoantibodies found in autoimmune hepatitis patients are antinuclear antibodies (ANAs), anti-smooth-muscle antibodies (directed at actin, vimentin and skeletin), antibodies to F-actin, anti-LKM, antibodies to "soluble liver antigen/liver pancreas antigen" (SLA/LP autoantibodies), antibodies to α-actinin, antibodies to liver-specific asialoglycoprotein receptor ("hepatic lectin").

1908. Which of the following statements about anti-soluble liver antigen is false?
Harrison's 20th Ed. Chapter 334 Page 2396

A. Associated with a more severe disease course
B. Present in nonhepatic autoimmune disorders
C. Target of anti-SLA is tRNP$^{(Ser)Sec}$
D. Specific serologic marker for autoimmune liver diseases

Anti-SLA is serologic marker for autoimmune liver diseases, is associated with a more severe disease course, it is virtually absent in nonhepatic autoimmune disorders. Target of anti-SLA is a UGA serine tRNA-associated protein complex [tRNP$^{(Ser)Sec}$].

1909. In autoimmune hepatitis, immunoregulatory dysfunction of which of the following occurs?
Harrison's 20th Ed. Chapter 334 Page 2396

A. CD8+CD24+ regulatory T cells
B. CD8+CD25+ regulatory T cells
C. CD4+CD24+ regulatory T cells
D. CD4+CD25+ regulatory T cells

Immunoregulatory dysfunction characterized by decreased numbers of CD4+CD25+ regulatory T cells and decreased levels of scurfin, the protein product of FOXP3 gene occurs in autoimmune hepatitis.

1910. Scurfin is the protein product of which gene?
Nature Immunology. 2003;4:337-342

A. FOXP1 gene
B. FOXP2 gene
C. FOXP3 gene
D. FOXP4 gene

In autoimmune hepatitis, levels of scurfin are decreased. Scurfin is the protein product of FOXP3 gene that is a member of forkhead family of transcription factors.

1911. **Extrahepatic manifestation of autoimmune hepatitis is?**
   Harrison's 20th Ed. Chapter 334 Page 2396
   A. Arthritis
   B. Cutaneous vasculitis
   C. Glomerulonephritis
   D. All of the above

   Extrahepatic manifestations of autoimmune hepatitis include arthralgias, arthritis, cutaneous vasculitis and glomerulonephritis.

1912. **In the clinical presentation suggestive of acute viral hepatitis, which of the following point towards autoimmune hepatitis?**
   Harrison's 20th Ed. Chapter 334 Page 2396
   A. Young to middle-aged women
   B. Marked hyperglobulinemia (>2.5 g/dL)
   C. High-titer circulating ANAs
   D. All of the above

1913. **Poor prognostic sign in autoimmune hepatitis is?**
   Harrison's 20th Ed. Chapter 334 Page 2397
   A. Multilobular collapse histopathologically at initial presentation
   B. Failure of serum bilirubin to improve after 2 weeks of therapy
   C. Bridging necrosis or multilobular necrosis on liver biopsy
   D. All of the above

   Poor prognostic signs in autoimmune hepatitis are the presence of multilobular collapse at the time of initial presentation on histopathologically and failure of serum bilirubin to improve after 2 weeks of therapy.

1914. **Type 1 autoimmune hepatitis is associated with which HLA-DR serotype?**
   Harrison's 20th Ed. Chapter 334 Page 2397
   A. HLA-DR1
   B. HLA-DR2
   C. HLA-DR3
   D. None of the above

   Type I autoimmune hepatitis is associated with HLA-DR3 or HLA-DR4.

1915. **Type 2 autoimmune hepatitis is associated with which HLA haplotype?**
   Harrison's 20th Ed. Chapter 334 Page 2397
   A. HLA-DRB1
   B. HLA-DRB2
   C. HLA-DRB3
   D. HLA-DRB4

   Type II autoimmune hepatitis is linked to HLA-DRB1 & HLA-DQB1 haplotypes.

1916. **Feature of HLA-DR3 associated autoimmune hepatitis include?**
   N Engl J Med. 2006;354:54-66
   A. Early-onset
   B. Severe form
   C. In girls and young women
   D. All of the above

   HLA-DR3–associated disease is more common in the early-onset, severe form of autoimmune hepatitis, which often occurs in girls and young women.

1917. **Feature of HLA-DR4 associated autoimmune hepatitis include?**
   N Engl J Med. 2006;354:54-66
   A. Common in adults
   B. Extrahepatic manifestations
   C. Better response to corticosteroid therapy
   D. All of the above

   HLA-DR4 associated autoimmune hepatitis is more common in adults and associated with increased incidence of extrahepatic manifestations, milder disease & a better response to corticosteroid therapy.

1918. **Type I autoimmune hepatitis is associated with which of the following antibodies?**
   Harrison's 20th Ed. Chapter 334 Page 2397
   A. Antinuclear antibodies (ANA)
   B. Atypical perinuclear antineutrophilic cytoplasmic antibodies
   C. Antiactin antibodies
   D. All of the above

   Type I autoimmune hepatitis is associated with circulating ANAs, autoantibodies against actin, atypical perinuclear antineutrophilic cytoplasmic antibodies (pANCA) & SLA/LP autoantibodies. Antiactin antibodies are more specific for type 1 autoimmune hepatitis. Anti–LKM-1 & anti–LC-1 characterize type 2 disease.

1919. **Which of the following is the most specific autoantibody identified in type 1 autoimmune hepatitis?**
   N Engl J Med. 2006;354:54-66
   A. Antiactin antibodies
   B. SLA/LP autoantibodies
   C. Antinuclear antibodies (ANA)
   D. Anti-LKM1

   SLA/LP autoantibodies are the most specific autoantibody identified in type 1 autoimmune hepatitis but is found in only 10 to 30 percent of cases.

1920. **Type II autoimmune hepatitis is associated with which of the following antibodies?**
   Harrison's 20th Ed. Chapter 334 Page 2397
   A. Antinuclear antibodies (ANA)
   B. Antiactin antibodies
   C. Anti-LKM1
   D. Atypical perinuclear antineutrophilic cytoplasmic antibodies

1921. **Type II autoimmune hepatitis is associated with which of the following antibodies?**
   Harrison's 20th Ed. Chapter 334 Page 2397
   A. Antinuclear antibodies (ANA)
   B. Antiactin antibodies
   C. Anti-liver cytosol 1 (anti–LC-1)
   D. Atypical perinuclear antineutrophilic cytoplasmic antibodies

   Type II autoimmune hepatitis is associated not with ANA but with anti-LKM1. Also seen is autoantibody directed against liver cytosol formiminotransferase cyclodeaminase, a liver-specific 58-kD metabolic enzyme (anti-liver cytosol 1).

1922. **In type II autoimmune hepatitis, the anti-LKM1 antibody is directed against which cytochrome?**
   Harrison's 20th Ed. Chapter 334 Page 2397
   A. P450 2D6
   B. P450 2C9

C. P450 2C19
D. P450 3A

In type II autoimmune hepatitis, the anti-LKM1 antibody is directed against cytochrome P450 2D6 (CYP2D6).

1923. Anti-LKM antibody seen in Type II autoimmune hepatitis is also seen in which of the following?
Harrison's 20th Ed. Chapter 334 Page 2397

A. Drug-induced hepatitis
B. Chronic hepatitis C
C. Chronic hepatitis D
D. All of the above

Anti-LKM1 antibody seen in type II autoimmune hepatitis is seen in some patients with chronic hepatitis C. Anti-LKM2 is seen in drug-induced hepatitis & anti-LKM3 is seen in patients with chronic hepatitis D.

1924. Which of the following statements is false?
Harrison's 20th Ed. Chapter 334 Page 2397

A. Anti-LKM1 is seen in type II autoimmune hepatitis
B. Anti-LKM2 is seen in drug-induced hepatitis
C. Anti-LKM3 is seen in chronic hepatitis D
D. None of the above

1925. Type III autoimmune hepatitis is associated with which of the following antibodies?
Harrison's 20th Ed. Chapter 334 Page 2397

A. Antinuclear antibodies (ANA)
B. Antibodies to soluble liver antigen/liver pancreas antigen
C. Anti-LKM1
D. All of the above

Type III autoimmune hepatitis patients lack ANA and anti-LKM1 but have circulating antibodies to soluble liver antigen/liver pancreas antigen.

1926. Which of the following is false about histopathological features of liver in autoimmune hepatitis?
Harrison's 20th Ed. Chapter 334 Page 2397

A. Mononuclear-cell infiltrate
B. Interface hepatitis or piecemeal necrosis
C. Sparing of the biliary tree
D. None of the above

Autoimmune hepatitis is characterized by a mononuclear-cell infiltrate (plasma cells + eosinophils) invading the limiting plate (piecemeal necrosis or interface hepatitis). Biliary tree is generally spared and fibrosis is present.

1927. Which of the following feature goes against the diagnosis of autoimmune hepatitis?
Harrison's 20th Ed. Chapter 334 Page 2397

A. Female gender
B. Predominant aminotransferase elevation
C. Mitochondrial antibodies
D. Globulin level elevation

Features that favor diagnosis of autoimmune hepatitis include female gender, predominant aminotransferase elevation, globulin level elevation, presence of nuclear, smooth muscle, LKM1, and other autoantibodies, concurrent other autoimmune diseases, characteristic histologic features (interface hepatitis, plasma cells, rosettes), HLA DR3 or DR4 markers, & response to treatment. Features against the diagnosis are predominant alkaline phosphatase elevation, mitochondrial antibodies, markers of viral hepatitis, history of hepatotoxic drugs or excessive alcohol, histologic evidence of bile duct injury, or such atypical histologic features as fatty infiltration, iron overload, and viral inclusions. Antimitochondrial antibody (AMA) is the sine qua non of primary biliary cirrhosis (PBC) but may be observed in the so-called overlap syndrome with autoimmune hepatitis.

1928. Mainstay of management in autoimmune hepatitis is?
Harrison's 20th Ed. Chapter 334 Page 2398

A. Azathioprine
B. Glucocorticoid
C. Cyclosporine
D. Mycophenolate mofetil

Mainstay of management in autoimmune hepatitis is daily glucocorticoid therapy. Azathioprine alone is not effective in achieving remission. Patients refractory to this regimen may be treated with cyclosporine, tacrolimus, or mycophenolate mofetil.

1929. Severe autoimmune hepatitis is defined as?
Harrison's 20th Ed. Chapter 334 Page 2398

A. Serum AST ≥ 10 times upper limit of normal
B. Serum AST ≥ 5 times upper limit of normal and gamma-globulin level ≥ twice normal
C. Bridging necrosis or multiacinar necrosis on liver biopsy
D. All of the above

1930. Therapy for autoimmune hepatitis should continue for at least?
Harrison's 20th Ed. Chapter 334 Page 2398

A. 3 - 6 months
B. 6 - 12 months
C. 12 - 18 months
D. 18 - 24 months

Therapy for autoimmune hepatitis should continue for at least 12–18 months. After tapering and cessation of therapy, the likelihood of relapse is at least 50%. Majority of patients require therapy at maintenance doses indefinitely.

1931. Which of the following is useful in refractory autoimmune hepatitis?
Harrison's 20th Ed. Chapter 334 Page 2398

A. Infliximab
B. Rituximab
C. Cyclosporine, tacrolimus, or mycophenolate mofetil
D. All of the above

Alcoholic Liver Disease

1932. Alcoholic Liver Disease (ALD) includes?
Clin Liver Dis. 2016 ;20(3):445-456

A. Hepatic steatosis
B. Acute alcoholic hepatitis with or without cirrhosis
C. Hepatocellular carcinoma as a complication of cirrhosis
D. All of the above

1933. Which of the following is the major lesion in the pathology of alcoholic liver disease?
Harrison's 20th Ed. Chapter 335 Page 2399

A. Fatty liver
B. Alcoholic hepatitis
C. Cirrhosis
D. All of the above

Major lesions in the pathology of alcoholic liver disease are fatty liver, alcoholic hepatitis & cirrhosis.

1934. Which of the following is considered to be a precursor to cirrhosis?
Harrison's 20th Ed. Chapter 335 Page 2399

A. Fatty liver
B. NASH
C. Alcoholic hepatitis
D. All of the above

Alcoholic hepatitis is thought to be a precursor to cirrhosis.

1935. Fatty liver is present in what proportion of daily as well as binge drinkers?
Harrison's 20th Ed. Chapter 335 Page 2399

A. > 30%
B. > 50%
C. > 70%
D. > 90%

Fatty liver is present in >90% of daily as well as binge drinkers.

1936. Which of the following can predict individual susceptibility to alcoholic liver disease?
Harrison's 20th Ed. Chapter 335 Page 2399

A. Quantity of alcohol consumed per day
B. Total duration of alcohol consumed
C. Obesity
D. None of the above

There are no diagnostic tools that can predict individual susceptibility to alcoholic liver disease.

1937. One beer (12 oz), four ounces of wine or one ounce of 80% spirits contain how many grams of alcohol?
Harrison's 20th Ed. Chapter 335 Page 2399

A. ~ 8 grams
B. ~ 10 grams
C. ~ 12 grams
D. ~ 14 grams

One beer, four ounces of wine, or one ounce of 80% spirits all contain ~12 grams of alcohol.

1938. In men, what quantity of ethanol produces fatty liver?
Harrison's 20th Ed. Chapter 335 Page 2399 Table 335-1

A. 10 - 20 gm/day
B. 20 - 40 gm/day
C. 40 - 80 gm/day
D. 80 - 120 gm/day

In men, 40–80 gram/day of ethanol produces fatty liver.

1939. In men, what quantity & duration of ethanol consumption causes hepatitis or cirrhosis?
Harrison's 20th Ed. Chapter 335 Page 2399 Table 335-1

A. 80 gm/day for 5 - 10 years
B. 160 gm/day for 5 - 10 years
C. 80 gm/day for 10 - 20 years
D. 160 gm/day for 10 - 20 years

In men, 160 gm/day for 10-20 years of ethanol consumption causes hepatitis or cirrhosis.

1940. What proportion of alcoholics develop alcoholic liver disease?
Harrison's 20th Ed. Chapter 335 Page 2399 Table 335-1

A. 15%
B. 30%
C. 45%
D. 75%

Only 15% of alcoholics develop alcoholic liver disease.

1941. Which of the following statements about alcohol consumption is false?
Harrison's 20th Ed. Chapter 335 Page 2399 Table 335-1

A. Alcohol is a direct hepatotoxin
B. Men more susceptible to alcoholic liver injury than women
C. Alcohol injury does not require malnutrition
D. 15% of alcoholics develop alcoholic liver disease

Women are more susceptible to alcoholic liver disease than men.

1942. Alcohol stimulates lipogenesis by the upregulation of?
Clin Liver Dis. 2016 ;20(3):445-456

A. Sterol regulatory element-binding transcription factor 1a
B. Sterol regulatory element-binding transcription factor 1b
C. Sterol regulatory element-binding transcription factor 1c
D. All of the above

Alcohol stimulates lipogenesis by upregulation of sterol regulatory element-binding transcription factor 1c (SREBP-1c). Alcohol also downregulates the negative regulators of SREBP-1c, including 5' adenosine monophosphate-activated protein kinase (AMPK), Sirtuin 1, adiponectin, and signal transducer and activator of transcription 3 (STAT3).

1943. Which of the following about alcohol is false?
Clin Liver Dis. 2016;20(3):445-456

A. Alcohol downregulates PPAR-α
B. Alcohol activates the complement system (C3, C4)
C. Alcohol disrupts intestinal tight junction integrity, "leaky gut"
D. None of the above

1944. Which of the following about alcohol is false?
Clin Liver Dis. 2016;20(3):445-456

A. KRT7 is a marker of ductular reaction in liver disease
B. Prominin-1 (PROM1) is a marker of progenitor cells from liver
C. Plasma miRNA-155 correlates with alcohol induced liver inflammation
D. None of the above

1945. Which of the following is related to the genetic risk factors for alcoholic liver disease?
Harrison's 20th Ed. Chapter 335 Page 2399 Table 335-1, N Engl J Med. 2018;379:1251-61

A. ATP8B1
B. IL28B
C. PNPLA3
D. ORMDL3

Patatin-like phospholipase domain-containing protein 3 (PNPLA3, rs738409C>G) has been associated with alcoholic cirrhosis.

1946. Which of the following is considered as a strong genetic risk locus for both alcoholic cirrhosis and AH?
Gut Liver. 2017;11:173-188

A. Patatin-like phospholipase encoding 3 (PNPLA3)
B. Membrane bound O-acyltransferase domain containing 7 (MBOAT7)
C. Transmembrane 6 superfamily member 2 (TM6SF2)
D. All of the above

Both PNPLA3 & TM6SF2 are implicated in hepatic lipid trapping, while MBOAT7 mediates the transfer of fatty acid between phospholipids and lysophospholipids, a potent driver of hepatic inflammation.

1947. Cytochrome P-450 2E1 (CYP2E1) converts alcohol to?
Gut Liver. 2017;11:173-188

A. Acetate
B. Carbon dioxide
C. Free fatty acids
D. Acetaldehyde

In liver, there are two main pathways of alcohol metabolism, alcohol dehydrogenase and cytochrome P-450 2E1. They converts alcohol to acetaldehyde. Acetaldehyde subsequently is metabolized to acetate via acetaldehyde dehydrogenase.

1948. Which of the following accelerates progression of alcoholic liver disease to cirrhosis in chronic and excessive drinkers?
Harrison's 20th Ed. Chapter 335 Page 2399

A. Acute hepatitis B
B. Acute hepatitis C
C. Chronic hepatitis B
D. Chronic hepatitis C

Chronic infection with hepatitis C (HCV) is an important comorbidity in the progression of alcoholic liver disease to cirrhosis in chronic and excessive drinkers. Alcohol intake also decreases efficacy of interferon-based antiviral therapy in them.

1949. Which of the following initiates the pathogenic process in alcoholic liver injury?
Harrison's 20th Ed. Chapter 335 Page 2399

A. Fatty acid oxidation
B. Intestinal-derived endotoxin
C. Microbiome dysbiosis
D. Proinflammatory cytokines

In the pathogenesis of alcoholic liver injury, intestinal-derived endotoxin initiates a pathogenic process through toll-like receptor 4 and tumor necrosis factor α (TNF-α) that facilitates hepatocyte apoptosis & necrosis.

1950. Initial and most common histologic response to hepatotoxic stimuli is?
Harrison's 20th Ed. Chapter 335 Page 2399

A. Fatty liver
B. NASH
C. Steatohepatitis
D. All of the above

1951. Chronic alcohol ingestion lead to which of the following?
Harrison's 20th Ed. Chapter 335 Page 2399

A. Autoimmune response
B. Fibrotic response
C. Inflammatory response
D. All of the above

Hepatocyte injury and impaired regeneration following chronic alcohol ingestion are ultimately associated with stellate cell activation and collagen production, which are key events in fibrogenesis.

1952. Major enzyme responsible for alcohol metabolism is?
Harrison's 20th Ed. Chapter 335 Page 2399

A. Alcohol dehydrogenase
B. Alcohol reductase
C. Alcohol oxidase
D. All of the above

In fatty liver secondary to alcohol induced liver injury, accumulation of fat within the perivenular hepatocytes coincides with the location of alcohol dehydrogenase which is the major enzyme responsible for alcohol metabolism.

1953. Which of the following about Damage-Associated Molecular Patterns (DAMPs) is false?
Clin Liver Dis. 2016;20(3):445-456

A. Endogenous, hidden from extracellular environment
B. Activate cellular pattern recognition receptors
C. Result in sterile inflammation (inflammasome)
D. None of the above

1954. Steatosis is characterized by the accumulation of which of the following in hepatocytes?
Clin Liver Dis. 2016;20(3):445-456

A. Triglycerides
B. Phospholipids

C. Cholesterol esters
D. All of the above

Steatosis refers to accumulation of triglycerides, phospholipids, and cholesterol esters in hepatocytes.

1955. Which of the following hepatic pathologic features may be associated with progressive liver injury?
Harrison's 20th Ed. Chapter 335 Page 2399

A. Giant mitochondria
B. Perivenular fibrosis
C. Macrovesicular fat
D. All of the above

1956. Histologically, the earliest changes in alcoholic hepatitis are located predominantly in?
Harrison's 20th Ed. Chapter 335 Page 2399

A. Zone 1
B. Zone 2
C. Zone 3
D. All of the above

Histologically, the earliest changes in alcoholic hepatitis are located predominantly around the central vein i.e. centrilobular (perivenular) areas (zone 3 of Rappaport).

1957. The hallmark features of hepatocyte injury in alcoholic hepatitis are all except?
Harrison's 20th Ed. Chapter 335 Page 2400

A. Polymorphonuclear infiltrate
B. Ballooning degeneration
C. Mallory-Denk bodies
D. Fibrosis in perisinusoidal space of Disse

Hallmark of alcoholic hepatitis is hepatocyte injury characterized by ballooning degeneration, spotty necrosis, polymorphonuclear infiltrate, and fibrosis in the perivenular and perisinusoidal space of Disse. Mallory-Denk bodies are often present in florid cases but are neither specific nor necessary for substantiating diagnosis.

1958. Which of the following is false about Terry's nails?
Indian J Dermatol. 2017;62(3):309-311

A. Ground glass appearance of fingernails
B. No lunula
C. Frequent in severe liver disease
D. None of the above

Terry's nails (a type of leukonychia) refers to finger/toe nails that have a "ground glass" appearance, with no lunula (white crescent-shaped area of finger). It frequently occurs in hepatic failure, cirrhosis, DM, CHF, hyperthyroidism, malnutrition.

1959. Skin texture of cheeks & nasolabial folds in patient with alcohol-related liver disease is called?
Cleveland Clinic Journal of Medicine. 2009;76(10):601

A. Gooseberry skin
B. Cheese wind skin
C. Weather heat skin
D. Paper-money skin

Paper-money skin (or "Dollar-paper" markings) seen in alcoholic cirrhosis describes the condition in which the upper trunk is covered with many randomly scattered, needle-thin superficial capillaries.

1960. Which of the following are found in patients with liver disease?
Cleveland Clinic Journal of Medicine. 2009;76(10):601

A. Xanthelasma
B. Bier spots
C. "Paper-money" skin
D. All of the above

Bier spots are small, irregularly shaped, hypopigmented patches on the arms and legs. Bier spots are a sign of liver disease.

1961. In alcoholic hepatitis, which of the following can occur in the absence of cirrhosis?
Harrison's 20th Ed. Chapter 335 Page 2400

A. Portal hypertension
B. Ascites
C. Variceal bleeding
D. All of the above

In alcoholic hepatitis, portal hypertension, ascites, or variceal bleeding can occur in the absence of cirrhosis. Patients with alcoholic cirrhosis often exhibit clinical features identical to other causes of cirrhosis.

1962. In alcoholic hepatitis, AST: ALT ratio is?
Harrison's 20th Ed. Chapter 335 Page 2400

A. > 0.25
B. > 0.50
C. > 0.75
D. > 1

In alcoholic hepatitis, the AST : ALT ratio is >1. AST:ALT ratio is higher in pericentral hepatocytes than other regions in liver lobule & pericentral zone is more selectively affected in acute alcoholic hepatitis.

1963. In alcoholic hepatitis, AST and ALT are rarely more than?
Harrison's 20th Ed. Chapter 335 Page 2400

A. 100 IU/L
B. 200 IU/L
C. 300 IU/L
D. 400 IU/L

In alcoholic hepatitis, AST & ALT are usually elevated 2-7 fold. They are rarely >400 IU/L.

1964. Which of the following is a laboratory feature alcoholic fatty liver?
Harrison's 20th Ed. Chapter 335 Page 2400

A. Increased gamma-glutamyl transpeptidase (GGTP)
B. Hypertriglyceridemia,
C. Hypercholesterolemia
D. All of the above

1965. Which of the following in ultrasonography indicates serious liver injury with less potential for complete reversal?
Harrison's 20th Ed. Chapter 335 Page 2400

A. Portal vein flow reversal
B. Ascites
C. Intra-abdominal collaterals
D. All of the above

1966. Discriminant function (DF) formula predicting the outcome of severe alcoholic hepatitis is named after?
Harrison's 20th Ed. Chapter 335 Page 2400

A. Nathan
B. Cushin
C. Maddrey
D. George

The discriminant function (DF) formula of Maddrey is based on PT and bilirubin.

1967. Which of the following is the correct formula of Discriminant function (DF)?

Harrison's 20th Ed. Chapter 335 Page 2400

A. 2.6 x PT prolongation + total S. bilirubin in mg/dL
B. 3.6 x PT prolongation + total S. bilirubin in mg/dL
C. 4.6 x PT prolongation + total S. bilirubin in mg/dL
D. 5.6 x PT prolongation + total S. bilirubin in mg/dL

Modified Maddrey's discriminant function predicts prognosis in alcoholic hepatitis. It is calculated as 4.6 x [prothombin time - control value (seconds)] + serum bilirubin (mg/dL). A value >32 implies poor outcome with one month mortality > 50% if only supportive treatment is given. Cut off value of 32 &/or hepatic encephalopathy has been used as a threshold to consider corticosteroid treatment.

1968. Formula for assessment of prognosis of alcoholic hepatitis is?

Gut Liver. 2017;11:173-188

A. Age, Bilirubin, INR, Creatinine (ABIC) score
B. Model for end-stage liver disease (MELD) score
C. Glasgow alcoholic hepatitis score (GAHS)
D. All of the above

Besides the above ones and also the classical Child-Turcotte-Pugh (CTP) score, Asymmetric dimethylarginine (ADMA) score is the most recently proposed predictor of adverse clinical outcome in patients with severe alcoholic hepatitis.

1969. Variables included in Glasgow alcoholic hepatitis score (GAHS) are all except?

Gut Liver. 2017;11:173-188

A. Age
B. Hemoglobin
C. Bilirubin
D. BUN

Five variables included in GAHS are age, bilirubin, BUN, PT, and TLC. Glasgow Alcoholic Hepatitis score ≥ 9 requires treatment.

1970. MELD score is calculated based on all except?

N Engl J Med. 2009;361:1279-90

A. Prothrombin time
B. Serum albumin
C. Serum creatinine
D. Serum bilirubin

MELD score is based on a patient's prothrombin time, serum creatinine & bilirubin.

1971. Model for End-Stage Liver Disease (MELD) score was introduced in USA in year?

N Engl J Med. 2009;361:1279-90

A. 1995
B. 1998
C. 2002
D. 2005

In 2002, MELD score derived from measurements of serum bilirubin, international normalized ratio of prothrombin time and serum creatinine to evaluate pretransplantation renal function was introduced as an aid to organ allocation among candidates for liver transplantation.

1972. The presence of which of the following in alcoholic hepatitis predicts a dismal prognosis?

Harrison's 20th Ed. Chapter 335 Page 2400

A. Ascites
B. Variceal hemorrhage
C. Hepatorenal syndrome
D. All of the above

The presence of ascites, variceal hemorrhage, deep encephalopathy, or hepatorenal syndrome predicts a dismal prognosis in patients with alcoholic hepatitis.

1973. Severe alcoholic hepatitis is defined as a discriminant function of?

Harrison's 20th Ed. Chapter 335 Page 2400

A. > 24
B. > 28
C. > 30
D. > 32

1974. Severe alcoholic hepatitis is defined as an MELD of?

Harrison's 20th Ed. Chapter 335 Page 2400

A. > 20
B. > 30
C. > 40
D. > 50

Patients with severe alcoholic hepatitis are defined as a discriminant function >32 or MELD >20.

1975. Which of the following score is used to identify alcoholic hepatitis patients unresponsive to therapy?

Harrison's 20th Ed. Chapter 335 Page 2400

A. Sanyal score
B. Lille score
C. Thurz score
D. Mathurin score

A Lille score >0.45 uses pretreatment variables plus change in total bilirubin at day 7 of glucocorticoids to identify those patients unresponsive to therapy.

1976. Which of the following drugs has been approved by Food and Drug Administration for treatment of alcohol-use disorder?

N Engl J Med. 2018;379:1251-61

A. Naltrexone
B. Disulfiram
C. Acamprosate
D. All of the above

Three medications (naltrexone, disulfiram, and acamprosate) have been approved by the Food and Drug Administration for the treatment of alcohol-use disorder. Nalmefene has been approved in many European countries for the reduction of alcohol consumption.

1977. Which of the following about Naltrexone is false?

N Engl J Med. 2018;379:1251-61

A. Mu-opioid and kappa-opioid receptor antagonist
B. Reduces alcohol-related dopamine release in nucleus accumbens
C. Reduces the reward sensation
D. None of the above

Naltrexone is a mu-opioid & kappa-opioid receptor antagonist. It reduces alcohol-related dopamine release in nucleus accumbens thereby reducing the reward sensation, thus making patients less motivated to drink.

1978. Which of the following about Acamprosate is false?

N Engl J Med. 2018;379:1251-61

A. Acts as N-methyl-D-aspartate receptor antagonist
B. Acts as a modulator of GABA type A receptor

C. Reduces symptoms of protracted abstinence
D. None of the above

Acamprosate acts as N-methyl-D-aspartate receptor antagonist and a modulator of γ-aminobutyric acid (GABA) type A receptor and reduces symptoms of protracted abstinence. Acamprosate has no hepatic metabolism.

1979. Which of the following about Acamprosate is false?
N Engl J Med. 2018;379:1251-61
A. Mu-opioid and delta-opioid receptor antagonist
B. Kappa-opioid receptor partial agonist
C. No evidence of hepatotoxicity
D. None of the above

1980. Which of the following about Baclofen is false?
N Engl J Med. 2018;379:1251-61
A. Selective GABA type B receptor antagonist
B. Also used to control spasticity
C. No liver toxicity
D. None of the above

1981. Which of the following drugs has been tested in patients with alcohol-use disorder?
N Engl J Med. 2018;379:1251-61
A. Gabapentin
B. Ondansetron
C. Varenicline
D. All of the above

Four other treatments that have been tested in patients with alcohol-use disorder include gabapentin, ondansetron, topiramate, and varenicline.

1982. Acetaldehyde syndrome consists of?
N Engl J Med. 2018;379:1251-61
A. Facial flushing
B. Nausea, vomiting
C. Tachycardia, hypotension
D. All of the above

Disulfiram inhibits acetaldehyde dehydrogenase, thus provoking acetaldehyde syndrome (facial flushing, nausea, vomiting, tachycardia, and hypotension) when disulfiram is consumed with alcohol. Use of disulfiram is contraindicated in patients with liver cirrhosis, especially in those with synthetic dysfunction.

1983. Which of the following is used as a pharmaceutical approaches to treat alcohol use disorders (AUD)?
N Engl J Med. 2018;379:1251-61
A. Baclofen
B. Disulfiram
C. Nalmefene
D. All of the above

Pharmaceutical approaches to treat AUD include baclofen, disulfiram, naltrexone and nalmefene. FDA-approved disulfiram & naltrexone are contraindicated in ALD patients due to possible hepatotoxicity. Nalmefene, a μ- and δ-opioid receptor antagonist and κ-opioid receptor partial-agonist was approved for AUD by FDA, but safety data in patients with ALD is limited.

1984. Which of the following is advocated for severe alcoholic hepatitis?
Harrison's 20th Ed. Chapter 335 Page 2400
A. Glucocorticoids
B. Thiamine
C. Proton pump inhibitors
D. All of the above

Patients with severe alcoholic hepatitis, Women with encephalopathy in particular, should be given prednisone, 40 mg/day, or prednisolone, 32 mg/day, for 4 weeks, followed by a steroid taper.

1985. Use of which of the following improves survival in severe alcoholic hepatitis?
Harrison's 20th Ed. Chapter 335 Page 2400
A. Pentoxifylline
B. Propylthiouracil
C. Infliximab
D. Colchicine

1986. Pentoxifylline improves survival in severe alcoholic hepatitis primarily due to a decrease in development of?
Harrison's 20th Ed. Chapter 335 Page 2400
A. Pancreatitis
B. Encephalopathy
C. Hepatorenal syndrome
D. All of the above

The nonspecific TNF inhibitor, pentoxifylline (orally absorbed nonselective phosphodiesterase inhibitor) improves survival in severe alcoholic hepatitis was primarily due to a decrease in the development of hepatorenal syndrome.

1987. Use of Infliximab in severe alcoholic hepatitis was stopped due to the increased risk of?
N Engl J Med. 2018;379:1251-61
A. Bone marrow suppression
B. Seizure
C. Infection
D. Jaundice

Use of Infliximab in severe alcoholic hepatitis was stopped due to the increased risk of increased deaths secondary to infection and renal failure.

1988. Most liver transplantation centers require alcoholics to have documented abstinence of at least?
N Engl J Med. 2018;379:1251-61
A. 3 months
B. 6 months
C. 9 months
D. 12 months

Most transplantation centers currently require patients with a history of alcohol abuse to have documented abstinence of at least 6 months before undergoing transplantation ("6-month abstinence rule").

Nonalcoholic Fatty Liver Disease and Nonalcoholic Steatohepatitis

1989. Accumulation of which of the following occurs within hepatocytes in hepatic steatosis?
Harrison's 20th Ed. Chapter 336 Page 2401

A. Cholesterol
B. Chylomicrons
C. Triglyceride
D. All of the above

Accumulation of triglyceride occurs within hepatocytes in hepatic steatosis.

1990. Which of the following statements about chronic hepatic steatosis is false?
Harrison's 20th Ed. Chapter 336 Page 2401

A. Risk of developing cirrhosis is extremely low
B. May become complicated by NASH
C. NAFLD-related cirrhosis may produce primary liver cancer
D. None of the above

Isolated hepatic steatosis is entirely benign. The risk of death from liver disease increases by a factor of 50 to 80 for patients with nonalcoholic steatohepatitis who have F3 or F4 fibrosis.

1991. "Cryptogenic" ALT elevations increase with which of the following?
Harrison's 20th Ed. Chapter 336 Page 2401

A. Alcohol consumption
B. Malnutrition
C. Body mass index
D. All of the above

"Cryptogenic" ALT elevations increase with body mass index. Serum ALT elevations that cannot be explained by excessive alcohol consumption, other known causes of fatty liver disease, viral hepatitis, drug-induced or congenital liver diseases are termed "cryptogenic".

1992. Nonalcoholic Steatohepatitis (NASH) is defined by a constellation of features that include?
Cleveland Clinic Journal of Medicine. 2017;84(4):273

A. Steatosis
B. Lobular & portal inflammation
C. Liver cell injury (hepatocyte ballooning)
D. All of the above

NAFLD remains a diagnosis of exclusion of other liver diseases.

1993. Which of the following can be a consequence of Nonalcoholic steatohepatitis?
N Engl J Med. 2017;377:2063-72

A. Can regress to isolated steatosis
B. Can smolder at a relatively constant level of activity
C. Can cause progressive fibrosis leading to cirrhosis (F4 fibrosis)
D. Any of the above

NASH is a potentially progressive type of nonalcoholic fatty liver disease (NAFLD). Nonalcoholic steatohepatitis is a dynamic condition that can regress to isolated steatosis, smolder at a relatively constant level of activity, or cause progressive fibrosis that leads to cirrhosis (F4 fibrosis). Nonalcoholic steatohepatitis is the sum of injury and repair responses triggered by lipotoxicity.

1994. Which of the following promote the development of nonalcoholic steatohepatitis?
N Engl J Med. 2017;377:2063-72

A. PDZ domain–containing protein
B. SCR homology 2 domain-containing leukocyte protein
C. Toll-interleukin 1 receptor domain-containing adapter protein
D. Patatin-like phospholipase domain–containing 3 (PNPLA3)

Polymorphisms in patatin-like phospholipase domain - containing 3 (PNPLA3) and transmembrane 6 superfamily, member 2 (TM6SF2) promote development of nonalcoholic steatohepatitis and related liver damage (cirrhosis, primary liver cancer).

1995. PNPLA3 encodes which of the following?
N Engl J Med. 2017;377:2063-72

A. Adipocytokine leptin (LEPR)
B. Adiponutrin
C. Adiponectin
D. Kisspeptin

PNPLA3 encodes adiponutrin, a lipase that regulates both triglyceride and retinoid metabolism. PNPLA3 polymorphisms (I148M) are strongly associated with hepatic steatosis, steatohepatitis, fibrosis & cancer.

1996. Hepatic cirrhosis develops in what percentage of individuals with NAFLD?
Harrison's 20th Ed. Chapter 336 Page 2401

A. ~ 1%
B. ~ 3%
C. ~ 6%
D. ~ 9%

Hepatic cirrhosis develops in about 6% of individuals with NAFLD. The risk for advanced liver fibrosis is highest in individuals with NASH who are older than 45–50 years of age and overweight/obese or afflicted with type 2 diabetes.

1997. Prevalence of hepatitis C-related cirrhosis in the United States is?
Harrison's 20th Ed. Chapter 336 Page 2401

A. ~ 0.1%
B. ~ 0.5%
C. ~ 1%
D. ~ 1.8%

Prevalence of hepatitis C-related cirrhosis in the United States is about 0.5%.

1998. Which of the following have been well documented in children?
Harrison's 20th Ed. Chapter 336 Page 2401

A. NAFLD
B. NASH
C. NAFLD-related cirrhosis
D. All of the above

NAFLD, NASH and NAFLD-related cirrhosis are well documented in children. As in adults, obesity and insulin resistance are the main risk factors for pediatric NAFLD.

1999. Hyperinsulinemia promotes which of the following?
Harrison's 20th Ed. Chapter 336 Page 2401

A. Lipid uptake
B. Fat synthesis
C. Fat storage
D. All of the above

Hyperglycemia in insulin resistance promotes pancreas to produce more insulin. Hyperinsulinemia promotes lipid uptake, fat synthesis and fat storage. This results in hepatic triglyceride accumulation (steatosis).

2000. Which of the following damage hepatocytes?
Harrison's 20th Ed. Chapter 336 Page 2402

A. Fatty acids
B. Diacylglycerols
C. Reactive oxygen species
D. All of the above

Triglyceride per se is not hepatotoxic. Its precursors (fatty acids and diacylglycerols) and metabolic by-products (reactive oxygen species) may damage hepatocytes leading to hepatocyte lipotoxicity, cell death and consequent cell healing and repair efforts. NASH is the morphologic manifestation of lipotoxicity and resultant wound healing responses or futile repair.

2001. One drink is defined as having how much ethanol?
Harrison's 20th Ed. Chapter 336 Page 2402

A. 5 grams
B. 10 grams
C. 14 grams
D. 18 grams

One drink is defined as having 10 grams of ethanol equivalent to one can of beer, 4 ounces of wine or 1.5 ounces (one shot) of distilled spirits.

2002. NAFLD risk factors include?
Harrison's 20th Ed. Chapter 336 Page 2402

A. Body mass index
B. Hyperuricemia/gout
C. Systemic hypertension
D. All of the above

NAFLD risk factors include increased body mass index, insulin resistance/type 2 diabetes mellitus, systemic hypertension, dyslipidemia, hyperuricemia/gout, cardiovascular disease in the patient or family members.

2003. NAFLD is associated with which of the following?
Harrison's 20th Ed. Chapter 336 Page 2403

A. Obstructive sleep apnea
B. Thyroid dysfunction
C. Chronic pain syndrome
D. All of the above

2004. Which of the following is an acceptable first-line test for diagnosis of NASH?
Harrison's 20th Ed. Chapter 336 Page 2403

A. Ultrasound scan
B. Computed tomography (CT)
C. Magnetic resonance imaging (MRI)
D. Liver biopsy

Ultrasound is an acceptable first-line test. Liver biopsy is the gold standard for establishing the severity of liver injury and fibrosis.

2005. Which of the following differentiates individuals with NASH from those with simple steatosis or normal livers?
Hepatology. 2004;40(2):459-66

A. D8/18
B. F8/18
C. J8/18
D. K8/18

Serum levels of keratins 8 and 18 (K8/18) are epithelial cytoskeletal proteins that undergo cleavage during programmed cell death (apoptosis). Both cleaved and full-length K8/18 are released into blood as hepatocytes die. Serum levels of K8/18 differentiate individuals with NASH from those with simple steatosis or normal livers more reliably than do serum aminotransferase levels.

2006. Which of the following tests must be done in every patient of NAFLD?
Cleveland Clinic Journal of Medicine. 2017;84(4):273

A. Viral hepatitis panel
B. Antinuclear antibody (ANA)
C. Antismooth muscle antibody (ASMA)
D. All of the above

2007. Which of the following tests must be done in every patient of NAFLD?
Cleveland Clinic Journal of Medicine. 2017;84(4):273

A. Iron studies
B. Alpha-1 antitrypsin level
C. Ceruloplasmin level
D. All of the above

Initial evaluation of a patient with suspected NAFLD should include a thorough serologic evaluation to exclude coexisting causes of chronic liver disease. Tests include: viral hepatitis panel, antinuclear antibody (ANA), antismooth muscle antibody (ASMA), antimitochondrial antibody (AMA), iron studies, alpha-1 antitrypsin level, and ceruloplasmin level. Liver biopsy is the gold standard for diagnosing steatohepatitis and fibrosis.

2008. Which of the following improve necroinflammation associated with NASH?
Cleveland Clinic Journal of Medicine 2017;84(4):273

A. Vitamin E
B. Thiazolidinediones
C. Obeticholic acid
D. All of the above

Pentoxifylline and obeticholic acid improve fibrosis, while vitamin E, thiazolidinediones, and obeticholic acid improve necroinflammation associated with NASH.

2009. Which is the best dietary regimen for patients with NAFLD?
World J Gastroenterol. 2014;20(26):8341-8350

A. Chinese diet
B. Lebanese diet
C. Mediterranean diet
D. Japanese diet

Mediterranean diet seems to be the best dietary regimen for patients with NAFLD.

2010. Which of the following stimulate hepatic lipid accumulation and progression in NASH?
World J Gastroenterol. 2014;20(26):8341-8350

A. Choline
B. High-protein diets rich in isoflavones
C. Antioxidants
D. Fructose

Saturated fat & fructose stimulate hepatic lipid accumulation & progression in NASH. Unsaturated fat, choline, antioxidants and high-protein diets rich in isoflavones have a preventive effect. Among polyunsaturated fatty acids, n-3 fatty acids reduce the accumulation of triglycerides & ameliorate hepatic steatosis.

Cirrhosis and its Complications

2011. Reversal of fibrosis in cirrhosis liver can be achieved with treatment in which of the following diseases?
Harrison's 20th Ed. Chapter 337 Page 2405

A. Chronic hepatitis C
B. Hemochromatosis
C. Alcoholic liver disease
D. All of the above

Upon successful treatment of chronic hepatitis C, hemochromatosis and alcoholic liver disease liver fibrosis can be reversed.

2012. The cardinal pathologic features of cirrhosis liver are?
Harrison's 20th Ed. Chapter 337 Page 2405

A. Irreversible chronic injury of hepatic parenchyma
B. Extensive fibrosis
C. Formation of regenerative nodules
D. All of the above

The cardinal pathologic features reflect irreversible chronic injury of the hepatic parenchyma and include extensive fibrosis in association with the formation of regenerative nodules.

2013. The pathologic features of cirrhosis liver result from?
Harrison's 20th Ed. Chapter 337 Page 2405

A. Hepatocyte necrosis
B. Destruction of the supporting reticulin network
C. Distortion of the vascular bed
D. All of the above

The pathologic features result from hepatocyte necrosis, collapse of the supporting reticulin network with subsequent connective tissue deposition, distortion of the vascular bed, and nodular regeneration of remaining liver parenchyma.

2014. Central event leading to hepatic fibrosis in cirrhosis liver is?
Harrison's 20th Ed. Chapter 337 Page 2405

A. Activation of the hepatic stellate cell
B. Activation of the CD 8+ cells
C. Activation of Kupffer cells
D. All of the above

The central event leading to hepatic fibrosis is activation of the hepatic stellate cell resulting in the formation of increased amounts of collagen and other components of the extracellular matrix.

2015. Alcohol induced liver injury refers to?
Harrison's 20th Ed. Chapter 337 Page 2405

A. Alcoholic cirrhosis
B. Alcoholic fatty liver
C. Alcoholic hepatitis
D. All of the above

Alcohol-induced liver injury includes consequences resulting from chronic alcohol ingestion like alcoholic fatty liver, alcoholic hepatitis and alcoholic cirrhosis.

2016. Alcoholic cirrhosis is also called?
Harrison's 20th Ed. Chapter 337 Page 2405

A. Gaucher's cirrhosis
B. Johnson's cirrhosis
C. Gilbert's cirrhosis
D. Laennec's cirrhosis

Alcoholic cirrhosis, historically referred to as Laennec's cirrhosis is the most common type of cirrhosis encountered in North America, western Europe and South America.

2017. Use of excessive alcohol can contribute to liver damage in patients with?
Harrison's 20th Ed. Chapter 337 Page 2405

A. Hepatitis C
B. Hemochromatosis
C. Fatty liver disease related to obesity
D. All of the above

Use of excessive alcohol can contribute to liver damage in patients with other liver diseases like hepatitis C, hemochromatosis and fatty liver disease related to obesity.

2018. Hepatic fibrosis secondary to chronic alcohol use is?
Harrison's 20th Ed. Chapter 337 Page 2405

A. Centrilobular
B. Pericellular
C. Periportal
D. Any of the above

Chronic alcohol use can produce fibrosis in the absence of accompanying inflammation and/or necrosis. Fibrosis can be centrilobular, pericellular, or periportal.

2019. The diameter of nodules in alcoholic cirrhosis is?
Harrison's 20th Ed. Chapter 337 Page 2405

A. < 0.5 mm
B. < 1 mm
C. < 2 mm
D. < 3 mm

In alcoholic cirrhosis, nodules are usually <3 mm in diameter (micronodular). With cessation of alcohol use, larger nodules may form, resulting in a mixed micronodular and macronodular cirrhosis.

2020. Ethanol is mainly absorbed in?
Harrison's 20th Ed. Chapter 337 Page 2405

A. Stomach
B. Small intestine
C. Large intestine
D. All of the above

Ethanol is mainly absorbed by small intestine and to a lesser degree through stomach.

2021. Which of the following initiates alcohol metabolism?
Harrison's 20th Ed. Chapter 337 Page 2405

A. Cytosolic alcohol dehydrogenase (ADH)
B. Microsomal ethanol-oxidizing system (MEOS)
C. Peroxisomal catalase
D. Gastric alcohol dehydrogenase (ADH)

Gastric alcohol dehydrogenase (ADH) initiates alcohol metabolism.

2022. Enzyme system for metabolism of alcohol in the liver is?
Harrison's 20th Ed. Chapter 337 Page 2405

A. Cytosolic alcohol dehydrogenase (ADH)
B. Microsomal ethanol oxidizing system (MEOS)
C. Peroxisomal catalase
D. All of the above

Three enzyme systems metabolize alcohol in liver. These are cytosolic ADH, the microsomal-oxidizing system (MEOS), and peroxisomal catalase.

2023. Which of the following is a hepatic consequence of intake of ethanol?
Harrison's 20th Ed. Chapter 440 Page 3238

A. Increases intracellular accumulation of triglycerides
B. Impairment of protein synthesis, glycosylation, and secretion
C. Production of excess collagen and extracellular matrix
D. All of the above

2024. Ethanol is oxidized to acetaldehyde by?
Harrison's 20th Ed. Chapter 337 Page 2405

A. Cytosolic alcohol dehydrogenase (ADH)
B. Microsomal-oxidizing system (MEOS)
C. Peroxisomal catalase
D. Gastric alcohol dehydrogenase (ADH)

Majority of ethanol oxidation occurs via ADH to form acetaldehyde.

2025. Which out of the following is a highly reactive molecule?
Harrison's 20th Ed. Chapter 337 Page 2405

A. Alcohol
B. Acetaldehyde
C. Acetate
D. All of the above

2026. Acetaldehyde is metabolized to acetate by?
Harrison's 20th Ed. Chapter 337 Page 2405

A. Succinic semialdehyde dehydrogenase
B. α-Aminoadipic semialdehyde synthase
C. Aldehyde dehydrogenase
D. All of the above

Ethanol oxidation occurs via ADH to form acetaldehyde which is metabolized to acetate by aldehyde dehydrogenase (ALDH). Acetaldehyde combines with proteins to form protein-acetaldehyde adducts that lead to hepatocyte damage like interference with specific enzyme activities (microtubular formation & hepatic protein trafficking), Kupffer cell activation. As a result, profibrogenic cytokines are produced that initiate and perpetuate stellate cell activation, with the resultant production of excess collagen and extracellular matrix.

2027. Aldehyde dehydrogenase is also expressed by?
Harrison's 20th Ed. Chapter 440 Page 3238

A. Cardiomyocytes
B. Hematopoietic precursors (stem cells)
C. Renal mesangial cells
D. Synovial fibroblasts

At high doses, cyclophosphamide eliminates mature lymphocytes but spares hematopoietic precursors (stem cells), because they express the enzyme aldehyde dehydrogenase, which hydrolyzes cyclophosphamide.

2028. In alcoholic cirrhosis, clinical findings include?
Harrison's 20th Ed. Chapter 337 Page 2406

A. Palmar erythema
B. Spider angiomas
C. Lacrimal gland enlargement
D. All of the above

2029. In alcoholic cirrhosis, clinical findings include all except?
Harrison's 20th Ed. Chapter 337 Page 2406

A. Clubbing of fingers
B. Muscle wasting
C. Signs of virilization in women
D. Xanthoma

2030. Which of the following findings are associated with alcoholism but are not specifically related to cirrhosis?
Harrison's 20th Ed. Chapter 337 Page 2406

A. Palmar erythema
B. Spider angiomas
C. Gynecomastia
D. Dupuytren's contractures

Frequent findings in alcoholic cirrhosis include jaundice, palmar erythema, spider angiomas, parotid and lacrimal gland enlargement, clubbing of fingers, splenomegaly, muscle wasting, and ascites with or without peripheral edema. Increased peripheral formation of estrogen due to diminished hepatic clearance of the precursor androstenedione leads to gynecomastia, testicular atrophy and decreased body hair in men. In women, signs of virilization or menstrual irregularities may occur. Dupuytren's contractures resulting from fibrosis of the palmar fascia with resulting flexion contracture of digits are associated with alcoholism but are not specifically related to cirrhosis.

2031. Which of the following is false about palmar erythema?
Harrison's 20th Ed. Chapter 337 Page 2406

A. Occurs in patients of alcoholic cirrhosis
B. Erythema is peripheral over the palm with central pallor
C. Frequently found during pregnancy
D. None of the above

Spider angiomata and palmar erythema occur in both acute and chronic liver disease. These manifestations may be especially prominent in persons with cirrhosis but can develop in normal individuals and are frequently found during pregnancy.

2032. Anemia in alcoholic cirrhosis may be due to?
Harrison's 20th Ed. Chapter 337 Page 2406

A. Acute/chronic GI blood loss
B. Coexistent folic acid & vitamin B_{12} deficiency
C. Hypersplenism
D. All of the above

2033. Anemia in alcoholic cirrhosis may be due to?
Harrison's 20th Ed. Chapter 337 Page 2406

A. Psychogenic factors
B. Direct suppressive effect of alcohol on bone marrow
C. Deficiency of iron
D. All of the above

Anemia results from acute & chronic gastrointestinal blood loss, coexistent folic acid & vitamin B12 deficiency, hypersplenism, & suppressive effect of alcohol on bone marrow.

2034. Zieve's syndrome in alcoholics is best related to?
Harrison's 20th Ed. Chapter 337 Page 2406

- A. Diarrhea
- B. Myocardial infarction
- C. Hemolytic anemia
- D. Pneumonia

ZS is an acute metabolic condition that can occur in severe alcoholic hepatitis and during withdrawal from prolonged alcohol abuse. It consists of hemolytic anemia (spur cells and acanthocytes), hyperlipoproteinemia, jaundice, and abdominal pain. The underlying cause is liver delipidization.

2035. Zieve's syndrome in alcoholics is best related to?
Harrison's 20th Ed. Chapter 337 Page 2406

- A. Acanthocytes
- B. Dacrocytes
- C. Schistocytes
- D. Echinocytes

A unique form of hemolytic anemia (with spur cells and acanthocytes) called Zieve's syndrome can occur in patients with severe alcoholic hepatitis.

2036. Acanthocyte is best related to?
Harrison's 20th Ed. Chapter 428 Page 3137

- A. Chorea
- B. Seizure
- C. Blindness
- D. Mania

Chorea-acanthocytosis (neuroacanthocytosis) is a progressive and typically fatal autosomal recessive disorder that is characterized by chorea coupled with red cell abnormalities on peripheral blood smear (acanthocytes).

2037. Acanthocytosis is best related to?
Harrison's 20th Ed. Chapter 109 Page 810

- A. Pelger-Huet anomaly
- B. Chediak-Higashi syndrome
- C. McLeod phenotype
- D. Severe uremia

The Kell protein is very large (720 amino acids) and its secondary structure contains many different antigenic epitopes. The immunogenicity of Kell is third behind the ABO and Rh systems. The absence of the Kell precursor protein (controlled by a gene on X) is associated with acanthocytosis, shortened RBC survival and a progressive form of muscular dystrophy that includes cardiac defects. This rare condition is called the McLeod phenotype.

2038. Acanthocytes reflect which of the following?
Harrison's 20th Ed. Chapter 58 Page 379, N Engl J Med. 2018;379:774

- A. Renal disease
- B. Abetalipoproteinemia
- C. Splenectomy
- D. All of the above

Acanthocytes are spiculated red cells with the spikes irregularly distributed. This process tends to be irreversible and reflects underlying renal disease, abetalipoproteinemia or splenectomy. Spur-cell anemia is associated with a poor prognosis and is definitively treated by liver transplantation.

2039. Apart from acanthocytosis, which of the following is a feature of abetalipoproteinemia?
Harrison's 20th Ed. Chapter 438 Page 3221

- A. Steatorrhea
- B. Pigmentary retinopathy
- C. Progressive ataxia
- D. All of the above

Abetalipoproteinemia is a rare autosomal dominant hereditary disorder characterized by steatorrhea, pigmentary retinopathy, acanthocytosis and progressive ataxia.

2040. Laboratory finding unusual in alcoholic cirrhosis is?
Harrison's 20th Ed. Chapter 335 Page 2400

- A. Hemolytic anemia
- B. Hyperbilirubinemia
- C. Elevated serum alkaline phosphatase
- D. Serum AST levels > 400 units

Hemolytic anemia due to effects of hypercholesterolemia or erythrocyte membranes resulting in unusual spurlike projections (acanthocytosis) may occur. Hyperbilirubinemia is found in association with elevated serum alkaline phosphatase levels. Levels of serum AST are frequently elevated, but levels > 400 units are unusual.

2041. The ratio of serum activities of AST and ALT is called as?
Clin Biochem Rev. 2013;34:117

- A. Rathbone ratio
- B. Josephine ratio
- C. Langworthy ratio
- D. De Ritis ratio

De Ritis ratio of AST to ALT has much clinical utility in detecting the cause of injury to the liver.

2042. Which of the following about AST and ALT is false?
Clin Biochem Rev. 2013;34:117

- A. ALT is only present in hepatocyte cytoplasm
- B. AST is present in both hepatocyte cytoplasm & mitochondria
- C. 80% of total AST activity in human liver is contributed by Mitochondrial AST
- D. None of the above

2043. Which of the following is false about alcoholic cirrhosis?
Harrison's 20th Ed. Chapter 337 Page 2406

- A. Serum alanine aminotransferase (ALT) elevated
- B. Serum aspartate aminotransferase (AST) elevated
- C. AST levels > ALT levels, usually by a 2:1 ratio
- D. None of the above

2044. In alcoholic liver disease, AST levels > ALT are due to?
Harrison's 20th Ed. Chapter 337 Page 2406

- A. Greater inhibition of ALT synthesis by ethanol
- B. Greater production of AST by ethanol
- C. Greater clearance of ALT by ethanol
- D. Lesser clearance of AST by ethanol

In alcoholic liver disease & in contrast to viral hepatitis, serum AST is usually disproportionately elevated relative to ALT (AST/ALT ratio >2) due to proportionally greater inhibition of ALT synthesis by ethanol which may be partially reversed by pyridoxal phosphate.

2045. Which of the following about alcoholic cirrhosis is true?
Harrison's 20th Ed. Chapter 337 Page 2406

- A. Glucocorticoids are helpful in severe alcoholic hepatitis & encephalopathy
- B. Survival benefit has been reported for S-adenosyl methionine in alcoholic cirrhosis

C. Diuretics, sedatives, aspirin, acetaminophen should be used with caution
D. All of the above

Glucocorticoids in moderately large doses for 4 weeks are helpful in patients with severe alcoholic hepatitis and encephalopathy but have no role in the treatment of established alcoholic cirrhosis. S-adenosyl methionine decreases proinflammatory cytokines and has survival benefit in alcoholic cirrhosis. Diuretics, sedatives, aspirin, acetaminophen should be used with caution.

2046. In patients with severe alcoholic hepatitis, treatment with glucocorticoids is restricted to patients with a discriminant function (DF) value of?

Harrison's 20th Ed. Chapter 337 Page 2406

A. > 24
B. > 28
C. > 30
D. > 32

In patients with severe alcoholic hepatitis, treatment with glucocorticoids is restricted to patients with a discriminant function (DF) value of >32.

2047. Which of the following medications is approved for treating alcoholism by reducing craving?

Harrison's 20th Ed. Chapter 337 Page 2407

A. Pentoxifylline
B. Acamprosate calcium
C. Colchicine
D. Penicillamine

Tiapride is a dopamine antagonist. Acamprosate reduces craving for alcohol, helps restore balance of excitatory & inhibitory neurotransmission in nucleus accumbens by blocking GABA receptors and Glutamate receptors and activating GABA-A receptors. Naltrexone is an opioid antagonist.

2048. In alcoholics, which concomitant hepatitis infection accelerates development of alcoholic cirrhosis?

Harrison's 20th Ed. Chapter 337 Page 2407

A. Acute hepatitis A
B. Acute hepatitis B
C. Chronic hepatitis B
D. Chronic hepatitis C

Concomitant chronic hepatitis C virus (HCV) infection significantly accelerates development of alcoholic cirrhosis. Of patients exposed to the hepatitis C virus (HCV), about 80% develop chronic hepatitis C and of those about 20–30% will develop cirrhosis over 20–30 years. Of adult patients exposed to hepatitis B, about 5% develop chronic hepatitis B and about 20% of those patients will go on to develop cirrhosis.

2049. Steatosis is present in patients with which HCV genotype?

Harrison's 20th Ed. Chapter 337 Page 2407

A. 1
B. 2
C. 3
D. 4

In patients with HCV genotype 3, steatosis is often present.

2050. Nonalcoholic steatohepatitis (NASH) is nowadays diagnosed as what was earlier diagnosed as?

Harrison's 20th Ed. Chapter 337 Page 2407

A. Autoimmune cholangiopathy
B. Cardiac cirrhosis
C. Cryptogenic cirrhosis
D. Autoimmune hepatitis

Many patients who were thought to have cryptogenic cirrhosis in fact have nonalcoholic steatohepatitis.

2051. Which of the following presentation result from both hepatocellular insufficiency and portal hypertension?

Harrison's 20th Ed. Chapter 337 Page 2407

A. Ascites
B. Jaundice
C. Coagulopathy
D. Splenomegaly

2052. Which of the following presentation result from both hepatocellular insufficiency and portal hypertension?

Harrison's 20th Ed. Chapter 337 Page 2407

A. Splenomegaly
B. Jaundice
C. Coagulopathy
D. Hepatic encephalopathy

Jaundice, edema, coagulopathy, and certain metabolic abnormalities are due to loss of functioning hepatocellular mass. Gastroesophageal varices and splenomegaly are due to portal hypertension. Ascites & hepatic encephalopathy result from both hepatocellular insufficiency & portal hypertension.

2053. Which of the following is a cause of chronic cholestatic syndrome?

Harrison's 20th Ed. Chapter 337 Page 2407

A. Primary biliary cirrhosis (PBC)
B. Autoimmune cholangitis (AIC)
C. Primary sclerosing cholangitis (PSC)
D. All of the above

Causes of chronic cholestatic syndromes are primary biliary cirrhosis (PBC), autoimmune cholangitis, primary sclerosing cholangitis (PSC) and idiopathic adulthood ductopenia.

2054. Histopathologic features of chronic cholestasis are all except?

Harrison's 20th Ed. Chapter 337 Page 2407

A. Copper deposition
B. Xanthomatous transformation of hepatocytes
C. Iron deposition
D. Biliary fibrosis

Histopathologic features of chronic cholestasis are cholate stasis, copper deposition, xanthomatous transformation of hepatocytes, and biliary fibrosis. There may also be chronic portal inflammation, interface activity and chronic lobular inflammation. Ductopenia is a result of this progressive disease as patients develop cirrhosis.

2055. Stauffer's syndrome refers to intrahepatic cholestasis specifically associated with?

J Gen Intern Med. 2006;21(7): 11-C13

A. Sarcoidosis
B. Carcinoma pancreas
C. Renal cell cancer
D. Halothane

Non-metastatic (paraneoplastic) hepatic dysfunction in patients suffering from renal cell carcinoma is known as Stauffer's syndrome. It is characterized by elevated AlkP, ESR, α-2-globulin, and γ-glutamyl transferase, thrombocytosis, prolongation of prothrombin time, and hepatosplenomegaly, in the absence of hepatic metastasis and jaundice.

2056. Primary biliary cholangitis (PBC) is characterized by?
Harrison's 20th Ed. Chapter 337 Page 2408

A. Fibrous obliteration of intrahepatic bile ductules
B. Fibrous obliteration of larger extrahepatic ducts
C. Fibrous obliteration of intrahepatic bile ductules and larger extrahepatic ducts both
D. None of the above

PBC is characterized by portal inflammation & necrosis of cholangiocytes in small and medium-sized bile ducts.

2057. Which of the following about primary biliary cholangitis (PBC) is false?
N Engl J Med. 2005;353:1261-73

A. Most prevalent in northern Europe
B. Slowly progressive autoimmune disease of liver
C. Primarily affects men
D. Peak incidence is in fifth decade of life

Among patients with symptomatic disease, 90% are women between age 35 to 60 years.

2058. Which of the following represent the pathological Stage I of PBC?
Harrison's 20th Ed. Chapter 337 Page 2408

A. Chronic nonsuppurative destructive cholangitis
B. Reduction in number of bile ducts and proliferation of smaller bile ductules
C. Decrease in interlobular ducts, loss of liver cells, and expansion of periportal fibrosis into a network of connective tissue scars
D. Micronodular or macronodular cirrhosis

PBC is divided morphologically into 4 stages. Stage I is termed chronic nonsuppurative destructive cholangitis. It is a necrotizing inflammatory process of portal triads characterized by destruction of medium & small bile ducts, a dense infiltrate of acute & chronic inflammatory cells, mild fibrosis & occasionally, bile stasis. In stage II, inflammatory infiltrate becomes less prominent, number of bile ducts are reduced & smaller bile ductules proliferate. Over months to years there is a decrease in interlobular ducts, loss of liver cells & expansion of periportal fibrosis into a network of connective tissue scars marking stage III. Stage IV represents cirrhosis - micronodular or macronodular.

2059. Antimitochondrial antibody (AMA) found in primary biliary cirrhosis is of which type of immunoglobulin?
Harrison's 20th Ed. Chapter 337 Page 2408

A. IgG
B. IgM
C. IgA
D. IgE

A circulating IgG antimitochondrial antibody (AMA) is detected in ~90% of patients with PBC and only rarely in other forms of liver disease.

2060. Which of the following is an autoreactive mitochondrial antigen in primary biliary cholangitis?
Harrison's 20th Ed. Chapter 337 Page 2408

A. Pyruvate dehydrogenase complex (PDC)
B. 2-oxoglutarate dehydrogenase complex (OGDC)
C. Branched-chain 2-oxoacid dehydrogenase complex
D. All of the above

In PBC, circulating IgG antimitochondrial autoantibodies (AMA) recognize inner mitochondrial membrane proteins identified as enzymes of the pyruvate dehydrogenase complex (PDC), branched chain 2-oxoacid dehydrogenase complex (BCOADC), and 2-oxoglutarate dehydrogenase complex (OGDC).

2061. T cells infiltrating the liver in primary biliary cholangitis are specific for?
N Engl J Med. 2005;353:1261-73

A. Pyruvate dehydrogenase E2 complex (PDC-E2)
B. E3-binding protein (E3-BP)
C. Ketoglutaric acid dehydrogenase E2 complex (OGDC-E2)
D. Branched-chain 2-oxo-acid dehydrogenase E2 complex (BCKD-E2)

The major autoantigen in PBC (90%) is 74-kDa E2 component of PDC, dihydrolipoamide acetyltransferase. Antibodies are directed to a region essential for binding of a lipoic acid cofactor and inhibit the overall enzymatic activity of the PDC. Other AMA autoantibodies in PBC patients are directed to similar constituents of BCOADC and OGDC and also inhibit their enzymatic function.

2062. In PBC, pruritus is most bothersome in?
Harrison's 20th Ed. Chapter 337 Page 2408

A. Morning
B. Afternoon
C. Evening
D. Night

Pruritus is seen in approximately 50% of PBC patients. Pruritus is most bothersome in evening.

2063. Features unique to PBC include all except?
Harrison's 20th Ed. Chapter 337 Page 2408

A. Hypopigmentation
B. Xanthelasma
C. Xanthomata
D. Bone pain

Features unique to PBC include hyperpigmentation, xanthelasma, xanthomata & bone pain. The first three are related to the altered cholesterol metabolism seen in PBC.

2064. In PBC, hyperpigmentation is evident on?
Harrison's 20th Ed. Chapter 337 Page 2408

A. Trunk
B. Face
C. Areas of exfoliation and lichenification
D. All of the above

In PBC, hyperpigmentation is evident on trunk and arms and in areas of exfoliation and lichenification.

2065. Which of the following about primary biliary cholangitis (PBC) is true?
N Engl J Med. 2005;353:1261-73

A. Antimitochondrial antibodies are present in ~90%
B. Antimitochondrial antibodies are detectable years before clinical signs appear
C. Autoantibodies recognize three to five inner mitochondrial membrane proteins
D. All of the above

2066. Which of the following about primary biliary cholangitis (PBC) is true?
N Engl J Med. 2005;353:1261-73

A. Fatigue & pruritus are the commonest presenting symptoms
B. Pruritus precedes onset of jaundice by months to years

C. Pruritus is usually worse at night and is exacerbated by contact with wool, other fabrics, or heat
D. All of the above

In PBC, the earliest symptom is pruritus, which may be either generalized or limited initially to palms and soles. Fatigue is a prominent early symptom.

2067. Which of the following is true for "autoimmune cholangitis"?
Harrison's 19th Ed. 2061

A. Histological features similar to PBC
B. Negative AMA
C. Antinuclear or smooth-muscle antibodies present
D. All of the above

In autoimmune cholangitis, histological features are similar to PBC. The AMA titre is negative. Antinuclear or smooth-muscle antibodies are present.

2068. Asymptomatic patients of PBC are initially detected by?
Harrison's 20th Ed. Chapter 337 Page 2408

A. Elevated serum alkaline phosphatase levels
B. Elevated AST levels
C. Elevated ALT levels
D. All of the above

Most patients with PBC are asymptomatic, and the disease is initially detected by elevated serum alkaline phosphatase levels during routine screening.

2069. Which of the following is increased in patients of PBC?
Harrison's 20th Ed. Chapter 337 Page 2408

A. γ-glutamyl transpeptidase
B. Alkaline phosphatase (ALP)
C. IgM Immunoglobulins
D. All of the above

Laboratory findings in PBC show cholestatic liver enzyme abnormalities with an elevation in γ-glutamyl transpeptidase and alkaline phosphatase (ALP) along with mild elevations in aminotransferases (ALT and AST). Immunoglobulins, particularly IgM, are typically increased.

2070. Which of the following is false about ursodiol therapy in PBC?
Harrison's 20th Ed. Chapter 337 Page 2408

A. Dose is 13 to 15 mg/kg per day
B. Should be given with food
C. As a single dose daily
D. None of the above

Ursodiol is given in doses of 13 to 15 mg/kg per day, with food and as a single dose daily.

2071. Which of the following drugs is useful in treatment of PBC patients with an inadequate response to UDCA?
Harrison's 20th Ed. Chapter 337 Page 2408

A. Aniticholic acid
B. Afoticholic acid
C. Obeticholic acid
D. Neoticholic acid

In 2016, obeticholic acid was approved for use in PBC patients with an inadequate response to UDCA.

2072. Drugs used to treat pruritus in PBC include all except?
Harrison's 20th Ed. Chapter 337 Page 2408

A. Cholestyramine
B. Naltrexone
C. Rifampin
D. Tetracycline

Rifampin, opiate antagonists (naloxone or naltrexone), ondansetron, plasmapheresis, and ultraviolet light have been tried for control of pruritus with varying results. Cholestyramine, an oral bile salt sequestering resin, may be helpful in doses of 12 to 16 gm/day to decrease both pruritus and hypercholesterolemia.

2073. The only established "cure" in the treatment of primary biliary cholangitis is?
Harrison's 20th Ed. Chapter 337 Page 2408

A. Liver transplantation
B. Long term Cyclosporine therapy
C. Long term Tacrolimus therapy
D. All of the above

Ursodiol therapy may not prevent ultimate progression of PBC and the only established 'cure' is liver transplantation.

2074. Secondary biliary cirrhosis (SBC) is characterized by?
Harrison's 20th Ed. Chapter 339 Page 2431

A. Fibrous obliteration of intrahepatic bile ductules
B. Fibrous obliteration of larger extrahepatic ducts
C. Fibrous obliteration of intrahepatic bile ductules and larger extrahepatic ducts both
D. None of the above

Biliary cirrhosis results from injury to or prolonged obstruction of either the intrahepatic or extrahepatic biliary system. It is associated with impaired biliary excretion, destruction of hepatic parenchyma, and progressive fibrosis. Primary biliary cirrhosis (PBC) is characterized by chronic inflammation and fibrous obliteration of intrahepatic bile ductules. Secondary biliary cirrhosis (SBC) is the result of longstanding obstruction of the larger extrahepatic ducts.

2075. Which of the following about Primary Sclerosing Cholangitis (PSC) is false?
Harrison's 20th Ed. Chapter 337 Page 2408

A. Chronic cholestatic syndrome
B. Obliteration of intrahepatic biliary tree
C. Obliteration of extrahepatic biliary tree
D. None of the above

PSC is a chronic cholestatic syndrome that is characterized by diffuse inflammation and fibrosis involving the entire biliary tree (intra- and extrahepatic), resulting in chronic cholestasis.

2076. Pathologic change occurs in PSC is?
Harrison's 20th Ed. Chapter 337 Page 2408

A. Bile duct proliferation
B. Ductopenia
C. Fibrous cholangitis (pericholangitis)
D. All of the above

Pathologic changes that can occur in PSC show bile duct proliferation as well as ductopenia and fibrous cholangitis (pericholangitis).

2077. Which of the following antibody is seen frequently in Primary Sclerosing Cholangitis (PSC)?
Harrison's 20th Ed. Chapter 337 Page 2409

A. Anti-DNA antibody
B. Cryoglobulins
C. Perinuclear antineutrophil cytoplasmic antibody (p-ANCA)
D. Antiphospholipid antibody

Perinuclear antineutrophil cytoplasmic antibody (p-ANCA), is positive in ~65% of patients of PSC.

2078. Which of the following is seen frequently in Primary Sclerosing Cholangitis (PSC)?
Harrison's 20th Ed. Chapter 337 Page 2409

A. Hodgkin's lymphoma
B. Ulcerative colitis (UC)
C. Azoospermia
D. Amenorrhea

Over 50% of patients with PSC also have ulcerative colitis (UC). PSC occurs less often in patients with CD. ~5% of patients with UC have PSC, but 50–75% of patients with PSC have IBD. IBD and PSC are commonly pANCA positive.

2079. Typical cholangiographic findings in PSC is?
Harrison's 20th Ed. Chapter 337 Page 2409

A. Multiple calculi in biliary tree
B. Multifocal stricturing & beading of biliary tree
C. Diffuse fibrotic narrowing of biliary tree
D. All of the above

Typical cholangiographic findings in PSC are multifocal stricturing and beading with intervening segments of normal or dilated ducts involving both the intrahepatic and extrahepatic biliary tree. Scarring prevents the intrahepatic ducts from dilating.

2080. Primary or idiopathic sclerosing cholangitis may be associated with?
Harrison's 20th Ed. Chapter 339 Page 2431

A. Autoimmune pancreatitis
B. Multifocal fibrosclerosis syndromes
C. Riedel's struma
D. All of the above

Primary or idiopathic sclerosing cholangitis may be associated with autoimmune pancreatitis; multifocal fibrosclerosis syndromes (retroperitoneal, mediastinal, and/or periureteral fibrosis), Riedel's struma or pseudotumor of the orbit.

2081. Which of the following has biochemical & cholangiographic features indistinguishable from PSC?
Harrison's 20th Ed. Chapter 339 Page 2431

A. Immunoglobulin G1 - associated cholangitis
B. Immunoglobulin G2 - associated cholangitis
C. Immunoglobulin G3 - associated cholangitis
D. Immunoglobulin G4 - associated cholangitis

Immunoglobulin G4–associated cholangitis is a recently described biliary disease of unknown etiology that presents with biochemical and cholangiographic features indistinguishable from PSC. Often associated with autoimmune pancreatitis & other fibrosing conditions but not inflammatory bowel disease, it is characterized by elevated serum IgG4 and infiltration of IgG4-positive plasma cells in bile ducts and liver tissue. Glucocorticoids and/or azathioprine are helpful.

2082. Independent predictor of a bad prognosis in PSC is?
Harrison's 20th Ed. Chapter 339 Page 2432

A. Age
B. Serum bilirubin concentration
C. Liver histologic changes
D. All of the above

Independent predictors of a bad prognosis in PSC are age, serum bilirubin concentration, liver histologic changes and splenomegaly. Cholangiocarcinoma is a dreaded consequence.

2083. Patients of PSC are more vulnerable to which of the following malignancies?
Harrison's 20th Ed. Chapter 319 Page 2269

A. Gallbladder polyp
B. Cervical cancer
C. Endometrial cancer
D. All of the above

Gallbladder polyps in patients with PSC have a high incidence of malignancy and cholecystectomy is recommended, even if a mass lesion is <1 cm in diameter.

2084. Which of the following malignancy is most commonly associated with PSC?
Harrison's 20th Ed. Chapter 337 Page 2409

A. Cholangiocarcinoma
B. Carcinoma pancreas
C. Carcinoma gallbladder
D. Ampullary cancer

Cholangiocarcinoma is most commonly associated with PSC and is exceptionally difficult to diagnose because its appearance is often identical to that of PSC. PSC patients have a 10–15% lifetime risk of developing cholangiocarcinoma.

2085. Cholangiography is normal in which variant of PSC?
Harrison's 20th Ed. Chapter 319 Page 2269

A. Pauci primary sclerosing cholangitis
B. Small duct primary sclerosing cholangitis
C. Hereditary sclerosing cholangitis
D. Drug induced sclerosing cholangitis

Cholangiography is normal in small duct primary sclerosing cholangitis - a variant of PSC. This variant is sometimes referred to as "pericholangitis" and involves small-caliber bile ducts. It has similar biochemical and histologic features to classic PSC and has significantly better prognosis than classic PSC, although it may evolve into classic PSC.

2086. Histopathologically, which of the following is helpful in making the diagnosis of PSC?
Harrison's 20th Ed. Chapter 337 Page 2409

A. Bile duct proliferation
B. Ductopenia
C. Periductal fibrosis
D. Xanthomatous transformation of hepatocytes

2087. Which of the following has cholangiographic appearance similar to that of PSC?
Harrison's 20th Ed. Chapter 339 Page 2432

A. AIDS cholangiopathy
B. Traumatic biliary injury
C. Chronic pancreatitis
D. All of the above

AIDS cholangiopathy is a condition, usually due to infection of the bile duct epithelium with CMV or cryptosporidia, which has a cholangiographic appearance similar to that of PSC. These patients usually present with greatly elevated serum alkaline phosphatase levels (mean, 800 IU/L), but the bilirubin is often near normal. These patients do not typically present with jaundice.

2088. Diagnosis of PSC is best made with?
Harrison's 20th Ed. Chapter 337 Page 2409

A. Ultrasound
B. MRCP
C. CT Scan
D. Liver biopsy

Primary sclerosing cholangitis is characterized by the destruction and fibrosis of larger bile ducts. Diagnosis of PSC is made with cholangiography (MRCP or ERCP), which demonstrates the pathognomonic segmental strictures.

2089. Which of the following is efficacious in PSC?
Harrison's 20th Ed. Chapter 337 Page 2409, Harrison's 20th Ed. Chapter 339 Page 2433

A. Glucocorticoids
B. Methotrexate
C. Cyclosporine
D. UDCA

Glucocorticoids, methotrexate, and cyclosporine have not been shown to be efficacious in PSC. UDCA in high dosage (20 mg/kg) improves serum liver tests, but an effect on survival has not been documented. Ultimate treatment is liver transplantation except when complicated by cholangiocarcinoma.

2090. "Nutmeg liver" is the term used to describe liver in?
Clin Liver Dis. 2002;6(4):947-67

A. Cardiac cirrhosis
B. Primary Biliary Cirrhosis
C. Secondary Biliary Cirrhosis
D. None of the above

In right heart failure, hepatic sinusoids become dilated & engorged with blood, along with hepatic ischemia from poor perfusion leading to necrosis of centrilobular hepatocytes with fibrosis in central areas. Centrilobular fibrosis extends outward in a characteristic stellate pattern from central vein.

2091. In "nutmeg liver", gross examination of liver shows which of the following?
Clin Liver Dis. 2002;6(4):947-67

A. Nodules on the surface of liver
B. Alternating red and pale areas
C. Pyramid like elevations on surface of liver
D. Brownish black discoloration of liver

In nutmeg liver, gross examination shows alternating red (congested) & pale (fibrotic) areas.

2092. Levels of which of the following is characteristically elevated in cardiac cirrhosis?
Harrison's 20th Ed. Chapter 337 Page 2409

A. S. Bilirubin
B. SGOT
C. SGPT
D. S. Alkaline phosphatase

ALP levels are characteristically elevated in cardiac cirrhosis, Aminotransferases may be normal or slightly increased with AST usually higher than ALT.

2093. Which of the following is false in cardiac cirrhosis?
Harrison's 20th Ed. Chapter 337 Page 2409

A. Pericentral fibrosis
B. Unlikely that patients will develop variceal hemorrhage
C. Unlikely that patients will develop encephalopathy
D. None of the above

2094. Inherited metabolic liver disease that can progress to cirrhosis is?
Harrison's 20th Ed. Chapter 337 Page 2409

A. Hemochromatosis
B. Wilson's disease
C. Cystic fibrosis
D. All of the above

Inherited metabolic liver diseases that can progress to cirrhosis include hemochromatosis, Wilson's disease, α_1 antitrypsin deficiency, and cystic fibrosis.

2095. Which of the following points is against the diagnosis of Budd-Chiari syndrome?
Harrison's 20th Ed. Chapter 337 Page 2409

A. Tender hepatomegaly
B. Intractable ascites
C. Right-sided heart failure
D. Centrilobular congestion & sinusoidal dilatation on liver biopsy

In Budd-Chiari syndrome, liver is grossly enlarged, tender & severe intractable ascites is present. Signs & symptoms of heart failure are notably absent. Hepatic venography or liver biopsy showing centrilobular congestion & sinusoidal dilatation in absence of right heart failure characterize Budd-Chiari syndrome.

2096. Toxicity of which of the following vitamins can cause veno-occlusive disease of liver?
Sherlock

A. A
B. D
C. E
D. K

2097. Acute Budd-Chiari syndrome has all the features except?
Sherlock

A. Abdominal pain
B. Jaundice
C. Ascites
D. Caudate lobe hypertrophy

2098. Initial investigation of choice in suspected Budd-Chiari syndrome is?
Sherlock

A. USG abdomen
B. Doppler studies
C. CT abdomen
D. MR angiography

2099. Portal hypertension is defined as elevation of hepatic venous pressure gradient (HVPG) to?
Harrison's 20th Ed. Chapter 337 Page 2410

A. > 2 mm Hg
B. > 3 mm Hg
C. > 4 mm Hg
D. > 5 mm Hg

Portal hypertension is defined as elevation of hepatic venous pressure gradient (HVPG) to >5 mm Hg. Varices may develop but do not bleed if HVPG is <12 mm Hg. HVPG is equal to wedged hepatic venous pressure (portal venous pressure) minus free hepatic venous pressure (intra-abdominal pressure).

2100. In variceal hemorrhage, mortality associated with each episode of bleeding is?
Harrison's 20th Ed. Chapter 337 Page 2410

A. 10 - 20%
B. 20 - 30%
C. 30 - 40%
D. 40 - 50%

Mortality associated with each episode of variceal bleeding is 20–30%. Even if the patient survives an initial episode of variceal bleeding, probability of another episode is high. Rebleeding rate without treatment is 70% within 1 year. The mortality rate with rebleeding is 33%.

2101. Portal vein is formed by the confluence of splenic vein with?
Harrison's 20th Ed. Chapter 337 Page 2410

A. Superior mesenteric vein
B. Inferior mesenteric vein
C. Gastric vein
D. All of the above

Portal vein is formed by the confluence of superior mesenteric and splenic veins.

2102. Which of the following is a posthepatic cause of portal hypertension?
Harrison's 20th Ed. Chapter 337 Page 2410

A. Portal vein thrombosis
B. Veno-occlusive disease
C. Splenic vein thrombosis
D. All of the above

2103. Which of the following is a posthepatic cause of portal hypertension?
Harrison's 20th Ed. Chapter 337 Page 2410

A. Budd-Chiari syndrome (BCS)
B. Veno-occlusive disease
C. Chronic right-sided cardiac congestion
D. All of the above

2104. Which of the following accounts for most cases of portal hypertension?
Harrison's 20th Ed. Chapter 337 Page 2410

A. Prehepatic
B. Intrahepatic
C. Posthepatic
D. Any of the above

Intrahepatic causes of portal hypertension account for over 95% of cases of portal hypertension and are represented by the major forms of cirrhosis.

2105. Esophageal varices are present in what percentage of compensated and decompensated cirrhosis?
Gastroenterol Hepatol (N Y). 2006;2(2):124-133

A. 10 & 40%
B. 20 & 50%
C. 30 & 60%
D. 40 & 70%

Esophageal varices are present in 30% of patients with compensated cirrhosis and in up to 60% of those with decompensated cirrhosis (with evidence of ascites or encephalopathy).

2106. Budd-Chiari syndrome is an example of?
Harrison's 20th Ed. Chapter 337 Page 2410

A. Presinusoidal obstruction
B. Sinusoidal obstruction
C. Post-sinusoidal obstruction
D. Any of the above

Postsinusoidal obstruction may also occur outside the liver at the level of the hepatic veins (Budd-Chiari syndrome), the inferior vena cava so that the liver parenchyma is exposed to elevated venous pressures.

2107. Which of the following is a presinusoidal cause of portal hypertension?
Harrison's 20th Ed. Chapter 337 Page 2410

A. Schistosomiasis
B. Chronic right-sided cardiac congestion
C. Cirrhosis liver
D. All of the above

Presinusoidal causes of portal hypertension include congenital hepatic fibrosis and schistosomiasis. Sinusoidal causes are related to cirrhosis from various causes.

2108. When cirrhosis is complicated by portal hypertension, the increased resistance is?
Harrison's 20th Ed. Chapter 337 Page 2410

A. Presinusoidal
B. Sinusoidal
C. Post-sinusoidal
D. All of the above

Portal hypertension (>10 mm Hg) mostly results from increased resistance to portal blood flow. When hepatic cirrhosis is complicated by portal hypertension, increased resistance is usually sinusoidal.

2109. 'Symmers' clay-pipe stem fibrosis in liver is due to?
Harrison's 20th Ed. Chapter 229 Page 1638

A. Brucellosis
B. Toxoplasmosis
C. Echinococcosis
D. Schistosomiasis

Intrahepatic presinusoidal causes of portal hypertension include congenital hepatic fibrosis and schistosomiasis. Schistosomiasis alone results in pure fibrotic lesions in liver. Cirrhosis occurs when other nutritional or infectious agents (hepatitis B or C virus) are involved. It is characteristically periportal (Symmers' clay pipe-stem fibrosis).

2110. Portal vein obstruction may occur in association with?
Harrison's 20th Ed. Chapter 337 Page 2410

A. Cirrhosis
B. Abdominal trauma
C. Pancreatitis
D. All of the above

Portal vein obstruction may be idiopathic or occur in association with cirrhosis, infection, pancreatitis, or abdominal trauma.

2111. Portal vein thrombosis may develop in?
Harrison's 20th Ed. Chapter 337 Page 2410

A. Polycythemia vera
B. Deficiencies of protein C, protein S, or antithrombin III
C. Factor V Leiden
D. All of the above

Idiopathic portal vein thrombosis may develop in hypercoagulable states like polycythemia vera, essential thrombocythemia, deficiencies of protein C / protein S / antithrombin III, resistance to activated protein C (factor V Leiden) & mutation of prothrombin gene (G20210A).

2112. Primary complication of portal hypertension is?
Harrison's 20th Ed. Chapter 337 Page 2410

A. Gastroesophageal varices with hemorrhage
B. Ascites
C. Hypersplenism
D. All of the above

Three primary complications of portal hypertension are gastroesophageal varices with hemorrhage, ascites, and hypersplenism.

2113. On screening of histologically confirmed cirrhosis cases, what proportion of patients have esophageal varices?
Harrison's 20th Ed. Chapter 337 Page 2410
- A. One - fourth
- B. One - third
- C. One - half
- D. Three - fourth

On screening of histologically confirmed cirrhosis cases, one - third of patients have esophageal varices.

2114. In cirrhosis, factor that predicts the risk of esophageal variceal bleeding is?
Harrison's 20th Ed. Chapter 337 Page 2410
- A. Severity of cirrhosis
- B. Wedged-hepatic vein pressure
- C. Tense ascites
- D. All of the above

In cirrhosis, factors that predict risk of esophageal variceal bleeding include severity of cirrhosis (Child's class, MELD score), height of wedged-hepatic vein pressure, size of varix, location of varix, endoscopic stigmatas (red wale signs, hematocystic spots, diffuse erythema, bluish color, cherry red spots, or white-nipple spots and tense ascites.

2115. Marker of the presence of cirrhosis in a patient being followed for chronic liver disease is?
Harrison's 20th Ed. Chapter 337 Page 2410
- A. Progressive decrease in platelet count
- B. Progressive increase in platelet count
- C. Progressive decrease in lymphocyte count
- D. Progressive increase in lymphocyte count

Progressive decrease in platelet count serves as a marker of the presence of cirrhosis in a patient being followed for chronic liver disease. A low-normal platelet count can be the first clue to progression to cirrhosis.

2116. Marker of the presence of cirrhosis in a patient being followed for chronic liver disease is?
Harrison's 20th Ed. Chapter 337 Page 2410
- A. Appearance of an enlarged spleen
- B. Development of ascites
- C. Hepatic encephalopathy
- D. All of the above

Progressive decrease in platelet count, appearance of enlarged spleen, development of ascites, encephalopathy, and/or esophageal varices with or without bleeding serve as markers of the presence of cirrhosis in a patient being followed for chronic liver disease.

2117. The risk of variceal hemorrhage is related to?
Harrison's 20th Ed. Chapter 337 Page 2410
- A. Size of varices
- B. Appearance of varices
- C. Severity of liver dysfunction
- D. All of the above

Risk of variceal hemorrhage is related to size of varices (varices ≤ 5 mm in diameter have a 7% risk of bleeding in 2 years, while those >5 mm have a 30% risk of bleeding within 2 years), appearance of the varices (red wale sign i.e. red streaks of mucosa overlying varix) have an increased risk of hemorrhage & severity of liver dysfunction (high Child-Pugh score - B or C represents decompensated cirrhosis & is associated with an increased risk of bleeding).

2118. In liver disease, development of portal hypertension is revealed by the appearance of which of the following?
Harrison's 20th Ed. Chapter 337 Page 2410
- A. Splenomegaly
- B. Ascites
- C. Encephalopathy
- D. All of the above

In patients with liver disease, development of portal hypertension is revealed by the appearance of splenomegaly, ascites, encephalopathy, and/or esophageal varices.

2119. Which of the following statements about free and wedged hepatic vein pressure is false?
Harrison's 20th Ed. Chapter 337 Page 2410
- A. Wedged hepatic vein pressure is usually normal in presinusoidal portal hypertension
- B. Wedged hepatic vein pressure is elevated in sinusoidal portal hypertension
- C. Wedged hepatic vein pressure is elevated in postsinusoidal portal hypertension
- D. None of the above

Wedged hepatic vein pressure is elevated in sinusoidal and postsinusoidal portal hypertension, it is normal in presinusoidal portal hypertension.

2120. What level of portal hypertension threatens bleeding from gastroesophageal varices?
Harrison's 20th Ed. Chapter 337 Page 2410
- A. > 6 mm Hg
- B. > 8 mm Hg
- C. > 10 mm Hg
- D. > 12 mm Hg

Wedged and free hepatic vein pressures allow calculation of a wedged-to-free gradient, which is equivalent to the portal pressure. Average normal wedged-to-free gradient is 5 mm Hg, and patients with a gradient >12 mm Hg are at risk for variceal hemorrhage.

2121. Apart from propranolol, which other β-adrenergic blocker is used to reduce portal pressure?
Harrison's 20th Ed. Chapter 337 Page 2411
- A. Atenolol
- B. Nadolol
- C. Sotalol
- D. Carvedilol

β-adrenergic blockade with nonselective agents (propranolol or nadolol) reduces portal pressure through vasoconstrictive effects on both splanchnic arterial bed & portal venous system in combination with reduced cardiac output. Such therapy is effective in preventing both a first variceal bleed & subsequent episodes.

2122. Doses of propranolol to treat portal hypertension should aim to reduce the resting pulse rate by?
Gut Liver. 2007;1(2):159-164
- A. 5%
- B. 10%
- C. 25%
- D. 33%

In treatment of portal hypertension, especially variceal bleeding, reduction of resting pulse through β-adrenergic blockade with nonselective agents such as propranolol by 25% is reasonable.

2123. The goal of treatment in patients of portal hypertension is to reduce hepatic venous pressure gradient (HVPG) to?
Gut Liver. 2007;1(2):159-164
- A. <20 mm Hg or by 50% from baseline
- B. <15 mm Hg or by 40% from baseline

C. <12 mm Hg or by 20% from baseline
D. <6 mm Hg or by 10% from baseline

Treatment of patients with clinically significant sequelae of portal hypertension, especially variceal bleeding, is titrated to reduce the hepatic venous pressure gradient (HVPG = wedged hepatic venous pressure – free hepatic venous pressure) to <12 mm Hg or by 20% from baseline.

2124. "Caput medusae" is best related to?
N Engl J Med. 2005; 353:e19

A. Cardioesophageal junction
B. Rectum
C. Retroperitoneal space
D. Falciform ligament of liver

Major sites of portalsystemic collateral flow are veins around cardioesophageal junction (esophagogastric varices), rectum (hemorrhoids), retroperitoneal space & falciform ligament of liver (periumbilical or abdominal wall collaterals). Abdominal wall collaterals appear as tortuous epigastric vessels that radiate from umbilicus toward xiphoid & rib margins (caput medusae).

2125. Which of the following is false about Dieulafoy's lesion?
Harrison's 20th Ed. Chapter 315 Page 2197

A. Large-caliber arteriole beneath gastrointestinal mucosa
B. Bleeds through a pinpoint mucosal erosion
C. Most common on greater curvature of proximal stomach
D. Also called persistent caliber artery

Dieulafoy's lesion is seen most commonly on the lesser curvature of the proximal stomach.

2126. Gastric antral vascular ectasia is the cause of?
Harrison's 20th Ed. Chapter 315 Page 2198

A. Washermen stomach
B. Watermelon stomach
C. Windmill stomach
D. Windshield stomach

Watermelon stomach is seen in gastric antral vascular ectasia (GAVE).

2127. Which of the following should be the first-line treatment to control bleeding acutely?
Harrison's 20th Ed. Chapter 337 Page 2411

A. Somatostatin/octreotide
B. Balloon tamponade
C. Emergency portal-systemic nonselective shunts
D. Endoscopic intervention

Endoscopic intervention should be the first-line treatment to control bleeding acutely. Treatment of acute bleeding requires both fluid and blood-product replacement as well as prevention of subsequent bleeding with Endoscopic variceal ligation (EVL).

2128. Sengstaken-Blakemore tube has how many lumens?
Harrison's 20th Ed. Chapter 337 Page 2411

A. 1
B. 2
C. 3
D. 4

2129. Minnesota tube has how many lumens?
Harrison's 20th Ed. Chapter 337 Page 2411

A. 1
B. 2
C. 3
D. 4

Balloon tamponade of bleeding gastroesophageal varices may be accomplished with a triple-lumen (Sengstaken-Blakemore) or four-lumen (Minnesota) tube with esophageal and gastric balloons.

2130. "TIPS" stands for?
Harrison's 20th Ed. Chapter 337 Page 2411

A. Transcuteneous intrahepatic portosystemic shunt
B. Transvenous intrahepatic portosystemic shunt
C. Transjugular intrahepatic portosystemic shunt
D. Transarterial intrahepatic portosystemic shunt

Decompression procedure to lower portal pressure is accomplished without surgery through percutaneous placement of a portal-systemic shunt, termed transjugular intrahepatic portosystemic shunt (TIPS).

2131. Hepatic encephalopathy occurs in what proportion of patients after TIPS?
Harrison's 20th Ed. Chapter 337 Page 2411

A. 10%
B. 20%
C. 30%
D. 40%

Hepatic encephalopathy occur in 20% of patients after TIPS.

2132. Somatostatin and octreotide are?
Harrison's 20th Ed. Chapter 337 Page 2411

A. Generalized vasoconstrictors
B. Direct splanchnic vasoconstrictors
C. Direct systemic vasoconstrictors
D. None of the above

Somatostatin and its analogue, octreotide, are direct splanchnic vasoconstrictors.

2133. Which of the following agents is useful in the treatment of portal hypertensive gastropathy?
Harrison's 20th Ed. Chapter 337 Page 2411

A. Proton pump inhibitors
B. H2 receptor blockers
C. Sucralfate
D. None of the above

Congestive gastropathy due to the venous hypertension is a complication of portal hypertension. Nonselective beta-adrenergic blockade is sometimes effective. Proton pump inhibitors or other agents useful in the treatment of peptic disease are usually not helpful.

2134. Theories proposed for ascites include?
Gastroenterol Hepatol (NY). 2009;5(9):647-656

A. "Underfilling" theory
B. "Overflow" theory
C. "Peripheral arterial vasodilation" theory
D. All of the above

2135. Hepatic hydrothorax is more common on which side?
Harrison's 20th Ed. Chapter 337 Page 2412

A. Right side
B. Left side
C. Bilateral
D. Any of the above

Hepatic hydrothorax is more common on right side due to a rent in the diaphragm with free flow of ascitic fluid into the thoracic cavity.

2136. What does SAAG stand for?
Harrison's 20th Ed. Chapter 337 Page 2412

A. Serum ascites-to-albumin gradient
B. Serum albumin-to-ascites gradient
C. Serum albumin-to-anion gradient
D. Serum anion-to-albumin gradient

In cirrhosis, protein concentration of ascitic fluid is low (<1 g/dL). With the use of serum ascites-to-albumin gradient (SAAG), terms like exudative or transudative fluid have been replaced. Cirrhosis leading to portal hypertension leading to ascites, gradient between serum albumin level and ascitic fluid albumin level is >1.1 g/dL. When the gradient is <1.1 g/dL, infectious or malignant causes of ascites should be considered.

2137. There is an increased risk for developing which of the following when levels of ascitic fluid proteins are very low?
Harrison's 20th Ed. Chapter 337 Page 2412

A. Refractory ascites
B. Hepatic Encephalopathy
C. Spontaneous Bacterial Peritonitis (SBP)
D. Hepatocellular cancer

When levels of ascitic fluid proteins are very low, patients are at increased risk for developing SBP.

2138. What absolute level of polymorphonuclear leukocytes count suggests ascitic fluid infection?
Harrison's 20th Ed. Chapter 337 Page 2412

A. > 100/μL
B. > 150/μL
C. > 200/μL
D. > 250/μL

A high level of red blood cells in the ascitic fluid signifies a traumatic tap or perhaps a hepatocellular cancer or a ruptured omental varix. When the absolute level of polymorphonuclear leukocytes is >250/μL, ascitic fluid infection should be strongly considered.

2139. The recommended amount of sodium per day in the management of ascites is?
Harrison's 20th Ed. Chapter 337 Page 2412

A. < 2 gram
B. < 4 gram
C. < 6 gram
D. < 8 gram

< 2 gram of sodium per day is the recommended amount in the management of ascites.

2140. Which of the following about refractory ascites is false?
Gastroenterol Hepatol (NY). 2009;5(9):647-656

A. Ascites that does not recede despite sodium restriction and diuretic treatment
B. Ascites that recurs shortly after therapeutic paracentesis
C. Prognosis for patients with cirrhosis with ascites is poor
D. None of the above

Refractory ascites is defined as ascites that does not recede or that recurs shortly after therapeutic paracentesis, despite sodium restriction and diuretic treatment. To date, there is no approved medical therapy specifically for refractory ascites. Management is based on large-volume paracentesis (LVP) and transjugular intrahepatic portosystemic shunts (TIPS), which temporarily alleviate symptoms, but are not curative. The only curative treatment is liver transplantation.

2141. Maximal doses of spironolactone and furosemide are?
Gastroenterol Hepatol (NY). 2009;5(9):647-656

A. Spironolactone 100 mg/day & furosemide 160 mg/day
B. Spironolactone 200 mg/day & furosemide 160 mg/day
C. Spironolactone 300 mg/day & furosemide 160 mg/day
D. Spironolactone 400 mg/day & furosemide 160 mg/day

Maximal doses of spironolactone and furosemide are 400 mg/day and 160 mg/day respectively.

2142. Which of the following is used to determine the likelihood that a patient with ascites will respond to therapy?
Gastroenterol Hepatol (NY). 2009;5(9):647-656

A. U_{Cr}/P_{Cr} ratio
B. Fractional excretion of sodium (Fe_{Na})
C. Serum vasopressin (AVP) level
D. All of the above

Initial fractional excretion of sodium (FeNa) >0.2% may predict the development of refractory ascites in patients receiving diuretic therapy.

2143. Which of the following statements about spontaneous bacterial peritonitis (SBP) is false?
Harrison's 20th Ed. Chapter 337 Page 2413

A. Develops without obvious primary source of infection
B. Ascitic fluid has high concentrations of albumin
C. In ascitic fluid, >250 PMN/μL is diagnostic
D. Monomicrobial nonneutrocytic bacterascites is a variant of SBP

SBP is characterized by spontaneous infection of ascitic fluid in absence of intra-abdominal source of infection. Bacterial translocation is the presumed mechanism for development of SBP, with gut flora traversing the intestine into mesenteric lymph nodes, leading to bacteremia and seeding of the ascitic fluid.

2144. Which of the following statements about spontaneous bacterial peritonitis (SBP) is false?
Harrison's 20th Ed. Chapter 337 Page 2413, N Engl J Med. 2004;350:1646-54

A. Escherichia coli are most commonly isolated
B. A single organism is typically isolated
C. Anaerobes are found less frequently
D. Recurrent episodes are relatively uncommon

SBP involves translocation of bacteria from intestinal lumen to lymph nodes, with subsequent bacteremia & infection of ascitic fluid. After resolution, SBP frequently recurs, with an estimated 70% probability of recurrence at one year.

2145. Which of the following statements about spontaneous bacterial peritonitis (SBP) is false?
Harrison's 20th Ed. Chapter 337 Page 2413

A. Therapy is for 10 to 14 days
B. Prophylactic norfloxacin reduces recurrences
C. Primary prevention recommended in high-risk cirrhotics
D. Empirical coverage for anaerobes is necessary

In patients with variceal hemorrhage, frequency of SBP is significantly increased, and prophylaxis against SBP is recommended when a patient presents with upper GI bleeding. Patients who have had an episode(s) of SBP and recovered, once-weekly administration of antibiotics is used as prophylaxis for recurrent SBP.

2146. Hepatorenal syndrome (HRS) occurs in what percentage of patients with advanced cirrhosis or acute liver failure?
Harrison's 20th Ed. Chapter 337 Page 2413

A. ~ 5%
B. ~ 10%
C. ~ 20%
D. ~ 30%

HRS is a type of functional renal failure "without renal pathology" that occurs in ~10% of patients with advanced cirrhosis or acute liver failure.

2147. Which of the following about hepatorenal syndrome is false?
Harrison's 20th Ed. Chapter 337 Page 2413

- A. Splanchnic vasodilation
- B. Arteriovenous shunting
- C. Profound renal vasoconstriction
- D. None of the above

In HRS, kidneys are structurally normal but fail due to splanchnic vasodilation & arteriovenous shunting, resulting in profound renal vasoconstriction resulting from extreme underfilling of arterial circulation.

2148. Renal failure in cirrhosis is defined as serum creatinine above?
N Engl J Med. 2009;361:1279-90

- A. 1.2 mg/dL
- B. 1.3 mg/dL
- C. 1.4 mg/dL
- D. 1.5 mg/dL

Most studies & consensus conferences have defined renal failure in cirrhosis as a serum creatinine concentration above 1.5 mg /dL.

2149. Which of the following about hepatorenal syndrome is false?
Harrison's 20th Ed. Chapter 337 Page 2413

- A. Type I HRS is the more aggressive form
- B. Type I HRS carries a mortality rate of >90%
- C. HRS is seen in patients with refractory ascites
- D. None of the above

HRS is a unique form of prerenal ARF that complicates advanced cirrhosis and acute liver failure and is seen in in patients with refractory ascites. Type I HRS is the more aggressive form of the disease & carries a mortality rate of >90%.

2150. Type 1 HRS is characterized by doubling of serum creatinine level to > 2.5 mg/dL in?
N Engl J Med. 2009;361:1279-90

- A. < 2 weeks
- B. < 4 weeks
- C. < 6 weeks
- D. < 8 weeks

Type 1 HRS is characterized by a doubling of serum creatinine level to > 2.5 mg/dL in < 2 weeks. Type 2 is characterized by a stable or less rapidly progressive course than in type 1.

2151. Which of the following is true for type 1 hepatorenal syndrome?
N Engl J Med. 2004;350:1646-54

- A. Progressive oliguria
- B. Rapid rise of serum creatinine
- C. Common precipitating event is SBP
- D. All of the above

Type 1 hepatorenal syndrome is characterized by progressive oliguria and a rapid rise of the serum creatinine. A common precipitating event is spontaneous bacterial peritonitis (SBP).

2152. Which of the following is true for type 2 hepatorenal syndrome?
N Engl J Med. 2004;350:1646-54

- A. Most have refractory ascites
- B. Increase in serum creatinine is moderate
- C. No tendency of serum creatinine to progress over time
- D. All of the above

In type 2 hepatorenal syndrome, most patients have refractory ascites, increase in serum creatinine is moderate and has no tendency to progress over time.

2153. Type 2 HRS is mainly characterized by?
N Engl J Med. 2009;361:1279-90

- A. Hepatic encephalopathy
- B. Refractory ascites
- C. Hypotension
- D. All of the above

Type 1 hepatorenal syndrome has severe multiorgan dysfunction, which affects not only the kidneys but also the heart, systemic circulation, brain, adrenal glands, and liver, whereas the clinical course of patients with type 2 hepatorenal syndrome is mainly characterized by refractory ascites.

2154. Which of the following treatments have a role in hepatorenal syndrome?
Harrison's 20th Ed. Chapter 337 Page 2413

- A. Midodrine
- B. Octreotide
- C. Intravenous albumin
- D. All of the above

Currently, patients of HRS are treated with midodrine, an α-agonist, along with octreotide & IV albumin. The best therapy for HRS is liver transplantation.

2155. Which of the following is a vasoconstrictor drug?
N Engl J Med. 2009;361:1279-90

- A. Terlipressin
- B. Norepinephrine
- C. Midodrine
- D. All of the above

Best approach in management of HRS is administration of vasoconstrictor drugs. Treatment with renal vasodilators like dopamine or prostaglandins is ineffective.

2156. Long-term administration of which of the following reduces the risk of hepatorenal syndrome & improves survival?
N Engl J Med. 2009;361:1279-90

- A. Norfloxacin
- B. Eplerenone
- C. Torsemide
- D. Vitamin E

Long-term oral norfloxacin reduces risk of hepatorenal syndrome & improves survival.

2157. Which of the following statements about hepatorenal syndrome (HRS) is false?
Harrison's 20th Ed. Chapter 337 Page 2413

- A. Worsening azotemia
- B. Avid sodium retention
- C. Oliguria without identifiable causes of renal dysfunction
- D. Kidneys are structurally smaller

2158. Which of the following statements about hepatorenal syndrome (HRS) is false?
Harrison's 20th Ed. Chapter 337 Page 2413

- A. Urinalysis normal
- B. Renal biopsy is normal
- C. Kidneys can be used for renal transplantation
- D. Hypernatremia

2159. Which of the following statements about hepatorenal syndrome (HRS) is false?
Harrison's 20th Ed. Chapter 337 Page 2413

A. Treatment is usually unsuccessful
B. Vasodilator therapy with intravenous infusions of low dose dopamine is effective
C. TIPS can improve renal function
D. Treatment of choice is liver transplantation

2160. Which of the following is false about hepatic encephalopathy?
Harrison's 20th Ed. Chapter 337 Page 2413

A. More common in chronic liver disease
B. Essential for diagnosis of fulminant hepatic failure
C. Diagnosis of hepatic encephalopathy is clinical
D. None of the above

2161. Which of the following characteristics about hepatic encephalopathy is false?
Harrison's 20th Ed. Chapter 337 Page 2413

A. Disturbances in consciousness
B. Behavior & personality changes
C. Fluctuating neurologic signs
D. No electroencephalographic changes

2162. Which of the following statements about hepatic encephalopathy is false?
Harrison's 20th Ed. Chapter 337 Page 2413

A. Blood-brain barrier is intact
B. Ammonia is incriminated in its pathogenesis
C. Many patients have elevated blood ammonia levels
D. Mercaptans, short-chain fatty acids, & phenol are incriminated in its pathogenesis

2163. Which of the following is the most common predisposing factor for hepatic encephalopathy?
Harrison's 20th Ed. Chapter 337 Page 2413

A. Gastrointestinal bleeding
B. Increased dietary protein
C. Electrolyte disturbances
D. Injudicious use of CNS-depressing drugs

2164. Which of the following is the most common predisposing factor for hepatic encephalopathy?
Harrison's 20th Ed. Chapter 337 Page 2413

A. Gastrointestinal bleeding
B. Surgery
C. Superimposed acute viral hepatitis
D. Alcoholic hepatitis

2165. Which of the following is the most common predisposing factor for hepatic encephalopathy?
Harrison's 20th Ed. Chapter 337 Page 2413

A. Gastrointestinal bleeding
B. Extrahepatic bile duct obstruction
C. Constipation
D. Surgery

In chronic liver disease, encephalopathy is usually triggered by a medical complication such as gastrointestinal bleeding, over-diuresis, uremia, dehydration, electrolyte imbalance, infection, constipation or use of narcotic analgesics.

2166. Astrocytic glutamine synthetase converts ammonia & glutamate into?
N Engl J Med. 2016;375:1660-70

A. Inositol
B. Taurine
C. Arginine
D. Glutamine

At high levels, ammonia can cross blood–brain barrier, where astrocytic glutamine synthetase converts ammonia & glutamate into glutamine, which acts as an osmolyte & increases cerebral volume.

2167. Which of the following elements is a possible contributor to hepatic encephalopathy?
N Engl J Med. 2016;375:1660-70

A. Molybdenum
B. Manganese
C. Nickel
D. Silicon

A possible contributor to hepatic encephalopathy, particularly in patients with long-standing cirrhosis, is manganese toxicity. Mercaptans, short fatty acids, decreased glutaminergic synaptic function, lactate & dopamine metabolites have also been implicated.

2168. The MELD score determination does not include?
Harrison's 20th Ed. Chapter 338 Page 2416

A. Bilirubin
B. Urea
C. Creatinine
D. Prothrombin time

The MELD score is based on a mathematical model that includes bilirubin, creatinine and prothrombin time expressed as international normalized ratio (INR). The formula is $3.78 \times \log_e$ bilirubin (mg/100 mL) $\pm 11.2 \times \log_e$ international normalized ratio (INR) $\pm 9.57 \times \log_e$ creatinine (mg/100 mL) ± 6.43.

2169. Neurologic signs in hepatic encephalopathy includes all except?
Harrison's 20th Ed. Chapter 337 Page 2413

A. Rigidity
B. Decreased DTR
C. Extensor plantar signs
D. Seizures

2170. Earliest sign of hepatic encephalopathy is?
Harrison's 20th Ed. Chapter 337 Page 2413

A. EEG changes
B. Asterixis
C. Reversal of sleep/wake cycle
D. Deterioration in handwriting

The first signs of hepatic encephalopathy are subtle & nonspecific like change in sleep patterns, change in personality, irritability and mental dullness. Thereafter, confusion, disorientation, stupor and eventually coma supervene.

2171. Typical smell in fetor hepaticus is due to?
Br J Gen Pract. 2012;62(605):652-653, Harrison's 16th Ed. 1867

A. Mercaptans
B. Ammonia

C. Bilirubin
D. All of the above

Fetor hepaticus refers to the slightly sweet, ammoniacal odor that can develop in patients with liver failure, particularly if there is portal-venous shunting of blood around the liver.

2172. Mercaptans are derived from intestinal metabolism of?
Br J Gen Pract. 2012;62(605):652-653, Harrison's 16th Ed. 1867

A. Threonine
B. Methionine
C. Leucine
D. Isoleucine

Fetor hepaticus is a feature of severe liver disease; a sweet and musty smell both on the breath and in urine. It is caused by the excretion of dimethyl disulphide and methyl mercaptan (CH_3SH), arising from an excess of methionine.

2173. For diagnosis of hepatic encephalopathy, which of the following tests has most relevance?
Harrison's 20th Ed. Chapter 337 Page 2413

A. Elevated arterial ammonia level
B. Examination of the cerebrospinal fluid
C. Computed tomography of brain
D. MRI of brain

Elevated arterial ammonia levels have been shown to correlate with outcome in fulminant hepatic failure.

2174. In hepatic encephalopathy, risk of cerebral edema increases with arterial ammonia levels that exceed?
N Engl J Med. 2016;375:1660-70

A. 140 μg per deciliter
B. 240 μg per deciliter
C. 340 μg per deciliter
D. 440 μg per deciliter

The correlation between serum ammonia levels and severity of hepatic encephalopathy appears to be stronger in patients with fulminant hepatic failure, and the risk of cerebral edema increases with arterial ammonia levels that exceed 200 μmol per liter (340 μg per deciliter).

2175. In Greek, sterixis means?
N Engl J Med. 2016;375:1660-70

A. Movement
B. Regular
C. Fixed position
D. Happy

In Greek language sterixis, means "fixed position," The term "asterixis" with the prefix a, meaning "without" denoted an inability to keep outstretched arms and hands in place.

2176. Which of the following is characteristic of the earlier stages of hepatic encephalopathy?
N Engl J Med. 2016;375:1660-70

A. Reduced awareness of surroundings and stimuli
B. Yawning
C. Dozing off
D. All of the above

Reduced awareness of surroundings & stimuli, yawning and dozing off are characteristic of the earlier stages. New irritability & maniacal excitement have also been reported.

2177. Hepatologists have graded severity of hepatic encephalopathy by?
N Engl J Med. 2016;375:1660-70

A. Milan criteria
B. West Haven criteria
C. University of California, San Francisco (UCSF) criteria
D. CURB-65 criteria

2178. Which of the following is a scoring method to grade severity of hepatic encephalopathy?
N Engl J Med. 2016;375:1660-70

A. Full Outline of Unresponsiveness (FOUR) score
B. Glasgow coma score
C. Karnofsky performance scores
D. Agatston score

Full Outline of Unresponsiveness (FOUR) score is more discriminating than the West Haven grading system because it includes brainstem and respiration assessment, which are not further differentiated in the West Haven system.

2179. Restless tossing & muscle or limb twitching seen in progressive hepatic encephalopathy is termed?
N Engl J Med. 2016;375:1660-70

A. Flotation
B. Fragmentation
C. Hypermutation
D. Jactitations

Jactitations refers to restless tossing & muscle or limb twitching common with progressive hepatic encephalopathy and may merge with multifocal myoclonus. Abnormal movements such as dystonia, orofacial dyskinesias, and parkinsonian features favour the diagnosis of Wilson's disease, which in rare cases may be characterized by acute hepatic failure.

2180. Main practical use of EEG in assessing patients for hepatic encephalopathy is to rule out?
N Engl J Med. 2016;375:1660-70

A. Nonconvulsive status epilepticus
B. Multifocal myoclonus
C. Hysterical conversion reaction
D. All of the above

The main practical use of EEG in assessing patients for hepatic encephalopathy is to rule out nonconvulsive status epilepticus.

2181. Outcome in hepatic encephalopathy worsens when which of the following happens in EEG?
N Engl J Med. 2016;375:1660-70

A. Dyssynchronization of fast activity
B. Appearance of triphasic waves
C. Increased dysrhythmicity
D. Slower delta activity

The outcome worsens in the setting of hepatic encephalopathy, once triphasic waves appear. Triphasic-wave patterns appear as generalized, bilaterally synchronous, bifrontal periodic waves, with background slowing. They appear in grade 2 or 3 of hepatic encephalopathy but disappear in comatose state.

2182. Disorders that can mimic the clinical features of hepatic encephalopathy are all except?
N Engl J Med. 2016;375:1660-70

A. Acute alcohol intoxication
B. Sedative overdose

C. Delirium tremens
D. Encephalitis

2183. **Disorders that can mimic the clinical features of hepatic encephalopathy are all except?**

N Engl J Med. 2016;375:1660-70

A. Wernicke's encephalopathy
B. Korsakoff's psychosis
C. Subdural hematoma
D. Schizophrenia

2184. **Disorders that can mimic the clinical features of hepatic encephalopathy are all except?**

N Engl J Med. 2016;375:1660-70

A. Meningitis
B. Hypoglycemia
C. Hypocalcemia
D. Wilson's disease

2185. **Which of the following disease has hyperammonemia with neuropsychiatric symptoms resembling hepatic encephalopathy?**

Harrison's 20th Ed. Chapter 414 Page 3022

A. "Punch-drunk" syndrome
B. Hashimoto's encephalopathy
C. Citrullinemia type 2
D. Posterior reversible encephalopathy syndrome (PRES)

Citrullinemia type 2 usually presents with sudden onset between 20 & 50 years of age with recurring episodes of hyperammonemia with associated neuropsychiatric symptoms such as altered mental status, irritability, seizures or coma resembling hepatic encephalopathy.

2186. **Citrullinemia type 2 is caused by molecular defect in?**

Harrison's 20th Ed. Chapter 414 Page 3022

A. Dibasic transporter SLC7A7
B. Carnitine transporter OCTN2
C. Mitochondrial apartate/glutamate carrier 2 SLC25A13
D. Lysosomal cystine transporter

Citrullinemia type 2 (Citrin deficiency) is a recessive condition caused by deficiency of mitochondrial aspartate-glutamate carrier AGC2 (citrin). A defect in this transporter reduces availability of cytoplasmic aspartate to combine with citrullin impairing urea cycle & decreasing transfer of reducing equivalents from cytosol to mitochondria through malate-aspartate NADH shuttle. Mutation is in SLC25A13 gene. Presentation is recurring episodes of hyperammonemia with associated neuropsychiatric symptoms like altered mental status, irritability, seizures or coma resembling hepatic encephalopathy. Without therapy, most patients die due to cerebral edema within a few years of onset.

2187. **Which of the following is an ammonia scavenger?**

N Engl J Med. 2017; 376:186

A. Sodium butyrate
B. Glycerol phenylbutyrate
C. Sodium phenylacetate
D. All of the above

Various ammonia scavengers are sodium butyrate, glycerol phenylbutyrate, sodium phenylacetate and sodium benzoate.

2188. **Which of the following about lactulose is false?**

Harrison's 20th Ed. Chapter 337 Page 2413

A. Nonabsorbable
B. Disaccharide
C. Leads to colonic acidification
D. None of the above

The mainstay of treatment for encephalopathy is lactulose (25 mL twice daily). It is a nonabsorbable disaccharide, which results in colonic acidification. Consequent catharsis eliminates nitrogenous products in gut that are responsible for the development of encephalopathy.

2189. **Goal of lactulose therapy is to promote how many soft stools per day?**

Harrison's 20th Ed. Chapter 337 Page 2414

A. 2 - 3
B. 4 - 6
C. 6 - 8
D. 8 - 10

The goal of lactulose therapy is to promote 2 - 3 soft stools per day.

2190. **Which of the following has a role in the treatment of hepatic encephalopathy?**

Harrison's 20th Ed. Chapter 337 Page 2414

A. Azithromycin
B. Ritonavir
C. Rifaximin
D. Lumefantrine

Rifaximin (550 mg twice daily) is very effective in treating encephalopathy without the known side effects of neomycin (renal insufficiency and ototoxicity) or metronidazole (peripheral neuropathy). Rifaximin is a poorly absorbed rifampin derivative & is highly effective against noninvasive bacterial pathogens (toxigenic & enteroaggregative E. coli).

2191. **Supplementation of which of the following is recommended in patients with hepatic encephalopathy?**

Harrison's 20th Ed. Chapter 337 Page 2414

A. Copper
B. Zinc
C. Calcium
D. Magnesium

Zinc supplementation is at times helpful in patients with hepatic encephalopathy.

2192. **First clotting factor to be depleted in cirrhosis liver is?**

Harrison's 20th Ed. Chapter 337 Page 2414

A. Factor V
B. Factor VII
C. Factor VIII
D. Factor IX

2193. **In hepatic cirrhosis, which clotting factor is not reduced?**

Harrison's 20th Ed. Chapter 337 Page 2414

A. Factor II
B. Factor V
C. Factor VII
D. Factor XI

2194. **Reduction in levels of which clotting factor is not worsened by the coincident malabsorption of vitamin K?**

Harrison's 20th Ed. Chapter 337 Page 2414

A. Factor II
B. Factor V

C. Factor VII
D. Factor XI

Vitamin K–dependent clotting factors are Factors II, VII, IX, and X. Because of a decrease in hepatic mass, administration of parenteral vitamin K does not improve clotting factors or prothrombin time.

2195. Coagulopathy in liver disease results due to?
Harrison's 20th Ed. Chapter 337 Page 2414

A. Decreased synthesis of clotting factors
B. Impaired clearance of anticoagulants
C. Thrombocytopenia due to hypersplenism
D. All of the above

Coagulopathy is almost universal in patients with cirrhosis. There is decreased synthesis of clotting factors and impaired clearance of anticoagulants. Patients may have thrombocytopenia from hypersplenism due to portal hypertension.

2196. The triad of hepatopulmonary syndrome includes all except?
Harrison's 20th Ed. Chapter 329 Page 2335

A. Liver disease
B. Hypoxemia
C. Hypercarbia
D. Pulmonary arteriovenous shunting

Patients with long-standing cirrhosis and portal hypertension are prone to develop the hepatopulmonary syndrome, defined by the triad of liver disease, hypoxemia, and pulmonary arteriovenous shunting. The defect in oxygenation is due to a ventilation perfusion mismatch.

2197. Hepatopulmonary syndrome is manifested by?
Harrison's 20th Ed. Chapter 329 Page 2335

A. Hypoxemia
B. Platypnea
C. Orthodeoxia
D. All of the above

Hepatopulmonary syndrome is characterized by platypnea and orthodeoxia, representing shortness of breath and oxygen desaturation that occur paradoxically upon assuming an upright position. If the partial pressure of oxygen in arterial blood decreases by 5% or more or by 4 mm Hg (0.5 kPa) or more when the patient moves from a supine to an upright position (called orthodeoxia), he or she may describe worsening dyspnea (platypnea) related to further ventilation perfusion mismatch.

2198. Platypnea is a clinical presentation of?
Harrison's 20th Ed. Chapter 33 Page 227

A. Constrictive pericarditis
B. Budd-Chiari Syndrome
C. Left atrial myxoma
D. HOCM

Platypnea (dyspnea in upright position with relief in supine position) is also a feature of left atrial myxoma. Left atrial myxoma or hepatopulmonary syndrome should be considered when the patient complains of platypnea or dyspnea in upright position with relief in the supine position.

2199. Which of the following is not a part of hepatopulmonary syndrome?
N Engl J Med. 2008;358:2378-87

A. Liver disease
B. Pulmonary vascular dilatation
C. Pulmonary vascular constriction
D. Defect in oxygenation

Hepatopulmonary syndrome has three components - liver disease, pulmonary vascular dilatation, and a defect in oxygenation.

2200. The unique striking pathological feature of hepatopulmonary syndrome is?
N Engl J Med. 2008;358:2378-87

A. Gross dilatation of pulmonary pre- & capillary vessels
B. Absolute increase in number of dilated vessels
C. Pleural & pulmonary arteriovenous shunts
D. All of the above

The unique striking pathological feature of hepatopulmonary syndrome is gross dilatation of pulmonary precapillary & capillary vessels (15 to 100 μm diameter), coupled with an absolute increase in number of dilated vessels. Also, pleural and pulmonary arteriovenous shunts and portopulmonary venous anastomoses can be seen. in a healthy person, diameter of capillary ranges between 8 and 15 μm.

2201. Which of the following has clinical similarities to hepatopulmonary syndrome?
N Engl J Med. 2008;358:2378-87

A. Blue rubber bleb syndrome
B. Chiari malformation
C. Dandy-Walker malformations
D. Type 1 Abernethy malformation

Rare congenital cardiac disorders without liver injury in which either hepatic venous blood flow does not reach the lung or portal venous blood reaches the inferior vena cava without passing through the liver (Type 1 Abernethy malformation) have clinical similarities to hepatopulmonary syndrome. This provides support for the hypothesis that blood from the gut must cross liver to prevent pulmonary vascular dilatation.

Hepatocellular Carcinoma

2202. Which of the following statements is false?
N Engl J Med. 2011;365:1118-27

A. Liver cancer is the fifth most common cancer in men and the seventh in women
B. Highest incidence rates of liver cancer is in regions where infection with hepatitis B virus (HBV) is endemic
C. Hepatocellular carcinoma rarely occurs before 40 years of age
D. Hepatocellular carcinoma incidence reaches a peak at approximately 50 years of age

Hepatocellular carcinoma incidence reaches a peak at approximately 70 years of age. Rates of liver cancer among men are two to four times as high as the rates among women.

2203. Which of the following is associated with a reduced risk of hepatocellular carcinoma?
N Engl J Med. 2011;365:1118-27

A. Coffee drinking
B. Tea drinking
C. Alcohol drinking
D. Tobacco chewing

Studies conducted in Japan and southern Europe found that coffee drinking is associated with a reduced risk of hepatocellular carcinoma. Coffee drinking has also been associated with reduced insulin levels and a reduced risk of type 2 diabetes.

2204. Major risk factors for hepatocellular carcinoma (HCC) include infection with all except?
N Engl J Med. 2011;365:1118-27

A. HBV
B. HCV
C. HIV
D. Alcoholic liver disease

Major risk factors for HCC include infection with HBV or HCV, alcoholic liver disease & nonalcoholic fatty liver disease. Less common causes include hereditary hemochromatosis, alpha 1-antitrypsin deficiency, autoimmune hepatitis, some porphyrias, and Wilson's disease.

2205. Liver cancer comprises of?
Harrison's 20th Ed. Chapter 78 Page 578

A. Hepatocellular carcinoma
B. Intrahepatic cholangiocarcinoma
C. Epithelioid hemangiothelioma
D. All of the above

Liver cancer comprises of hepatocellular carcinoma, intrahepatic cholangiocarcinoma, fibrolamellar HCC, mixed HCCiCCA, epithelioid hemangiothelioma, and pediatric cancer hepatoblastoma.

2206. HCC is less common in cirrhosis associated with?
Harrison's 20th Ed. Chapter 78 Page 578

A. Alcohol abuse
B. Metabolic syndrome
C. Alpha-1 antitrypsin deficiency
D. Hemochromatosis

2207. HCC is less common in cirrhosis associated with?
Harrison's 20th Ed. Chapter 78 Page 578

A. Autoimmune hepatitis
B. Wilson's disease
C. Cholestatic liver disorders
D. All of the above

HCC is less common in cirrhosis associated with alpha-1 antitrypsin deficiency, autoimmune hepatitis, Wilson's disease, and cholestatic liver disorders.

2208. Factor associated with an increased risk of developing HCC is?
Harrison's 20th Ed. Chapter 78 Page 578

A. Hepatitis B or C chronic infection
B. Cirrhosis from any cause
C. Nonalcoholic steatohepatitis (NASH)
D. All of the above

Factor associated with an increased risk of developing HCC include hepatitis, alcohol, autoimmune chronic active hepatitis, cryptogenic cirrhosis and NASH/NAFL. Less common association is with primary biliary cirrhosis and several metabolic diseases including hemochromatosis, Wilson disease, alpha$_1$-antitrypsin deficiency, tyrosinemia, porphyria cutanea tarda, glycogenesis types 1 and 3, citrullinemia, and orotic aciduria.

2209. Predictors of liver cancer development among cirrhotic patients include?
Harrison's 20th Ed. Chapter 78 Page 579

A. Platelet count of <100,000/mm^3
B. Presence of portal hypertension
C. Higher degree of liver stiffness on transient elastography (TE)
D. All of the above

Predictors of liver cancer development among cirrhotic patients is associated with liver disease severity i.e. platelet count of <100,000/mm^3, presence of portal hypertension, degree of liver stiffness as measured by transient elastography (TE), and liver gene signatures capturing the cancer field effect.

2210. Which country has the highest incidence of HCC globally?
Harrison's 20th Ed. Chapter 78 Page 579 Figure 78-2

A. Sudan
B. Egypt
C. Mongolia
D. China

Mongolia has the highest incidence of HCC globally, with 78 cases per 100,000 inhabitants.

2211. Which country has the highest prevalence of HCV infection?
Harrison's 20th Ed. Chapter 78 Page 579 Figure 78-2

A. Sudan
B. Egypt
C. Mongolia
D. China

2212. Aflatoxin B$_1$ is the cause of development of HCC in which country?
Harrison's 20th Ed. Chapter 78 Page 579 Figure 78-2

A. Sudan
B. Egypt

C. Mongolia
D. China

2213. HCC occurrence with HCV infection is greater if?
Harrison's 20th Ed. Chapter 78 Page 579

A. Advanced hepatic fibrosis is present
B. HCV genotype is 1b
C. Polymorphism that activates EGF receptor is present
D. All of the above

2214. Which polymorphism is strongly associated with fatty and alcoholic chronic liver diseases & HCC occurrence?
Harrison's 20th Ed. Chapter 78 Page 580

A. GPIV T13254C
B. PI A2
C. PNPLA3
D. MTHFR C677T

Patatin-like phospholipase domain-containing protein 3 (PNPLA3) polymorphism is strongly associated with fatty and alcoholic chronic liver diseases and HCC occurrence.

2215. Aflatoxin B_1 is related to which of the following pathogen?
Harrison's 20th Ed. Chapter 78 Page 580

A. Aspergillus
B. Nocardia
C. Candida
D. Cryptococcus

Aflatoxin B_1 is a product of the Aspergillus fungus. It is a most potent ubiquitous natural chemical carcinogen producing signature mutations in p53 (mutation of arginine to serine at codon 249) and leads to hepatocellular carcinoma.

2216. Which of the following predispose to HCC development?
Harrison's 20th Ed. Chapter 78 Page 580

A. Infection with adeno-associated virus 2
B. Tobacco
C. Aflatoxin B_1
D. All of the above

2217. Which of the following about HCC is false?
Harrison's 20th Ed. Chapter 78 Page 580

A. Inflammation-associated cancer
B. Mutations in telomere reverse transcriptase (TERT) gene
C. Wnt/β-catenin pathway activation
D. All of the above

In HCC, the most common mutations are in the telomerase reverse transcriptase (TERT) promoter, TP53, CTNNB1, ARID2, ARID1A and AXIN1 genes.

2218. Which of the following genes is mutated in HCC?
Harrison's 20th Ed. Chapter 78 Page 580

A. HER2
B. PIK3CA
C. BRAF
D. None of the above

Solid tumors such as EGFR, HER2, PIK3CA, BRAF, or KRAS are rarely mutated in HCC.

2219. HCV infection & alcohol abuse are significantly associated with which mutation?
Harrison's 20th Ed. Chapter 78 Page 581

A. MLL4
B. CTNNB1
C. CCNE1
D. TP53

HBV integrates into the genome of driver genes, like TERT promoter, MLL4 & cyclin E1 (CCNE1). HCV infection & alcohol abuse are significantly associated with CTNNB1 mutations. TP53 mutations are the most frequent alterations with a specific hotspot of mutation (R249S) in patients with aflatoxin B1 exposure.

2220. Serum "quad" test consists of all except?
Harrison's 20th Ed. Chapter 456 Page 3367

A. α-fetoprotein
B. β human chorionic gonadotropin
C. Inhibin-A
D. Conjugated estriol

Serum "quad" test consists of α-fetoprotein, β human chorionic gonadotropin, inhibin-A & unconjugated estriol.

2221. α-fetoprotein is found in patients of?
Harrison's 20th Ed. Chapter 74 Page 553

A. Germ cell tumor
B. Medullary cancer of the thyroid
C. Hodgkin's disease
D. All of the above

2222. Use of which of the following is associated with a reduced risk of HCC?
Harrison's 20th Ed. Chapter 78 Page 581

A. Coffee consumption
B. Statins
C. Metformin
D. All of the above

2223. Which of the following is recommended as a method of surveillance for HCC?
Harrison's 20th Ed. Chapter 78 Page 581

A. Ultrasonography
B. Computed tomography (CT)
C. Magnetic resonance imaging (MRI)
D. All of the above

2224. Which of the following imaging modality is most recommended for hepatocellular carcinoma surveillance?
Harrison's 20th Ed. Chapter 78 Page 581, N Engl J Med. 2011;365:1118-27

A. Ultrasonographic imaging
B. Computed tomography (CT)
C. Magnetic resonance imaging (MRI)
D. All of the above

CT and MRI are not generally recommended for hepatocellular carcinoma surveillance. Their sensitivity, specificity, and positive and negative predictive values for this purpose are unknown, and their use is associated with high cost as well as possible harm.

2225. Which of the following is of no use in the diagnosis of HCC?
Harrison's 20th Ed. Chapter 78 Page 581

A. Triphasic CT
B. Gadolinium-enhanced MRI
C. Ultrasound
D. PET imaging

Positron emission tomography (PET)-scan performs poorly for early diagnosis.

2226. Serum biomarker that identifies patients with HCC is?
Harrison's 20th Ed. Chapter 78 Page 581

A. Alpha-fetoprotein (AFP)
B. L3 fraction of AFP (AFP-L3)
C. Des-γ carboxyprothrombin (DCP)
D. All of the above

AFP levels ≥ 400 ng/dL are highly suspicious, but not diagnostic of HCC according to guidelines.

2227. Which of the following is a protein induced by vitamin K absence?
J Adv Res. 2013;4(6):539-546

A. PIVKA-I
B. PIVKA-II
C. PIVKA-III
D. PIVKA-IV

Prothrombin induced by vitamin K absence-II (PIVKA-II) is also known as Des-gamma carboxyprothrombin (DCP) is an abnormal prothrombin protein that is increased in the sera of patients with HCC. This protein is increased in as many as 80% of HCC patients but may also be elevated in patients with vitamin K deficiency. It is always elevated after Coumadin use. It may predict for portal vein invasion.

2228. Radiological diagnosis of HCC with a high degree of confidence is established if on contrast-enhanced imaging techniques?
Harrison's 20th Ed. Chapter 78 Page 581

A. Lesion is ≥2 cm in diameter
B. Vascular uptake of the nodule in the arterial phase
C. Washout in the portal venous or delayed phases
D. All of the above

The above radiological pattern captures the hypervascular nature characteristic of HCC and the diagnostic specificity is ~95–100% and a biopsy is not necessary.

2229. For HCC, the most accepted staging system is?
Harrison's 20th Ed. Chapter 78 Page 582

A. Anderson-Clinic-Liver Cancer (ACLC) Classification
B. Barcelona-Clinic-Liver Cancer (BCLC) Classification
C. Cleveland-Clinic-Liver Cancer (CCLC) Classification
D. Detroit-Clinic-Liver Cancer (DCLC) Classification

For HCC, the most accepted staging system is the Barcelona-Clinic-Liver Cancer (BCLC) Classification, which is endorsed by U.S. and European clinical practice guidelines.

2230. Which of the following treatments have improved survival in HCC?
Harrison's 20th Ed. Chapter 78 Page 582

A. Surgical resection, liver transplantation
B. Radiofrequency (RF) ablation, chemoembolization
C. Systemic therapies
D. All of the above

2231. Which of the following drugs is used for systemic therapy of HCC?
Harrison's 20th Ed. Chapter 78 Page 582

A. Sorafenib
B. Regorafenib
C. Lenvatinib
D. All of the above

Agents used for systemic therapy in HCC include sorafenib, regorafenib, lenvatinib, cabozantinib, & ramucirumab. Sorafenib is the standard of care systemic therapy for HCC.

2232. TACE stands for?
N Engl J Med. 2011;365:1118-27

A. Transarterial catheter embolization
B. Transarterial cryoembolization
C. Transarterial chemoembolization
D. Transarterial cavity embolization

Transarterial chemoembolization (TACE) is useful in intermediate-stage hepatocellular carcinoma. TACE improves survival among patients with preserved liver function, particularly those with Child-Pugh class A cirrhosis who do not have extrahepatic metastases, vascular invasion, or prominent cancer-related symptoms.

2233. A typical interval between HCV-associated transfusion and subsequent HCC is approximately?
Harrison's 20th Ed. Chapter 332 Page 2362

A. 10 years
B. 20 years
C. 30 years
D. 40 years

A typical interval between HCV-associated transfusion and subsequent HCC is approximately 30 years. HCV-associated HCC patients tend to have more frequent and advanced cirrhosis, but in HBV-associated HCC, only half the patients have cirrhosis; the remainder having chronic active hepatitis.

2234. Worldwide, chronic HBV infection accounts for what percentage of all cases of hepatocellular carcinoma?
N Engl J Med. 2011;365:1118-27

A. ~25%
B. ~50%
C. ~75%
D. ~100%

Worldwide, chronic HBV infection accounts for ~50% of all cases of hepatocellular carcinoma and virtually all childhood cases.

2235. What percentage of patients with HBV-related hepatocellular carcinoma have cirrhosis?
N Engl J Med. 2011;365:1118-27

A. ~25%
B. ~50%
C. ~75%
D. ~100%

HBV can cause hepatocellular carcinoma in the absence of cirrhosis. However, majority (70 to 80%) of patients with HBV-related hepatocellular carcinoma have cirrhosis.

2236. Which of the following is a paraneoplastic syndrome in HCC?
N Engl J Med. 2011;365:1118-27

A. Erythrocytosis
B. Hypercalcemia
C. Hypercholesterolemia
D. All of the above

Most paraneoplastic syndromes in HCC are biochemical abnormalities without associated clinical consequences. They include hypoglycemia, erythrocytosis, hypercalcemia, hypercholesterolemia, dysfibrinogenemia, carcinoid syndrome, increased thyroxin-binding globulin, changes in secondary sex characteristics (gynecomastia, testicular atrophy & precocious puberty) & porphyria cutanea tarda.

2237. Which of the following estimations are useful in the surveillance for hepatocellular carcinoma?

N Engl J Med. 2011;365:1118-27

- A. Serum alpha-fetoprotein (AFP)
- B. Des-gamma-carboxyprothrombin (DCP)
- C. Lens culinaris agglutinin-reactive fraction of AFP (AFP-L3)
- D. All of the above

Combined measurement of alpha-fetoprotein, with des-gamma-carboxyprothrombin or lectin-bound alpha-fetoprotein, provide limited additional benefit as compared with the measurement of alpha-fetoprotein alone.

2238. Which of the following imaging feature is diagnostic of hepatocellular carcinoma?

N Engl J Med. 2011;365:1118-27

- A. Focal hepatic mass >2 cm in diameter in cirrhotics
- B. Areas of early arterial enhancement
- C. Areas of delayed washout
- D. All of the above

In patients with cirrhosis and a focal hepatic mass larger than 2 cm in diameter, areas of early arterial enhancement and delayed washout in venous or delayed phase of four-phase multidetector CT or in dynamic contrast-enhanced MRI have high predictive value for HCC.

2239. Child-Pugh scoring system uses how many clinical measures of liver disease?

N Engl J Med. 2011;365:1118-27

- A. 3
- B. 4
- C. 5
- D. 6

The Child-Pugh scoring system uses five clinical measures of liver disease.

2240. How many points in Child-Pugh scoring system denote class A disease?

N Engl J Med. 2011;365:1118-27

- A. 5 or 6 points
- B. 7 to 9 points
- C. 10 to 15 points
- D. 16 to 20 points

A sum of 5 or 6 points Child-Pugh scoring system indicate class A disease, 7 to 9 points class B, and 10 to 15 points class C, or the most severe disease.

Liver Transplantation

2241. Who pioneered liver transplantation?
Harrison's 20th Ed. Chapter 338 Page 2414

A. PW Angus
B. Thomas Starzl
C. JA Fishman
D. KF Murray

Pioneered in 1960s by Thomas Starzl at the University of Colorado and, later, at the University of Pittsburgh and by Roy Calne in Cambridge, England, liver transplantation is now performed routinely worldwide. Success measured as 1-year survival has improved from 30% in the 1970s to 90% today.

2242. Routine candidates for liver transplantation are patients with?
Harrison's 20th Ed. Chapter 338 Page 2415

A. Alcoholic cirrhosis
B. Chronic viral hepatitis
C. Primary hepatocellular malignancies
D. All of the above

Routine candidates for liver transplantation are patients with alcoholic cirrhosis, chronic viral hepatitis, and primary hepatocellular malignancies.

2243. Currently, which of the following is the most common indications for liver transplantation in adults?
Harrison's 20th Ed. Chapter 338 Page 2415

A. Fulminant hepatitis
B. Primary sclerosing cholangitis
C. Chronic hepatitis C
D. Primary biliary cirrhosis

Currently, chronic hepatitis C & alcoholic liver disease are the most common indications for liver transplantation, accounting for over 40% of all adult candidates who undergo the procedure.

2244. Which of the following is false about chronic HCV patients after transplantation?
Harrison's 20th Ed. Chapter 338 Page 2415

A. Reinfection in the donor organ is universal
B. Allograft cirrhosis develops in 20–30% at 5 years
C. Cirrhosis occur at a higher frequency beyond 5 years
D. None of the above

2245. Patients with which of the following nonmetastatic primary hepatobiliary tumors have undergone liver transplantation?
Harrison's 20th Ed. Chapter 338 Page 2415

A. Cholangiocarcinoma
B. Hepatoblastoma
C. Angiosarcoma
D. All of the above

Patients with nonmetastatic primary hepatobiliary tumors like primary hepatocellular carcinoma (HCC), cholangiocarcinoma, hepatoblastoma, angiosarcoma, epithelioid hemangioendothelioma, and multiple or massive hepatic adenomata have undergone liver transplantation.

2246. Which of the following hepatic malignancies have a likelihood of recurrence after liver transplantation?
Harrison's 20th Ed. Chapter 338 Page 2415

A. Hepatoblastoma
B. Angiosarcoma
C. Epithelioid hemangioendothelioma
D. Cholangiocarcinoma

2247. Arteriohepatic dysplasia, with paucity of bile ducts, and congenital malformations, including pulmonary stenosis is called?
Harrison's 20th Ed. Chapter 338 Page 2415, Table 338-1

A. Alagille's syndrome
B. Byler's disease
C. Caroli's disease
D. Budd-Chiari syndrome

2248. Intrahepatic cholestasis, progressive liver failure, mental and growth retardation is called?
Harrison's 20th Ed. Chapter 338 Page 2415, Table 338-1

A. Alagille's syndrome
B. Byler's disease
C. Caroli's disease
D. Budd-Chiari syndrome

2249. Multiple cystic dilatations of the intrahepatic biliary tree is called?
Harrison's 20th Ed. Chapter 338 Page 2415, Table 338-1

A. Alagille's syndrome
B. Byler's disease
C. Caroli's disease
D. Budd-Chiari syndrome

2250. The most common indication for transplantation in children is?
Harrison's 20th Ed. Chapter 338 Page 2415

A. Congenital hepatic fibrosis
B. Biliary atresia
C. Crigler-Najjar disease type I
D. Neonatal hepatitis

The most common indication for transplantation in children is biliary atresia.

2251. Postoperative anticoagulation after liver transplantation is essential for which disease?
Harrison's 20th Ed. Chapter 338 Page 2415

A. Autoimmune hepatitis
B. Budd-Chiari syndrome
C. Caroli's disease
D. Nonalcoholic steatohepatitis

Postoperative anticoagulation is essential in patients who undergo transplantation for hepatic vein thrombosis (Budd-Chiari syndrome, underlying myeloproliferative disorders).

2252. Which of the following is not an absolute contraindication for liver transplantation?
Harrison's 20th Ed. Chapter 338 Page 2415

A. Advanced age (>70 years)
B. Metastatic malignancy

C. Active drug abuse
D. Active alcohol abuse

Absolute contraindications for transplantation include life-threatening systemic diseases, uncontrolled extrahepatic bacterial or fungal infections, preexisting advanced cardiovascular or pulmonary disease, multiple uncorrectable life-threatening congenital anomalies, metastatic malignancy, and active drug or alcohol abuse. Advanced age (>70 years) should be considered a relative contraindication.

2253. Cadaver donor livers for liver transplantation are procured primarily from victims of?
Harrison's 20th Ed. Chapter 338 Page 2416

A. Head trauma
B. Jail deaths
C. Suicide deaths
D. Voluntary donors

Cadaver donor livers for transplantation are procured primarily from victims of head trauma.

2254. Which of the following about cadaver donor livers for liver transplantation is false?
Harrison's 20th Ed. Chapter 338 Page 2416

A. Compatibility in ABO blood group is essential
B. Human leukocyte antigen (HLA) matching is not required
C. University of Wisconsin (UW) solution used for preservation
D. None of the above

2255. University of Wisconsin (UW) solution is rich in?
Harrison's 20th Ed. Chapter 338 Page 2416

A. Lactobiotin
B. Parobionate
C. Raffinose
D. Sobrinose

The use of University of Wisconsin (UW) solution is rich in lactobionate & raffinose. It permits extension of cold ischemic time up to 20 hours, preferably 12 hours.

2256. UNOS stands for?
Harrison's 20th Ed. Chapter 338 Page 2416

A. United Network for Organ Selection
B. United Network for Organ Sharing
C. United Network for Organ Surgery
D. United Network for Organ Substitution

UNOS stands for United Network for Organ Sharing. It was adopted in 2002. It is designed to allocate available organs based on regional considerations and recipient acuity.

2257. Liver recipients with what MELD scores experienced higher post-transplantation mortality rates?
Harrison's 20th Ed. Chapter 338 Page 2416

A. < 15
B. < 20
C. < 25
D. < 30

Liver recipients with MELD scores <15 experienced higher post-transplantation mortality rates. The MELD scale is continuous, with 34 levels ranging between 6 and 40. Donor organs usually do not become available unless the MELD score exceeds 20.

2258. Model for End-Stage Liver Disease (MELD) scale uses which of the following variables?
Harrison's 20th Ed. Chapter 338 Page 2416 Table 338-3

A. Bilirubin (mg/100 mL)
B. International normalized ratio (INR)
C. Creatinine (mg/100 mL)
D. All of the above

$MELD = 3.78 \times \log_e \text{bilirubin (mg/100 mL)} \pm 11.2 \times \log_e \text{international normalized ratio (INR)} \pm 9.57 \times \log_e \text{creatinine (mg/100 mL)} + 6.43$

2259. Which of the following is an important predictor of survival in liver transplantation candidates?
Harrison's 20th Ed. Chapter 338 Page 2416

A. Serum sodium
B. Serum potassium
C. Serum uric acid
D. Serum creatinine

In 2016, MELD score was modified to include serum sodium which is another important predictor of survival in liver transplantation candidates (MELD-Na score). MELD-Na = MELD + 1.59 x (135 – Na [mEq/L]). There is an increase in mortality by 5% for each millimole decrease in serum sodium between 125 and 140 mmol/L

2260. Pediatric End-Stage Liver Disease (PELD) scale uses which of the following variables?
Harrison's 20th Ed. Chapter 338 Page 2416 Table 338-3

A. Albumin
B. Bilirubin
C. INR
D. All of the above

For children <18 years of age, the Pediatric End-Stage Liver Disease (PELD) scale is used. This scale is based on albumin, bilirubin, INR, growth failure, and age.

2261. The highest priority (status 1) for liver transplantation is?
Harrison's 20th Ed. Chapter 338 Page 2416 Table 338-3

A. Severe acute alcoholic hepatitis
B. Hepatic vein thrombosis
C. Fulminant hepatic failure
D. Primary hepatocellular carcinoma (HCC)

Highest priority (status 1) is reserved for patients with fulminant hepatic failure or primary graft nonfunction.

2262. Disease-specific MELD exceptions include?
Harrison's 20th Ed. Chapter 338 Page 2417

A. Hepatocellular carcinoma (HCC)
B. Portopulmonary hypertension
C. Hepatopulmonary syndrome
D. All of the above

2263. What is the risk of death to the healthy donor in living donor transplantation?
Harrison's 20th Ed. Chapter 338 Page 2417

A. 0.02 - 0.04%
B. 0.06 - 0.1%
C. 0.2 - 0.4%
D. 0.6 - 1.3%

2264. For living donor transplantation, characteristics of the donor includes?
Harrison's 20th Ed. Chapter 338 Page 2417

A. 18 - 60 years old
B. Compatible blood type with the recipient

C. Related genetically or emotionally to the recipient
D. All of the above

Donors for living donor transplantation should be 18 - 60 years old; have a compatible blood type with recipient; have no chronic medical problems or history of major abdominal surgery; should be related genetically or emotionally to recipient; and normal clinical, biochemical, and serologic evaluations.

2265. Which of the following anastomosis is performed last in liver transplantation?

Harrison's 20th Ed. Chapter 338 Page 2417

A. Caval
B. Portal vein
C. Hepatic artery
D. Common bile duct

Caval, portal vein, hepatic artery, and bile duct anastomoses are performed in succession, the last by end-to-end suturing of the donor and recipient common bile ducts.

2266. Which immunosuppressive agent can be given after liver transplantation?

Harrison's 20th Ed. Chapter 338 Page 2417

A. Cyclosporine
B. Tacrolimus
C. Mycophenolic acid
D. All of the above

2267. Which of the following is true about Cyclosporine?

Harrison's 20th Ed. Chapter 338 Page 2417

A. Isolated from Streptomyces tsukubaensis
B. Calcineurin inhibitor (CNI)
C. Nonnucleoside purine metabolism inhibitor
D. Monoclonal antibodies to T cells

Cyclosporine is a calcineurin inhibitor (CNI). It blocks early activation of T cells & is specific for T cell functions that result from the interaction of T cell with its receptor and that involve the calcium-dependent signal transduction pathway. Activity of cyclosporine leads to inhibition of lymphokine gene activation, blocking interleukins 2, 3, and 4, tumor necrosis factor α, and other lymphokines. Cyclosporine also inhibits B cell functions. This process occurs without affecting rapidly dividing cells in the bone marrow, thus reducing frequency of posttransplantation systemic infections.

2268. Which of the following is a macrolide lactone antibiotic?

Harrison's 20th Ed. Chapter 338 Page 2417

A. Cyclosporine
B. Tacrolimus
C. Mycophenolic acid
D. Rapamycin

Tacrolimus is a macrolide lactone antibiotic isolated from a Japanese soil fungus, Streptomyces tsukubaensis.

2269. Which of the following side effects are not present with use of Tacrolimus, but present with use of Cyclosporine?

Harrison's 20th Ed. Chapter 338 Page 2417

A. Nephrotoxicity
B. Hypertension
C. Hirsutism
D. Diabetes mellitus

Tacrolimus does not cause hirsutism or gingival hyperplasia.

2270. Which of the following is used occasionally to help boost tacrolimus levels?

Harrison's 20th Ed. Chapter 338 Page 2418

A. Carbamazepine
B. Rifampin
C. Itraconazole
D. Phenobarbital

Drugs that inhibit cytochrome P450 increase cyclosporine and tacrolimus blood levels. Itraconazole is used occasionally to help boost tacrolimus levels.

2271. Which of the following is a nonnucleoside purine metabolism inhibitor?

Harrison's 20th Ed. Chapter 338 Page 2418

A. Cyclosporine
B. Tacrolimus
C. Mycophenolic acid
D. Rapamycin

Mycophenolic acid, a nonnucleoside purine metabolism inhibitor derived as a fermentation product from several Penicillium species.

2272. Induction or maintenance of immunosuppression in renal dysfunction, which of the following is preferred?

Harrison's 20th Ed. Chapter 338 Page 2418

A. Cyclosporine
B. Tacrolimus
C. Mycophenolic acid
D. Antithymocyte globulin (ATG, thymoglobulin)

2273. Hemolytic uremic syndrome can be associated with?

Harrison's 20th Ed. Chapter 338 Page 2419

A. Cyclosporine
B. Tacrolimus
C. OKT3
D. All of the above

Hemolytic uremic syndrome can be associated with cyclosporine, tacrolimus, or OKT3.

2274. Hepatic artery thrombosis in post-transplantation period is an adverse effect of?

Harrison's 20th Ed. Chapter 338 Page 2419

A. OKT3
B. Sirolimus
C. Antithymocyte globulin
D. Cyclosporine

2275. Which of the following neoplasms appear at increased frequency after liver transplantation?

Harrison's 20th Ed. Chapter 338 Page 2420

A. Carcinoma pancreas
B. Squamous cell carcinoma
C. Carcinoma of lung
D. Carcinoma esophagus

De novo neoplasms appear at increased frequency after liver transplantation, particularly squamous cell carcinomas of the skin.

2276. Which of the following accounts for most of the mortality after liver transplantation?
Harrison's 20th Ed. Chapter 338 Page 2420

A. Hepatic complications
B. Renal failure
C. Cardiovascular disease
D. Cerebrovascular disease

Hepatic complications account for most of the mortality after liver transplantation.

2277. Rejection of the transplanted liver begins how many weeks after surgery?
Harrison's 20th Ed. Chapter 338 Page 2420

A. 1 - 2 weeks
B. 2 - 3 weeks
C. 3 - 4 weeks
D. 4 - 5 weeks

Rejection of the transplanted liver occurs in a proportion of patients, beginning 1–2 weeks after surgery, despite the use of immunosuppressive drugs.

2278. Morphologic features of acute rejection after liver transplantation include?
Harrison's 20th Ed. Chapter 338 Page 2420

A. Mixed portal cellular infiltrate
B. Bile duct injury
C. Endothelial inflammation ("endothelialitis")
D. All of the above

2279. Morphologic features of acute rejection after liver transplantation include?
Harrison's 20th Ed. Chapter 338 Page 2420

A. Progressive cholestasis
B. Vanishing bile duct syndrome
C. Hepatic fibrosis
D. All of the above

Morphologically, chronic rejection after liver transplantation is characterized by progressive cholestasis, focal parenchymal necrosis, mononuclear infiltration, vascular lesions and fibrosis. Also, vanishing bile duct syndrome more common in patients undergoing liver transplantation for autoimmune liver disease.

2280. Survival rate for patients undergoing liver transplantation is?
Harrison's 20th Ed. Chapter 338 Page 2420

A. 55 - 70%
B. 75 - 80%
C. 85 - 90%
D. 95 - 99%

2281. The 5-year survival rate for patients undergoing liver transplantation is?
Harrison's 20th Ed. Chapter 338 Page 2420

A. ~ 40%
B. ~ 50%
C. ~ 60%
D. ~ 70%

Failures within the first 3 months are due to technical complications, postoperative infections, and hemorrhage. Transplant failures after the first 3 months are due to infection, rejection, or recurrent disease (malignancy or viral hepatitis).

2282. Feature of which of the following overlap with those of rejection or posttransplantation bile duct injury?
Harrison's 20th Ed. Chapter 338 Page 2420

A. Autoimmune hepatitis
B. Primary sclerosing cholangitis
C. Primary biliary cirrhosis
D. All of the above

2283. Which of the following do not recur after liver transplantation?
Harrison's 20th Ed. Chapter 338 Page 2420

A. Wilson's disease
B. α1-antitrypsin deficiency
C. Hemophiliacs
D. All of the above

2284. Which of the following recur after liver transplantation?
Harrison's 20th Ed. Chapter 338 Page 2420

A. Hemochromatosis
B. Budd-Chiari syndrome
C. Cholangiocarcinoma
D. All of the above

Diseases of the Gallbladder and Bile Ducts

2285. Electrolyte composition of hepatic bile resembles that of?
Harrison's 20th Ed. Chapter 339 Page 2422

A. Cerebrospinal fluid
B. Blood plasma
C. Lymph
D. Ascitic fluid

Hepatic bile is an isotonic fluid with an electrolyte composition resembling blood plasma.

2286. Total solute concentration of hepatic bile is?
Harrison's 20th Ed. Chapter 339 Page 2422

A. 1 - 2 gram/dL
B. 2 - 3 gram/dL
C. 3 - 4 gram/dL
D. 4 - 5 gram/dL

2287. Total solute concentration of gallbladder bile is?
Harrison's 20th Ed. Chapter 339 Page 2422

A. 5 - 10 gram/dL
B. 10 - 15 gram/dL
C. 15 - 20 gram/dL
D. 20 - 25 gram/dL

The electrolyte composition of gallbladder bile differs from that of hepatic bile because most of the inorganic anions, chloride, and bicarbonate are removed by reabsorption across gallbladder epithelium. As a result of water reabsorption, total solute concentration of bile increases from 3–4 gram/dL in hepatic bile to 10–15 gram/dL in gallbladder bile.

2288. Which of the following is the most abundant solute component of bile?
Harrison's 20th Ed. Chapter 339 Page 2422

A. Bile acids
B. Lecithin and other phospholipids
C. Unesterified cholesterol
D. Albumin

Major solute components of bile are bile acids (80%), lecithin and phospholipids (16%), and unesterified cholesterol (4%).

2289. Human cystic bile does not contain?
World J Gastroenterol 2013;19(42):7341-7360

A. Vitamins
B. Mineral salts
C. Trace elements
D. Triglycerides

Human cystic bile is virtually free of triglycerides.

2290. In the lithogenic state, the cholesterol level in bile can be?
Harrison's 20th Ed. Chapter 339 Page 2422

A. 8 - 10%
B. 12 - 18%
C. 18 - 30%
D. 30 - 40%

In the lithogenic state, the cholesterol value can be 8–10%.

2291. The total daily basal secretion of hepatic bile is?
Harrison's 20th Ed. Chapter 339 Page 2422

A. ~ 50 - 100 mL
B. ~ 100 - 250 mL
C. ~ 250 - 400 mL
D. ~ 500 - 600 mL

The total daily basal secretion of hepatic bile is ~500–600 mL.

2292. Which of the following is synthesized de novo in hepatocyte?
Harrison's 20th Ed. Chapter 339 Page 2422

A. Phospholipids
B. Primary bile acids
C. Cholesterol
D. All of the above

Phospholipids, portion of primary bile acids & some cholesterol are synthesized de novo in hepatocyte.

2293. Which of the following is a secretin-mediated and cyclic AMP–dependent mechanism?
Harrison's 20th Ed. Chapter 339 Page 2422

A. Active transport of bile acids from hepatocytes into bile canaliculi
B. Active transport of other organic anions
C. Cholangiocellular secretion
D. All of the above

Cholangiocellular secretion is a secretin-mediated and cyclic AMP dependent mechanism that results in the secretion of a sodium- and bicarbonate-rich fluid into the bile ducts.

2294. Which of the following is located on the apical plasma membrane of the hepatocyte?
Harrison's 20th Ed. Chapter 339 Page 2422

A. Na+/taurocholate cotransporter (NTCP, SLC10A1)
B. Organic anion–transporting proteins (OATPs)
C. Anionic conjugate export pump (MRP2, ABCC2)
D. All of the above

2295. Which of the following is a solute carrier (SLC) transporter on basolateral (sinusoidal) end of hepatocyte?
Harrison's 20th Ed. Chapter 339 Page 2422

A. OAT (Organic anion transporter)
B. OCT (Organic cation transporter)
C. NTCP (Na+/taurocholate co-transporting polypeptide)
D. All of the above

2296. Which of the following is an ATP-binding cassette transporter?
Harrison's 20th Ed. Chapter 339 Page 2422

A. MRP2 (Multidrug resistance protein 2)
B. BSEP (Bile salt export pump)
C. BRCP (Breast cancer resistance protein)
D. All of the above

On the basolateral (sinusoidal) end of hepatocyte, Na+/taurocholate cotransporter (NTCP, SLC10A1) and the organic anion–transporting proteins (OATPs) are present. On the canalicular apical plasma membrane of hepatocyte, "export pumps" (ATP-binding cassette transport proteins) are present. Bile salt export pump (BSEP, ABCB11); the anionic conjugate export pump (MRP2, ABCC2), which mediates the canalicular excretion of various amphiphilic conjugates formed by phase II conjugation (e.g., bilirubin mono- and diglucuronides and drugs); the multidrug export pump (MDR1, ABCB1) for hydrophobic cationic compounds; and the phospholipid export pump (MDR3, ABCB4).

2297. The solute carrier (SLC) families encode membrane proteins that have been identified as?

Current Pharmaceutical Design. 2010;16(2):224

- A. Passive transporters
- B. Ion coupled transporters
- C. Exchangers
- D. All of the above

The two most commonly studied membrane transporters include members of the ATP-binding cassette transporters and solute carriers (SLCs). Their prototype representative is organic anion transporting polypeptides (OATP) which mediate the sodium-independent transport.

2298. Which of the following is not a primary bile acid?

Harrison's 20th Ed. Chapter 339 Page 2423

- A. Cholic acid
- B. Chenodeoxycholic acid
- C. Deoxycholate
- D. All of the above

2299. The primary bile acids are synthesized from?

Harrison's 20th Ed. Chapter 339 Page 2423

- A. Lipopolysaccharide
- B. Cholesterol
- C. Secondary bile acids
- D. Heme

The primary bile acids are cholic acid and chenodeoxycholic acid (CDCA), are synthesized from cholesterol in the liver, conjugated with glycine or taurine, and secreted into the bile. Bile acid synthesis is a major pathway for hepatic cholesterol catabolism. Bile acids are biological detergents that facilitate intestinal absorption of lipids and fat-soluble vitamins.

2300. Which of the following is not a secondary bile acid?

Harrison's 20th Ed. Chapter 339 Page 2423

- A. Deoxycholate
- B. Ursodeoxycholic acid
- C. Lithocholate
- D. All of the above

Secondary bile acids are deoxycholate and lithocholate. They are formed in colon as bacterial metabolites of the primary bile acids. Ursodeoxycholic acid (UDCA), a stereoisomer of CDCA, is also a secondary bile acid found in low concentration.

2301. Which of the following is a secondary bile acid?

World J Gastroenterol. 2013;19(42):7341-7360

- A. Lithocholic acid
- B. Ursodeoxycholic acid
- C. Sulfolithocholic acid
- D. All of the above

Biliary secondary bile acids are deoxycholic, lithocholic, ursodeoxycholic and sulfolithocholic acids.

2302. Whose name is associated with the discovery of bile acids?

World J Gastroenterol. 2013;19(42):7341-7360

- A. Shaffer
- B. Strecker
- C. Trauner
- D. Crawford

In 1848 Strecker discovered bile acids.

2303. In healthy subjects, the ratio of glycine to taurine conjugates in bile is?

Harrison's 20th Ed. Chapter 339 Page 2423

- A. ~1:1
- B. ~2:1
- C. ~3:1
- D. ~4:1

In healthy subjects, the ratio of glycine to taurine conjugates in bile is ~3:1.

2304. Molecular aggregates (micelles) are formed above what level of critical concentration of bile acids?

Harrison's 20th Ed. Chapter 339 Page 2423

- A. ~1 mM
- B. ~2 mM
- C. ~3 mM
- D. ~4 mM

2305. Which of the following is false about bile acids?

Harrison's 20th Ed. Chapter 339 Page 2423

- A. Detergent-like molecules
- B. Above a concentration of ~2 mM form micelles
- C. Facilitate normal intestinal absorption of dietary fats
- D. None of the above

2306. Passive diffusion for unconjugated bile acids occurs in?

Harrison's 20th Ed. Chapter 339 Page 2423

- A. Jejunum
- B. Ileum
- C. Colon
- D. All of the above

2307. Active transport mechanism for conjugated bile acids occurs in?

Harrison's 20th Ed. Chapter 339 Page 2423

- A. Jejunum
- B. Proximal ileum
- C. Distal ileum
- D. Colon

Unconjugated, and to a lesser degree conjugated, bile acids are absorbed by passive diffusion along the entire gut. Active transport mechanism for conjugated bile acids (95%) occurs in distal ileum by apical sodium-dependent bile acid transporter (ASBT) located in the brush border membrane.

2308. Enterohepatic circulation includes which of the following?

Harrison's 20th Ed. Chapter 339 Page 2423

- A. Reabsorption of bile acids
- B. Reconjugation in hepatocytes
- C. Resecreted into bile
- D. All of the above

Enterohepatic circulation refers to the sequesnce of events i.e. reabsorption of bile acids, rapid reconjugation by hepatocytes, and resecretion into bile.

2309. The normal bile acid pool size is?
Harrison's 20th Ed. Chapter 339 Page 2423

A. ~ 2 - 4 gram
B. ~ 10 - 14 gram
C. ~ 20 - 40 gram
D. ~ 40 - 60 gram

The normal bile acid pool size is ~2 - 4 gram.

2310. Normally, the bile acid pool circulates how many times daily?
Harrison's 20th Ed. Chapter 339 Page 2423

A. ~ 2 - 3 times
B. ~ 3 - 5 times
C. ~ 5 - 10 times
D. ~ 10 - 12 times

Normally, the bile acid pool circulates ~5 - 10 times daily.

2311. Fecal loss of bile acids is about?
Harrison's 20th Ed. Chapter 339 Page 2423

A. 0.2 - 0.4 gram/day
B. 0.8 - 2.4 gram/day
C. 2.4 - 4.4 gram/day
D. 5.2 - 7.4 gram/day

Fecal loss of bile acids is ~ 0.2–0.4 gram/day. Normally, this fecal loss is compensated by an equal daily synthesis of bile acids by liver.

2312. The maximum rate of synthesis by bile acids by liver is?
Harrison's 20th Ed. Chapter 339 Page 2423

A. ~ 2 gram/day
B. ~ 3 gram/day
C. ~ 4 gram/day
D. ~ 5 gram/day

The maximum rate of synthesis by bile acids by liver is ~ 5 gram/day. Synthesis of BAs from cholesterol occurs either via the classical pathway (7α-hydroxylation of cholesterol; CYP7A1) or via the alternate pathway (CYP39A1 or CYP7B1). BAs induce FXR, which inhibits CYP7A1 transcription by activation of SHP (small heterodimer partner) and inhibition of HNF4α transactivation.

2313. Bile acids release fibroblast growth factor 19 (FGF19) in?
Harrison's 20th Ed. Chapter 339 Page 2423

A. Liver
B. Bile ducts
C. Intestine
D. All of the above

Bile acids in intestine release fibroblast growth factor 19 (FGF19) into circulation, which is transported to the liver.

2314. Rate-limiting enzyme that suppresses synthesis of bile acids is?
Harrison's 20th Ed. Chapter 339 Page 2423

A. CYP3A4
B. CYP24A1
C. CYP2C19
D. CYP7A1

Fibroblast growth factor 19 (FGF19) in liver suppresses synthesis of bile acids from cholesterol by inhibiting the rate-limiting enzyme cytochrome P450 7A1 (CYP7A1, cholesterol 7α-hydroxylase) and also promotes gallbladder relaxation.

2315. Which of the following is a acid sensor?
Harrison's 20th Ed. Chapter 339 Page 2423

A. Farnesoid X receptor (FXR)
B. Constitutive androstane receptor (CAR)
C. Pregnane X receptor (PXR)
D. All of the above

The nuclear receptor farnesoid X receptor (FXR) is the master regulator of bile acids (BAs) homeostasis since it transcriptionally drives modulation of BA synthesis, influx, efflux, and detoxification along the enterohepatic axis. FXR is encoded by NR1H4 gene. It is activated by bile acids. The hepatic BSEP (ABCB11) is upregulated by farnesoid X receptor (FXR), a bile acid sensor that also represses bile acid synthesis. FXR regulates the BSEP and MDR3 phospholipid flippase.

2316. Which of the following is a cholesterol transporter?
Harrison's 20th Ed. Chapter 339 Page 2423

A. ABCC2
B. ATP8B1
C. ABCG5/G8
D. ABCB4

ABCG5/G8 are two hemitransporters that function as a couple and constitute the canalicular cholesterol and phytosterol transporter.

2317. Liver X receptor (LXR) best relates to?
Harrison's 20th Ed. Chapter 339 Page 2423

A. Bile acid sensor
B. Oxysterol sensor
C. Intracellular microbial sensor
D. Calcium sensor

The expression of the cholesterol transporter, ABCG5/G8, is upregulated by the liver X receptor (LXR), which is an oxysterol sensor. LXR regulates ABCG5/G8 cholesterol transport protein. Oxysterols are potent regulators of cholesterol synthesis and lipid metabolism. Oxysterols are derived from cholesterol, and the intermediates of the cholesterol and bile acid synthesis pathways by either enzymatic or nonenzymatic oxidations. The most abundant oxysterol in circulation is 27-hydroxycholesterol.

2318. Which of the following nuclear receptors is involved in the regulation of lipogenesis?
Harrison's 20th Ed. Chapter 339 Page 2423

A. Peroxisome proliferator-activated receptors (PPARs)
B. Liver X receptors (LXRs)
C. Farnesoid X receptor (FXR)
D. All of the above

Peroxisome proliferator-activated receptors (PPARs), liver X receptors (LXRs), farnesoid X receptor (FXR) and hepatocyte nuclear factor 4α (HNF4α) are the nuclear receptors involved in the regulation of lipogenesis.

2319. Which of the following is a bile acid-activated nuclear receptor?
Harrison's 20th Ed. Chapter 339 Page 2423

A. Farnesoid X receptor (FXR)
B. Pregnane X receptor (PXR)
C. Vitamin D receptor (VDR)
D. All of the above

Bile acid-activated nuclear receptors, farnesoid X receptor (FXR), pregnane X receptor (PXR), & vitamin D receptor (VDR), play critical roles in regulation of key regulatory genes involved in bile acid metabolism in the liver and intestine.

2320. Cholecystokinin (CCK) is released from?
Harrison's 20th Ed. Chapter 339 Page 2423

A. Stomach mucosa
B. Duodenal mucosa

C. Jejunal mucosa
D. All of the above

2321. Which of the following is a function of cholecystokinin (CCK)?
Harrison's 20th Ed. Chapter 339 Page 2423

A. Powerful contraction of the gallbladder
B. Decreased resistance of the sphincter of Oddi (SOD)
C. Enhanced flow of biliary contents into duodenum
D. All of the above

Major factor controlling evacuation of gallbladder is the peptide hormone cholecystokinin (CCK), which is released from the duodenal mucosa in response to the ingestion of fats & amino acids.

2322. How much is the normal capacity of the gallbladder of bile?
Harrison's 20th Ed. Chapter 339 Page 2423

A. ~ 15 mL
B. ~ 30 mL
C. ~ 45 mL
D. ~ 60 mL

The normal capacity of the gallbladder is ~30 mL of bile.

2323. Phrygian cap best relates to?
Harrison's 20th Ed. Chapter 339 Page 2423

A. Agenesis of the gallbladder
B. Rudimentary or oversized "giant" gallbladders
C. Diverticula of the gallbladder
D. None of the above

In Phrygian cap, a partial or complete septum separates the fundus from the body.

2324. Which of the following about gallstones is false?
Harrison's 20th Ed. Chapter 339 Page 2423

A. Gallstone formation increases after age 50
B. Gallstones are formed because of abnormal bile composition
C. Cholesterol stones account for >90% of all gallstones in West
D. None of the above

2325. >50% content of cholesterol gallstones is?
Harrison's 20th Ed. Chapter 339 Page 2423

A. Cholesterol monohydrate
B. Cholesterol dinohydrate
C. Cholesterol trihydrate
D. Cholesterol tetrahydrate

Cholesterol gallstones usually contain >50% cholesterol monohydrate plus an admixture of calcium salts, bile pigments, proteins and fatty acids.

2326. Pigment stones contain how much cholesterol?
Harrison's 20th Ed. Chapter 339 Page 2423

A. < 20%
B. < 30%
C. < 40%
D. < 50%

Pigment stones are composed primarily of calcium bilirubinate. They contain <20% cholesterol.

2327. Gallstones forming secondary to chronic biliary infection are?
Harrison's 20th Ed. Chapter 339 Page 2423

A. Black colored
B. Brown colored
C. Yellow colored
D. White colored

Gallstones forming secondary to chronic biliary infection are brown colored.

2328. Black gallstones are associated with?
Surgical Clinics of North America. 2008;88(6):1175-1194

A. Chronic hemolytic states
B. Cirrhosis
C. Gilbert syndrome
D. All of the above

Pigment stones are formed by the precipitation of bilirubin in bile, with black stones associated with chronic hemolytic states, cirrhosis, Gilbert syndrome, or cystic fibrosis, and brown stones associated with chronic bacterial or parasitic infections.

2329. Which of the following about gallstones is false?
Harrison's 20th Ed. Chapter 339 Page 2423

A. More frequent in females
B. Major types include cholesterol and pigment stones
C. Hemolytic anemia causes gallstones
D. None of the above

2330. Mixed micelles consist of?
Harrison's 20th Ed. Chapter 339 Page 2423

A. Bile acids
B. Phospholipids (lecithin)
C. Cholesterol
D. All of the above

2331. Mixed micelles are formed due to the action of?
Harrison's 20th Ed. Chapter 339 Page 2423

A. Lipase
B. Bile acids
C. Cholecystokinin (CCK)
D. All of the above

Cholesterol & phospholipids are secreted into bile and are converted into mixed micelles consisting of bile acids, phospholipids, and cholesterol by the action of bile acids.

2332. Higher incidence of gallstones is reported in?
Harrison's 20th Ed. Chapter 339 Page 2423

A. Subtotal gastrectomy
B. Chronic hemolytic disease
C. Octreotide treatment
D. All of the above

2333. Which of the following favor cholesterol gallstone formation?
Harrison's 20th Ed. Chapter 339 Page 2424 Figure 339-1

A. ↑ Cholesterol
B. ↓ Bile acids
C. ↓ Lecithin
D. All of the above

2334. Which of the following favor cholesterol gallstone formation?
Harrison's 20th Ed. Chapter 339 Page 2424 Figure 339-1
- A. ↑ ABCG5/G8
- B. ↓ CYP7A1
- C. ↓ MDR3 (ABCB4)
- D. All of the above

2335. Which of the following is called phospholipid export pump?
Harrison's 20th Ed. Chapter 339 Page 2424 Figure 339-1
- A. Multidrug resistance protein 1 (MDR1)
- B. Multidrug resistance protein 2 (MDR2)
- C. Multidrug resistance protein 3 (MDR3)
- D. Multidrug resistance protein 4 (MDR4)

2336. Most important mechanism in the formation of lithogenic bile is?
Harrison's 20th Ed. Chapter 339 Page 2423
- A. High-caloric and cholesterol-rich diets
- B. Genetic factors
- C. Increased biliary secretion of cholesterol
- D. Gallbladder hypomotility

The most important mechanism in the formation of lithogenic (stone-forming) bile is increased biliary secretion of cholesterol.

2337. Increased biliary secretion of cholesterol may be due to?
Harrison's 20th Ed. Chapter 339 Page 2423
- A. Increased activity of HMG-CoA reductase
- B. High-caloric and cholesterol-rich diets
- C. Clofibrate
- D. All of the above

2338. Cholesterol crystal formation requires the presence of?
Surgical Clinics of North America. 2008;88(6):1175-1194
- A. Cholesterol supersaturation
- B. Accelerated nucleation
- C. Gallbladder hypomotility/bile stasis
- D. Any of the above

Cholesterol crystal formation requires the presence of one or more of the following: (a) cholesterol supersaturation, (b) accelerated nucleation, or (c) gallbladder hypomotility/bile stasis.

2339. Mutation in which of the following causes defective phospholipid secretion into bile?
Harrison's 20th Ed. Chapter 339 Page 2424
- A. CYP7A1
- B. MDR3 (ABCB4)
- C. ABCG5/G8
- D. All of the above

Mutations in the MDR3 (ABCB4) gene (encodes the phospholipid export pump in the canalicular membrane of the hepatocyte) may cause defective phospholipid secretion into bile, resulting in cholesterol supersaturation of bile and formation of cholesterol gallstones in the gallbladder and in the bile ducts.

2340. Which of the following state is associated with gallstones?
Harrison's 20th Ed. Chapter 339 Page 2424
- A. Hypersecretion of cholesterol
- B. Hyposecretion of bile acids
- C. Hyposecretion of phospholipids
- D. All of the above

2341. Which of the following state is associated with hypersecretion of cholesterol into bile?
Harrison's 20th Ed. Chapter 339 Page 2424
- A. Enhanced conversion of cholic acid to deoxycholic acid
- B. Gain of function of the cholesterol transporter ABCG5/G8
- C. Increased activity of HMG-CoA reductase
- D. All of the above

2342. Nucleating factor of cholesterol monohydrate crystals is?
Harrison's 20th Ed. Chapter 339 Page 2424
- A. Mucin
- B. Apolipoprotein A-I
- C. Apolipoprotein A-II
- D. All of the above

Cholesterol monohydrate crystal nucleation & crystal growth occur within the mucin gel layer.

2343. Condition associated with infrequent or impaired gallbladder emptying is?
Harrison's 20th Ed. Chapter 339 Page 2424
- A. Fasting
- B. Parenteral nutrition
- C. Pregnancy
- D. All of the above

The incidence of gallstones is increased in conditions associated with infrequent or impaired gallbladder emptying like fasting, parenteral nutrition, pregnancy and drugs that inhibit gallbladder motility.

2344. Biliary sludge contains which of the following?
Harrison's 20th Ed. Chapter 339 Page 2424
- A. Lecithin-cholesterol liquid crystals
- B. Cholesterol monohydrate crystals
- C. Calcium bilirubinate
- D. All of the above

Biliary sludge is a thick, mucous material that contains lecithin-cholesterol liquid crystals, cholesterol monohydrate crystals, calcium bilirubinate and mucin gels. Presence of biliary sludge implies supersaturation of bile with either cholesterol or calcium bilirubinate.

2345. Which of the following can occur to biliary sludge?
Harrison's 20th Ed. Chapter 339 Page 2424
- A. May disappear and not recur
- B. May disappear and reappear
- C. May form gallstones
- D. All of the above

2346. Gallbladder hypomotility is caused by?
Harrison's 20th Ed. Chapter 339 Page 2424
- A. Total parenteral nutrition
- B. Pregnancy
- C. Oral contraceptives, octreotide
- D. All of the above

2347. During pregnancy, gallbladder sludge develops in what proportion of women?
Harrison's 20th Ed. Chapter 339 Page 2425
- A. 2 - 3%
- B. 5 - 10%
- C. 10 - 20%
- D. 20 - 30%

During pregnancy, gallbladder sludge develops in 20 - 30% of women and gallstones in 5 - 12%. it is usually asymptomatic and resolves spontaneously after delivery.

2348. In persons with rapid weight reduction through dieting, gallstones develop in what proportion of persons?
Harrison's 20th Ed. Chapter 339 Page 2425

A. 2 - 3%
B. 5 - 10%
C. 10 - 20%
D. 20 - 30%

~10–20% of persons with rapid weight reduction through very-low-calorie dieting develop gallstones. 600 mg/day of UDCA is highly effective in preventing gallstone formation.

2349. Pigment stones develop in which of the following conditions?
Harrison's 20th Ed. Chapter 339 Page 2425 Table 339-1

A. Primary biliary cirrhosis
B. Alcoholic liver cirrhosis
C. Genetic defect of the CYP7A1 gene
D. Clofibrate therapy

2350. Pigment stones develop in which of the following conditions?
Harrison's 20th Ed. Chapter 339 Page 2425 Table 339-1

A. Pernicious anemia
B. Cystic fibrosis
C. Ileal disease, ileal resection or bypass
D. All of the above

2351. Which of the following is false about biliary sludge?
Harrison's 20th Ed. Chapter 339 Page 2425

A. Material of low echogenic activity
B. In the most dependent position of the gallbladder
C. Shifts with postural changes
D. Produces acoustic shadowing

On USG, biliary sludge has low echogenic activity. It forms a layer in the most dependent position of gallbladder. This layer shifts with postural changes but does not produce acoustic shadowing.

2352. Which of the following about biliary colic is false?
Harrison's 20th Ed. Chapter 339 Page 2426

A. Intermittent
B. May persist with severe intensity for 30 minutes to 5 hours
C. Nocturnal
D. Precipitated by eating a fatty meal

Biliary colic begins quite suddenly and may persist with severe intensity for 30 minutes to 5 hours, subsiding gradually or rapidly. It is steady rather than intermittent. Pain persisting beyond 5 hours should raise the suspicion of acute cholecystitis.

2353. Biliary colic pain may radiate to?
Harrison's 20th Ed. Chapter 339 Page 2426

A. Interscapular area
B. Right scapula
C. Shoulder
D. All of the above

2354. Patients with gallstones remaining asymptomatic for how many years are unlikely to develop symptoms during follow up?
Harrison's 20th Ed. Chapter 339 Page 2426

A. 5 years
B. 10 years
C. 15 years
D. 20 years

Patients with gallstones remaining asymptomatic for 15 years are unlikely to develop symptoms during further follow-up.

2355. Prophylactic cholecystectomy is recommended in?
Harrison's 20th Ed. Chapter 339 Page 2427

A. Gallstones >3 cm in diameter
B. Gallstones in a congenitally anomalous gallbladder
C. Young patients with silent gallstones
D. All of the above

2356. Which of the following about gallstone treatment is false?
Harrison's 20th Ed. Chapter 339 Page 2427

A. Radiolucent stones <10 mm dissolve with UDCA therapy
B. Pigment stones are not responsive to UDCA therapy
C. Dose of UDCA is 10–15 mg/kg per day
D. None of the above

2357. Ursodeoxycholic acid (UDCA) is recommended in which of the following conditions?
Harrison's 20th Ed. Chapter 339 Page 2427

A. Primary biliary cholangitis (PBC)
B. Primary Sclerosing Cholangitis
C. Cholangiocarcinoma
D. All of the above

2358. Chemical inflammation in acute cholecystitis best relates to?
Harrison's 20th Ed. Chapter 339 Page 2427

A. Isolecithin
B. Lysolecithin
C. Phylolecithin
D. All of the above

In acute cholecystitis, chemical inflammation is caused by the release of lysolecithin due to the action of phospholipase on lecithin in bile.

2359. Cholecystectomy is recommended in porcelain gallbladder because of the increased risk of?
Harrison's 20th Ed. Chapter 339 Page 2429

A. Perforation
B. Carcinoma
C. Chronic infection
D. All of the above

2360. Biliary obstruction due to extrinsic compression of the ducts is mostly because of?
Harrison's 20th Ed. Chapter 339 Page 2431

A. Carcinoma of the head of the pancreas
B. Lymphoma
C. Metastatic carcinoma
D. Hepatocellular carcinoma

2361. Low phospholipid-associated cholelithiasis (LPAC) is best related to?
Orphanet J Rare Dis. 2007; 2:29

A. ABCB1
B. ABCB2
C. ABCB3
D. ABCB4

Low phospholipid-associated cholelithiasis (LPAC) is characterized by the association of ABCB4 mutations and low biliary phospholipid concentration with symptomatic and recurring cholelithiasis.

Approach to the Patient with Pancreatic Disease

2362. The mortality rate of acute pancreatitis is?
Harrison's 20th Ed. Chapter 340 Page 2433

A. ~ 1%
B. ~ 2%
C. ~ 3%
D. ~ 4%

The incidence of acute pancreatitis is ~5 - 35 per 100,000 new cases per year worldwide, with a mortality rate of about 3%.

2363. In US, which of the following is the most common gastrointestinal diagnosis requiring hospitalization?
Harrison's 20th Ed. Chapter 340 Page 2433

A. Peptic ulcer disease
B. Ulcerative colitis
C. Acute pancreatitis
D. Acute cholecystitis

In USA, acute pancreatitis is the most common gastrointestinal diagnosis requiring hospitalization.

2364. How much of pancreas must be damaged before maldigestion of fat and protein is manifested?
Harrison's 20th Ed. Chapter 340 Page 2433

A. ~ 25%
B. ~ 50%
C. ~ 75%
D. ~ 90%

Pancreas has a large secretory reserve capacity. > 90% of pancreas must be damaged before maldigestion of fat & protein is manifested.

2365. Which of the following is the enzyme measurement of choice for diagnosis of acute pancreatitis?
Harrison's 20th Ed. Chapter 340 Page 2434 Table 340-1

A. Serum lipase
B. Serum lipase amylase
C. Urine amylase
D. Fecal elastase

Lipase is the single best enzyme to measure for the diagnosis of acute pancreatitis.

2366. In acute pancreatitis, serum amylase rises within?
Harrison's 20th Ed. Chapter 340 Page 2433

A. 24 hours
B. 36 hours
C. 48 hours
D. 72 hours

2367. In acute pancreatitis, serum amylase remains elevated for?
Harrison's 20th Ed. Chapter 340 Page 2433

A. 1 - 3 days
B. 3 - 7 days
C. 7 - 9 days
D. 9 - 14 days

In acute pancreatitis, the serum amylase is usually elevated within 24 hours of onset and remains so for 3 - 7 days. Levels usually return to normal within 7 days unless there is pancreatic ductal disruption, ductal obstruction, or pseudocyst formation.

2368. Patients with proven pancreatitis have spuriously low levels of amylase in?
Harrison's 20th Ed. Chapter 340 Page 2433

A. Incomplete ductal obstruction
B. Pseudocyst formation
C. Hypertriglyceridemia
D. All of the above

Serum amylase level may be normal if hypertriglyceridemia is present.

2369. Amylase is not found in which of the followng?
Harrison's 20th Ed. Chapter 340 Page 2433

A. Fallopian tubes
B. Thyroid
C. Tonsils
D. Cornea

In addition to pancreas & salivary glands, small quantities of amylase are found in the tissues of fallopian tubes, lung, thyroid, and tonsils.

2370. Hyperamylasemia is found in?
Harrison's 20th Ed. Chapter 340 Page 2436, Table 340-2

A. Acute Pancreatitis
B. Diabetic ketoacidosis
C. Perforated peptic ulcer
D. All of the above

2371. Hyperamylasemia is found in which of the following?
Harrison's 20th Ed. Chapter 340 Page 2436, Table 340-2

A. Carcinoma of lung
B. Carcinoma of esophagus
C. Breast carcinoma
D. All of the above

"Tumor" hyperamylasemia is seen in Carcinoma of lung, Carcinoma of esophagus, Breast carcinoma and ovarian carcinoma.

2372. Hyperamylasemia is found in which of the following?
Harrison's 20th Ed. Chapter 340 Page 2436, Table 340-2

A. Pregnancy
B. Aortic aneurysm
C. Morphine
D. All of the above

2373. Abdominal disorder that can simulate pancreatitis is?
Harrison's 20th Ed. Chapter 340 Page 2434

A. Intestinal obstruction
B. Intestinal infarction

C. Perforated peptic ulcer
D. All of the above

2374. Which of the following blood test is reliable for diagnosis of acute pancreatitis in patients with renal failure?
Harrison's 20th Ed. Chapter 340 Page 2434

A. Serum amylase
B. Serum lipase
C. Serum trypsinogen
D. None of the above

No single blood test is reliable for the diagnosis of acute pancreatitis in patients with renal failure. Trypsinogen, amylase & lipase are excreted by kidney therefore are elevated in renal failure.

2375. The recommended screening test for acute pancreatitis in renal disease is?
Harrison's 20th Ed. Chapter 340 Page 2434

A. Serum lipase
B. Serum amylase
C. Serum trypsinogen
D. None of the above

The recommended screening test for acute pancreatitis in renal disease is serum lipase. Also, serum lipase is the single best enzyme to measure for the diagnosis of acute pancreatitis.

2376. Serum amylase levels are elevated when creatinine clearance is less than?
Harrison's 20th Ed. Chapter 340 Page 2434

A. < 100 mL/minute
B. < 85 mL/minute
C. < 75 mL/minute
D. < 50 mL/minute

Serum amylase levels are elevated in patients with renal dysfunction when creatinine clearance is < 50 mL/minute. They are invariably <500 IU/L in the absence of acute pancreatitis.

2377. In acute pancreatitis, serum amylase values are highly specific if they are more than?
Harrison's 20th Ed. Chapter 340 Page 2434

A. Two times normal
B. Three times normal
C. Four times normal
D. Five times normal

In acute pancreatitis, serum amylase values > 3 times normal are highly specific.

2378. Which of the following is a finding of acute pancreatitis by Computed tomography (CT)?
Harrison's 20th Ed. Chapter 340 Page 2435

A. Enlargement of the pancreatic outline
B. Distortion of the pancreatic contour
C. Pancreatic fluid with different attenuation coefficient than normal pancreas
D. All of the above

The major benefit of CT in acute pancreatitis is the diagnosis of pancreatic necrosis in patients not responding to conservative management within 72 hours

2379. What is the incidence of post-ERCP pancreatitis?
Harrison's 20th Ed. Chapter 340 Page 2435

A. 1 - 5%
B. 5 - 10%
C. 10 - 15%
D. 15 - 20%

2380. Which of the following can be performed by endoscopic ultrasonography?
Harrison's 20th Ed. Chapter 340 Page 2435

A. HR imaging of pancreatic parenchyma and pancreatic duct
B. Pancreatic biopsy
C. Nerve-block anesthesia
D. All of the above

2381. Which of the following is not included in the endoscopic ultrasonographic criteria for chronic pancreatitis?
Harrison's 20th Ed. Chapter 340 Page 2436 Table 340-3

A. Main duct irregularity
B. Visible side branches
C. Main duct dilatation
D. Main duct not visible

2382. Which of the following is included in the endoscopic ultrasonographic criteria for chronic pancreatitis?
Harrison's 20th Ed. Chapter 340 Page 2436 Table 340-3

A. Echogenic strands
B. Echogenic foci
C. Lobular contour
D. All of the above

Criteria for ductal imaging includes: Stones, Hyperechoic main duct margins, Main duct irregularity, Main duct dilatation and Visible side branches. Criteria for parenchymal imaging includes: Echogenic strands, Echogenic foci, Lobular contour and Cyst. Presence of five or more of the nine criteria is highly predictive of chronic pancreatitis.

2383. Which of the following statements is false?
Harrison's 20th Ed. Chapter 340 Page 2436

A. Secondary ducts are not visualized in normal pancreas by MRI
B. Secretin-enhanced MRCP is better to evaluate ductal changes
C. T2 imaging can differentiate necrotic debris from fluid
D. T2 imaging can diagnose hemorrhage

2384. ERCP in today's time is meant for?
Harrison's 20th Ed. Chapter 340 Page 2436

A. Clarification of equivocal findings of imaging techniques
B. Primarily of therapeutic value
C. Should not be done for diagnostic purposes
D. All of the above

2385. Double-duct sign best relates to?
Harrison's 20th Ed. Chapter 340 Page 2436

A. Acute pancreatitis
B. Chronic pancreatitis
C. Pancreatic carcinoma
D. All of the above

Pancreatic carcinoma is characterized by stenosis or obstruction of either pancreatic duct or common bile duct. Double-duct sign is present when both ductal systems are abnormal.

2386. **In the Cambridge classification, mild chronic pancreatitis is defined as?**
World J Gastroenterol. 2008;14(8):1218-1221

A. Normal main pancreatic duct
B. > 3 abnormal side branches
C. No cysts
D. All of the above

2387. **In the Cambridge classification, severe chronic pancreatitis is defined as?**
World J Gastroenterol. 2008;14(8):1218-1221

A. Gross irregularity of main pancreatic duct
B. Intraductal calculus
C. Large cysts > 10 mm
D. All of the above

2388. **Which of the following can decrease the incidence of ERCP-induced pancreatitis?**
Harrison's 20th Ed. Chapter 340 Page 2436

A. Glucose-Insulin therapy
B. Methylprednisolone
C. Octreotide
D. Rectal indomethacin

Elevated serum amylase after ERCP occur in majority of patients and clinical pancreatitis in 5 to 10% of patients. Pancreatic duct stenting & rectal indomethacin can decrease incidence of ERCP-induced pancreatitis.

2389. **Which of the following is false about secretin test?**
Harrison's 20th Ed. Chapter 340 Page 2436

A. Pancreatic ductal secretory function test
B. Synthetic human secretin is given IV, 0.2 µg/kg as a bolus
C. Maximal bicarbonate concentration is most useful variable
D. None of the above

2390. **Normal value for the standard secretin test is?**
Harrison's 20th Ed. Chapter 340 Page 2436

A. Volume output > 2 mL / kg per hour
B. Bicarbonate concentration > 80 mmol / L
C. Bicarbonate output > 10 mmol / L in 1 hour
D. All of the above

In the standard assay, secretin is given IV in a dose of 0.2 µg/kg of synthetic human secretin as a bolus.

2391. **What solid fecal level of elastase-1 activity (FE-1) is definitive for pancreatic exocrine insufficiency (PEI)?**
Harrison's 20th Ed. Chapter 340 Page 2436

A. < 50 µg/gram
B. < 100 µg/gram
C. < 150 µg/gram
D. < 200 µg/gram

FE-1 levels >200 µg/gram are normal. Fecal levels <50 µg/gram are definitive for pancreatic exocrine insufficiency (PEI).

2392. **The newer lipase assays relate best to which of the following?**
Harrison's 20th Ed. Chapter 341 Page 2437

A. Trypsin
B. Chymotrypsin
C. Colipase
D. Phospholipase A_2

Lipase is the single best enzyme to measure for diagnosis of acute pancreatitis. The newer lipase assays have colipase as a cofactor and are fully automated.

2393. **Enzyme trypsinogen is present in which of the following?**
Harrison's 20th Ed. Chapter 341 Page 2437

A. Gallbladder
B. Pancreas
C. Intestine
D. All of the above

Pancreas is the only organ that contains trypsinogen.

2394. **"Sentinel loop" refers to a localized ileus of which part of intestine in acute pancreatitis?**
N Engl J Med. 1954; 251(13):497

A. Duodenum
B. Jejunum
C. Ileum
D. Colon

"Sentinel loop" refers to a localized ileus of jejunum in acute pancreatitis. A sentinel loop is a short segment of adynamic ileus close to an intra-abdominal inflammatory process. The sentinel loop sign may aid in localising the source of inflammation. For example, a sentinel loop in the upper abdomen may indicate pancreatitis, while one in the right lower quadrant may be due to appendicitis.

2395. **"Colon cutoff sign" refers to isolated distention of which part of intestine in acute pancreatitis?**
N Engl J Med. 2018; 378:1621

A. Ascending colon
B. Transverse colon
C. Descending colon
D. Sigmoid colon

Abrupt termination of gas within the descending colon is referred to as a colon cutoff sign. The colon cutoff sign is classically described in association with acute pancreatitis, when inflammation causes spasm or narrowing at the splenic flexure and isolated distention of transverse colon.

2396. **In chronic pancreatitis, pancreatic calcification on radiological examination is superimposed on which lumbar vertebra?**
World J Gastrointest Pathophysiol. 2014;5(3):252-270

A. I
B. II
C. III
D. IV

In chronic pancreatitis, radiographic pancreatic calcification is superimposed on 2nd lumbar vertebra.

Acute and Chronic Pancreatitis

2397. The quantity of pancreatic secretion per day is?
Harrison's 20th Ed. Chapter 341 Page 2437

A. 1000 - 1500 ml
B. 1500 - 3000 ml
C. 3000 - 4500 ml
D. About 5000 ml

2398. The pancreatic secretion contain about?
Harrison's 20th Ed. Chapter 341 Page 2437

A. 10 enzymes and zymogens
B. 20 enzymes and zymogens
C. 30 enzymes and zymogens
D. 40 enzymes and zymogens

2399. The pancreatic secretion is?
Harrison's 20th Ed. Chapter 341 Page 2437

A. Isosmotic alkaline
B. Isosmotic acidic
C. Hyposmotic alkaline
D. Hyposmotic acidic

Pancreas secretes 1500 - 3000 mL of isosmotic alkaline (pH > 8.0) fluid / day containing ~20 enzymes & zymogens.

2400. Which of the following about secretin is false?
Harrison's 20th Ed. Chapter 341 Page 2437

A. Gastric acid is a stimulus for release of secretin
B. Secretin is a peptide with 27 amino acids
C. pH threshold for release of secretin from duodenum & jejunum is 6.5
D. Secretin stimulates secretion of pancreatic juice rich in water & electrolytes

2401. Which of the following cells of the duodenal mucosa secrete secretin?
Harrison's 20th Ed. Chapter 341 Page 2437

A. S cells
B. T cells
C. U cells
D. V cells

Gastric acid is the stimulus for the release secretin from the duodenal mucosa (S cells) which in turn stimulates the secretion of water and electrolytes from pancreatic ductal cells.

2402. Ito cells are located in?
Harrison's 20th Ed. Chapter 341 Page 2437

A. Gastric antral mucosa
B. Proximal jejunal mucosa
C. Distal jejunal mucosa
D. Proximal ileal mucosa

Cholecystokinin (CCK) is released from the duodenal and proximal jejunal mucosa (Ito cells).

2403. Which of the following essential amino acids trigger release of Cholecystokinin (CCK)?
Harrison's 20th Ed. Chapter 341 Page 2437

A. Tryptophan
B. Phenylalanine
C. Methionine
D. All of the above

Essential amino acids - tryptophan, phenylalanine, valine and methionine trigger release of Cholecystokinin (CCK).

2404. Which of the following about cholecystokinin (CCK) is false?
Harrison's 20th Ed. Chapter 341 Page 2437

A. CCK evokes an enzyme-rich secretion from pancreas
B. Release of CCK is triggered by short-chain fatty acids
C. Release of CCK is triggered by essential amino acids
D. Release of CCK is triggered by gastric acid

Release of CCK from duodenum & jejunum is triggered by long-chain fatty acids, essential amino acids (tryptophan, phenylalanine, valine, methionine), and gastric acid itself.

2405. Which of the following statements is false?
Harrison's 20th Ed. Chapter 341 Page 2437

A. Bile salts stimulate pancreatic secretion
B. Parasympathetic nervous system exerts significant control over pancreatic secretion
C. Vasoactive intestinal peptide (VIP) is a CCK agonist
D. H_2O and HCO_3^- secretion by pancreas is dependent secretin and CCK

Vagal stimulation leads to release of VIP which is a secretin agonist.

2406. The quantity of bicarbonate from pancreas needed to neutralize gastric acid is?
Harrison's 20th Ed. Chapter 341 Page 2437

A. 20 to 30 mmol/day
B. 50 to 100 mmol/day
C. 120 to 300 mmol/day
D. About 500 mmol/day

2407. In acini and in ducts, which hormone causes the cells to add water and bicarbonate to pancreatic fluid?
Harrison's 20th Ed. Chapter 341 Page 2437

A. Insulin
B. Secretin
C. Somatostatin
D. Gastrin

Gastric acid is the stimulus for release of secretin which stimulates secretion of pancreatic juice rich in water and electrolytes. CCK evokes an enzyme-rich secretion from the pancreas.

2408. How much exocrine function of pancreas must be lost before secretin stimulation test is abnormal?
Harrison's 20th Ed. Chapter 341 Page 2437

A. ~ 15%
B. ~ 20%

C. ~ 40%
D. ~ 60%

Secretin stimulation test for assessing pancreatic exocrine function is abnormal when >60% of exocrine function has been lost.

2409. Which of the following is an inhibitory neuropeptide?
Harrison's 20th Ed. Chapter 341 Page 2437

A. Somatostatin
B. Neuropeptide Y
C. Calcitonin gene - related peptides
D. All of the above

2410. Pancreatic exocrine secretion is influenced by?
Harrison's 20th Ed. Chapter 341 Page 2437

A. Somatostatin
B. Neuropeptide Y
C. Calcitonin gene - related peptides
D. All of the above

Pancreatic exocrine secretion is influenced by inhibitory neuropeptides like somatostatin, pancreatic polypeptide, peptide YY, neuropeptide Y, enkephalin, pancreastatin, calcitonin gene–related peptides, glucagon, and galanin.

2411. Which of the following correlates best between stimulation with secretin and the pancreatic mass?
Harrison's 20th Ed. Chapter 341 Page 2437

A. Maximal sodium output
B. Maximal chloride output
C. Maximal acid output
D. Maximal bicarbonate output

2412. Bicarbonate in pancreatic secretion is related to?
Harrison's 20th Ed. Chapter 341 Page 2437

A. Insulin
B. Glucagon
C. Cystic fibrosis transmembrane conductance regulator
D. All of the above

2413. Which of the following plays an important role in ductal cell secretion?
Harrison's 20th Ed. Chapter 341 Page 2437

A. CCK
B. Secretin and VIP
C. Acetylcholine
D. All of the above

Bicarbonate enters the duct lumen through the sodium bicarbonate cotransporter with depolarization caused by chloride efflux through the cystic fibrosis transmembrane conductance regulator (CFTR). Secretin and VIP bind at the basolateral surface and cause an increase in secondary messenger intracellular cyclic AMP, and act on the apical surface of the ductal cells opening the CFTR in promoting secretion. CCK, acting as a neuromodulator, markedly potentiates the stimulatory effects of secretin. Acetylcholine also plays an important role in ductal cell secretion.

2414. Pancreas secretes which of the following enzymes?
Harrison's 20th Ed. Chapter 341 Page 2437

A. Amylolytic
B. Lipolytic
C. Proteolytic
D. All of the above

The pancreas secretes amylolytic, lipolytic, and proteolytic enzymes.

2415. The lipolytic enzymes secreted by pancreas are?
Harrison's 20th Ed. Chapter 341 Page 2437

A. Lipase
B. Phospholipase A
C. Cholesterol esterase
D. All of the above

Lipolytic enzymes secreted by pancreas include lipase, phospholipase A & cholesterol esterase.

2416. Which of the following about bile salts is false?
Harrison's 20th Ed. Chapter 341 Page 2437

A. Inhibit lipase in isolation
B. Colipase binds to lipase & prevents inhibition by bile salts
C. Activate phospholipase A and cholesterol esterase
D. None of the above

Bile salts inhibit lipase in isolation, but colipase of pancreatic secretion, binds to lipase and prevents this inhibition. Bile salts activate phospholipase A and cholesterol esterase.

2417. Which of the following statements is false?
Harrison's 20th Ed. Chapter 341 Page 2437

A. Bile salts inhibit lipase
B. Colipase binds to lipase
C. Bile salts activate phospholipase A & cholesterol esterase
D. None of the above

Bile salts inhibit lipase. Colipase in pancreatic secretion binds to lipase and prevents this inhibition. Bile salts activate phospholipase A and cholesterol esterase.

2418. Proteolytic enzymes secreted as inactive precursors are called?
Harrison's 20th Ed. Chapter 341 Page 2437

A. Zymogens
B. Proteogens
C. Amylogens
D. Chymogens

Proteolytic enzymes are secreted as inactive precursors called zymogens.

2419. Which of the following is an endopeptidase?
Harrison's 20th Ed. Chapter 341 Page 2437

A. Carboxypeptidases
B. Aminopeptidases
C. Chymotrypsin
D. Elastase

Proteolytic enzymes include endopeptidases, exopeptidases and elastase. Endopeptidases like trypsin & chymotrypsin act on internal peptide bonds of proteins and polypeptides. Exopeptidases are carboxypeptidases & aminopeptidases, which act on the free carboxyl- and amino-terminal ends of peptides, respectively.

2420. Enzyme that cleaves lysine-isoleucine bond of trypsinogen to form trypsin is?
Harrison's 20th Ed. Chapter 341 Page 2437

A. Duodenokinase
B. Enterokinase

C. Gastrokinase
D. Trypsokinase

2421. Bond that is cleaved to form trypsin from trypsinogen is?
Harrison's 20th Ed. Chapter 341 Page 2437

A. Lysine-isoleucine bond
B. Arginine-Threonine bond
C. Arginine-Lysine bond
D. Threonine-Lysine bond

2422. Enzyme enterokinase is found in?
Harrison's 20th Ed. Chapter 341 Page 2437

A. Gastric mucosa
B. Duodenal mucosa
C. Jejunal mucosa
D. Ileal mucosa

Enterokinase is an enzyme found in duodenal mucosa. It cleaves lysine-isoleucine bond of trypsinogen to form trypsin.

2423. Which of the following is the pH optima range of pancreatic enzymes?
Harrison's 20th Ed. Chapter 341 Page 2437

A. 7.1 to 7.2
B. 7.2 to 7.3
C. 7.3 to 7.4
D. 7.4 to 7.5

All pancreatic enzymes have pH optima in the alkaline range.

2424. Which of the following initiates pancreatic enzyme secretion?
Harrison's 20th Ed. Chapter 341 Page 2437

A. Acetylcholine
B. VIP
C. CCK
D. Secretin

The nervous system initiates pancreatic enzyme secretion. Neurologic stimulation is cholinergic, involving extrinsic innervation by vagus nerve & subsequent innervation by intrapancreatic cholinergic nerves. Stimulatory neurotransmitters are acetylcholine & gastrin-releasing peptides. These neurotransmitters activate calcium-dependent secondary messenger systems, resulting in the release of zymogens into pancreas duct.

2425. VIP in intrapancreatic nerves potentiates the effect of?
Harrison's 20th Ed. Chapter 341 Page 2437

A. Acetylcholine
B. Enterokinase
C. CCK
D. Secretin

VIP is present in intrapancreatic nerves and potentiates the effect of acetylcholine.

2426. In humans, receptors of which of the following are absent on acinar cells?
Harrison's 20th Ed. Chapter 341 Page 2437

A. Acetylcholine
B. Gastrin-releasing peptides
C. CCK
D. VIP

In contrast to other species, there are no CCK receptors on acinar cells in humans. CCK in physiologic concentrations stimulates pancreatic secretion by stimulating afferent vagal and intrapancreatic nerves.

2427. Which of the following can lyse and inactivate trypsin?
Harrison's 20th Ed. Chapter 341 Page 2437

A. Mesotrypsin
B. Chymotrypsin C
C. Enzyme Y
D. All of the above

Mesotrypsin, chymotrypsin C, and enzyme Y can also lyse and inactivate trypsin.

2428. Protease inhibitors are found in?
Harrison's 20th Ed. Chapter 341 Page 2438

A. Pancreatic acinar cells
B. Pancreatic secretions
C. a_1- and a_2-globulin fractions of plasma
D. All of the above

Protease inhibitors, that prevent autodigestion of pancreas, are found in the acinar cells, the pancreatic secretions, and the a_1- and a_2-globulin fractions of plasma.

2429. Autodigestion of the pancreas is prevented by which of the following?
Harrison's 20th Ed. Chapter 341 Page 2438

A. Low intracellular sodium in cytosol of acinar cell
B. Low intracellular potassium in cytosol of acinar cell
C. Low intracellular calcium in cytosol of acinar cell
D. Low intracellular chloride in cytosol of acinar cell

Low intracellular calcium in the cytosol of the acinar cell promotes the destruction of spontaneously activated trypsin.

2430. Kazal type 1 (SPINK1) is best related to?
Lancet 2008;371:143-52

A. Pancreatic hyperstimulation
B. Alcohol abuse
C. Anti-inflammatory cytokine
D. Serine protease inhibitor

Autodigestion of the pancreas is prevented by the packaging of proteases in precursor form and by the synthesis of protease inhibitors, i.e., pancreatic secretory trypsin inhibitor (PSTI) and serine protease inhibitor, kazal type 1 (SPINK1) that prevents conversion of trypsinogen to trypsin.

2431. SPINK1 is synthesised in?
Lancet 2008;371:143-52

A. Gallbladder
B. Duodenum
C. Stomach
D. Pancreas

Pancreas synthesises SPINK1, a specific trypsin inhibitor, the function of which can be lost by mutation. In pancreatic ductal cells, CFTR controls chloride and bicarbonate fluxes. SPINK1 and CFTR mutations together may cause pancreatitis.

2432. Which of the following is not a type of trypsinogen in human pancreatic juice?
Gastroenterology 2007;132:1557-1573

A. Telotrypsinogen
B. Cationic trypsinogen
C. Anionic trypsinogen
D. Mesotrypsinogen

Three different trypsinogens in human pancreatic juice have been designated according to their electrophoretic mobility, as cationic trypsinogen (PRSS1), anionic trypsinogen (PRSS2) & mesotrypsinogen (PRSS3). Compared with the anionic isoenzyme, cationic trypsinogen autoactivates more easily and is more resistant to autolysis.

2433. Which of the following is the most common PRSS1 mutation?
Gastroenterology 2007;132:1557-1573

A. R122A
B. R122C
C. R122H
D. R122K

R122H is the most common PRSS1 mutation observed worldwide. Mutations in PRSS1 gene are seen in most patients with hereditary pancreatitis.

2434. CFTR and SPINK1 genetic mutations causing acute pancreatitis are frequent in?
Lancet 2008;371:143-52

A. Thalassemia patients
B. HIV-positive patients
C. COPD patients
D. Leukemia patients

Genetic mutations such as those in CFTR and SPINK1 genes are frequent in HIV-positive patients with acute pancreatitis.

2435. CCK-releasing factor (CCK-RF) is present in?
Harrison's 20th Ed. Chapter 341 Page 2438

A. Stomach
B. Duodenum
C. Jejunum
D. All of the above

Duodenum contains a peptide CCK-releasing factor that is involved in stimulating CCK release.

2436. Which of the following statements is false?
Harrison's 20th Ed. Chapter 341 Page 2438

A. Serine proteases inhibit pancreatic secretion
B. Secretin activates bicarbonate secretion
C. CCK acts to increase pancreatic enzyme secretion
D. None of the above

Acidification of the duodenum releases secretin, which stimulates vagal and other neural pathways to activate pancreatic duct cells, which secrete bicarbonate. CCK in blood in physiologic concentrations acts primarily through neural pathways (vagal-vagal) leading to acetylcholine mediated pancreatic enzyme secretion. Serine proteases inhibit pancreatic secretion by inactivating CCK-releasing peptide in the lumen of the small intestine.

2437. Which of the following is the most common cause of acute pancreatitis?
Harrison's 20th Ed. Chapter 341 Page 2438

A. Gallstones
B. Alcohol
C. Drugs
D. ERCP

Cause of acute pancreatitis include gallstones (30-60%), alcohol (15-30%), ERCP (5-10%), hypertriglyceridemia (1.3-3.8%) and drug-related (0.1-2%).

2438. Risk factors for post-ERCP pancreatitis include?
Harrison's 20th Ed. Chapter 341 Page 2438

A. Sphincter of Oddi dysfunction
B. Age < 60 years
C. > 2 contrast injections into pancreatic duct
D. All of the above

Risk factors for post-ERCP pancreatitis include minor papilla sphincterotomy, sphincter of Oddi dysfunction, prior history of post-ERCP pancreatitis, age <60 years, >2 contrast injections into the pancreatic duct, and endoscopic trainee involvement.

2439. What level of hypertriglyceridemia causes acute pancreatitis?
Harrison's 20th Ed. Chapter 341 Page 2438

A. > 250 mg / dL
B. > 500 mg / dL
C. > 750 mg / dL
D. > 1000 mg / dL

Hypertriglyceridemia can cause acute pancreatitis in 1.3 - 3.8% of cases when serum triglyceride levels are usually > 1000 mg/dL. The goal is to reduce fasting plasma triglycerides to below 500 mg/dL to prevent the risk of acute pancreatitis.

2440. Deficiency of which of the following have an increased incidence of pancreatitis?
Harrison's 20th Ed. Chapter 341 Page 2438

A. ApoA-I
B. ApoB-100
C. ApoC-I
D. ApoC-II

Both LPL & apoC-II deficiency usually present in childhood with recurrent episodes of severe abdominal pain due to acute pancreatitis. Apolipoprotein CII activates lipoprotein lipase. Triglycerides of chylomicrons are hydrolyzed by LPL, and free fatty acids are released. ApoC-II, which is transferred to circulating chylomicrons from HDL, acts as a required cofactor for LPL in this reaction.

2441. Deficiency of which of the following poses an increased incidence of pancreatitis?
Harrison's 20th Ed. Chapter 341 Page 2438

A. Apolipoprotein CII
B. Apolipoprotein A-I
C. Apolipoprotein A-II
D. All of the above

Patients with deficiency of apolipoprotein CII have an increased incidence of pancreatitis. Apolipoprotein CII activates lipoprotein lipase, which is important in clearing chylomicrons from bloodstream.

2442. Which of the following statements is false?
Harrison's 20th Ed. Chapter 341 Page 2438

A. Hypertriglyceridemia can precede & cause pancreatitis
B. >80% patients of acute pancreatitis do not have hypertriglyceridemia
C. Patients with pancreatitis & hypertriglyceridemia have preexisting abnormalities in lipoprotein metabolism
D. Fasting Tg levels of < 500 mg/dL pose no risk of pancreatitis

Fasting Tg levels of < 300 mg/dL pose no risk of pancreatitis.

2443. Drugs that can elevate serum triglycerides include all except?
Harrison's 20th Ed. Chapter 341 Page 2438

A. Progesterone
B. Vitamin A
C. Thiazide diuretics
D. Beta-blockers

Drugs that can elevate serum Tg are estrogens, vitamin A, thiazides and propranolol.

2444. What percentage of acute pancreatitis are drug-related?
Harrison's 20th Ed. Chapter 341 Page 2439

A. 0.1 to 2%
B. 2 to 5%
C. 5 to 10%
D. About 15%

~ 0.1 - 2% of acute pancreatitis are drug-related.

2445. Which of the following statements about interstitial pancreatitis is false?
Harrison's 20th Ed. Chapter 341 Page 2439

A. Acute pancreatitis
B. Self-limited
C. Blood supply to pancreas maintained
D. None of the above

Pathologically, acute pancreatitis varies from interstitial pancreatitis (pancreas blood supply maintained), which is generally self-limited to necrotizing pancreatitis in which pancreas blood supply is interrupted and the extent of necrosis may correlate with severity of attack & its systemic complications.

2446. Which of the following is a proteolytic enzyme?
Harrison's 20th Ed. Chapter 341 Page 2439

A. Trypsinogen
B. Chymotrypsinogen
C. Proelastase
D. All of the above

Autodigestion is a currently accepted pathogenic theory of acute pancreatitis in which pancreatitis results when proteolytic enzymes (trypsinogen, chymotrypsinogen, proelastase) and lipolytic enzymes such as phospholipase A2 are activated in the pancreas acinar cell rather than in the intestinal lumen.

2447. Which of the following factors facilitate premature activation of trypsin?
Harrison's 20th Ed. Chapter 341 Page 2439

A. Oxidative stress
B. Direct trauma
C. Lysosomal calcium
D. All of the above

A number of factors (endotoxins, exotoxins, viral infections, ischemia, oxidative stress, lysosomal calcium and direct trauma) are believed to facilitate premature activation of trypsin.

2448. Activation, chemoattraction & sequestration of neutrophils in pancreas occur in which phase of pancreatitis?
Harrison's 20th Ed. Chapter 341 Page 2439

A. Phase 1
B. Phase 2
C. Phase 3
D. Phase 4

Pancreatitis evolves in three phases. Initial phase is characterized by intrapancreatic digestive enzyme activation & acinar cell injury. Second phase involves activation, chemoattraction & sequestration of neutrophils in pancreas resulting in intrapancreatic inflammatory reaction. Third phase is due to effects of activated proteolytic enzymes & cytokines released by inflamed pancreas on distant organs.

2449. Cathepsin B is best related to?
Harrison's 20th Ed. Chapter 341 Page 2439

A. Fat necrosis
B. Activation of elastase & phospholipase
C. Lysosomal hydrolases
D. Chemoattraction of neutrophils

Zymogen activation is mediated by lysosomal hydrolases (cathepsin B) which become co-localized with digestive enzymes in intracellular organelles leading to pancreatic acinar cell injury.

2450. In pancreatitis, cellular injury results in liberation of?
Harrison's 20th Ed. Chapter 341 Page 2439

A. Bradykinin peptides
B. Vasoactive substances
C. Histamine
D. All of the above

Cellular injury and death result in the liberation of bradykinin peptides, vasoactive substances, and histamine that can produce vasodilation, increased vascular permeability and edema with profound effects on many organs.

2451. Which of the following is an accurate predictor of severity & death when measured early in the course of acute pancreatitis?
Harrison's 20th Ed. Chapter 341 Page 2439

A. Bradykinin peptides
B. Vasoactive substances
C. Histamine
D. MCP-1 levels

Monocyte chemotactic protein (MCP-1) levels measured early in the course of acute pancreatitis are an accurate predictor of severity and death.

2452. Which of the following susceptibility gene is a determinant of occurrence of pancreatitis?
Harrison's 20th Ed. Chapter 341 Page 2439

A. PRSS1
B. CFTR
C. SPINK1
D. All of the above

Five genetic variants have been identified as being associated with susceptibility to pancreatitis. The genes that have been identified include (1) cationic trypsinogen gene (PRSSI), (2) pancreatic secretory trypsin inhibitor (SPINK1), (3) the cystic fibrosis transmembrane conductance regulator gene (CFTR), (4) the chymotrypsin C gene (CTRC) and (5) the calcium-sensing receptor (CASR).

2453. Which of the following is false about abdominal pain of acute pancreatitis?
Harrison's 20th Ed. Chapter 341 Page 2439

A. Colicky
B. Radiates to back
C. Radiate to chest, flanks, and lower abdomen
D. Located in epigastrium & periumbilical region

Abdominal pain of acute pancreatitis is steady & boring in character.

2454. Abdominal pain due to pancreatitis may have which of the following location?
Harrison's 20th Ed. Chapter 341 Page 2439

A. Right upper quadrant
B. Epigastric
C. Left upper quadrant
D. Any of the above

2455. Exudation of blood & plasma proteins into retroperitoneal space due to activated proteolytic enzymes in acute pancreatitis is termed as?
Harrison's 20th Ed. Chapter 341 Page 2439

A. Retroperitoneal abscess
B. Retroperitoneal tan
C. Retroperitoneal quinsy
D. Retroperitoneal burn

Exudation of blood & plasma proteins into retroperitoneal space due to activated proteolytic enzymes in acute pancreatitis is termed as retroperitoneal burn.

2456. Pleural effusion in acute pancreatitis is most frequently?
Harrison's 20th Ed. Chapter 341 Page 2439

A. Left-sided
B. Right-sided
C. Bilateral
D. Any of the above

Pleural effusion in acute pancreatitis is most frequently left-sided.

2457. Erythematous skin nodules in acute pancreatitis is due to?
Harrison's 20th Ed. Chapter 341 Page 2439

A. Vasculitis
B. Subcutaneous fat necrosis
C. Thromboembolism
D. All of the above

Erythematous skin nodules in acute pancreatitis is due to subcutaneous fat necrosis.

2458. Fat necrosis associated with pancreatic disease is seen in?
Harrison's 20th Ed. Chapter 341 Page 2439

A. Pancreatic carcinoma
B. Acute pancreatitis
C. Chronic pancreatitis
D. All of the above

Fat necrosis associated with pancreatic disease is secondary to circulating lipases and is seen in pancreatic carcinoma and acute & chronic pancreatitis.

2459. Cullen's sign of severe necrotizing pancreatitis is due to?
Harrison's 20th Ed. Chapter 341 Page 2439

A. Pancreatic pseudocyst
B. DIC
C. Intestinal ischemia
D. Hemoperitoneum

Cullen's sign in severe necrotizing pancreatitis refers to a faint blue discoloration around umbilicus as the result of hemoperitoneum.

2460. Turner's sign of severe necrotizing pancreatitis is due to?
Harrison's 20th Ed. Chapter 341 Page 2439

A. Tissue catabolism of hemoglobin
B. Pyoperitoneum
C. Intestinal ischemia
D. DIC

Turner's sign of severe necrotizing pancreatitis refers to a blue-red-purple or green-brown discoloration of flanks and reflects tissue catabolism of hemoglobin.

2461. Pearson syndrome is characterized by?
Harrison's 20th Ed. Chapter 472 Page 3483

A. Diabetes mellitus from pancreatic insufficiency
B. Pancytopenia
C. Lactic acidosis
D. All of the above

Pearson syndrome is characterized by diabetes mellitus from pancreatic insufficiency with pancytopenia & lactic acidosis, caused by large-scale sporadic deletion of several mtDNA genes. Kearns-Sayre syndrome (KSS), sporadic progressive external ophthalmoplegia (PEO) and Pearson syndrome are three disease phenotypes caused by large-scale mtDNA rearrangements including partial deletions or partial duplication.

2462. Which of the following about pancreatitis is false?
Harrison's 20th Ed. Chapter 341 Page 2439

A. Risk of acute pancreatitis is greater with gallstone <5 mm than larger stones
B. ~ 25% of acute pancreatitis will have recurrence
C. Cystic fibrosis is a cause of recurrent pancreatitis
D. None of the above

Gallstones with a diameter of ~ 5 mm can migrate in bile duct & trigger acute pancreatitis. Gallstones with diameter of >8 mm remain in gallbladder.

2463. Which of the following about acute pancreatitis is false?
Harrison's 20th Ed. Chapter 341 Page 2439

A. Pancreatic isoamylase & lipase remain elevated for 7-14 days
B. Serum amylase is higher in gallstone pancreatitis
C. Serum lipase higher in alcohol-associated pancreatitis
D. None of the above

2464. Patients with which of the following may have spurious elevations in serum amylase?
Harrison's 20th Ed. Chapter 341 Page 2439

A. Acidemia
B. Hyponatremia
C. Hyperkalemia
D. All of the above

Patients with acidemia (arterial pH <=7.32) may have spurious elevations in serum amylase.

2465. Which of the following is a significant risk factor for mortality in acute pancreatitis?
Harrison's 20th Ed. Chapter 341 Page 2439

A. Azotemia
B. Hemoconcentration
C. Hyperglycemia
D. All of the above

In acute pancreatitis, hemoconcentration may be the harbinger of more severe disease (pancreatic necrosis) whereas azotemia is a significant risk factor for mortality.

2466. Hyperglycemia in acute pancreatitis is due to?
Harrison's 20th Ed. Chapter 341 Page 2439

A. Decreased insulin release
B. Increased glucagon release
C. Increased output of adrenal glucocorticoids & catecholamines
D. All of the above

Hyperglycemia in acute pancreatitis is due to decreased insulin release, increased glucagon release and increased output of adrenal glucocorticoids and catecholamines.

2467. Hypocalcemia may occur in which of the following conditions?
Harrison's 20th Ed. Chapter 403 Page 2937

A. Burns
B. Tumor lysis
C. Pancreatitis
D. All of the above

Hypocalcemia may occur with severe tissue injury like burns, rhabdomyolysis, tumor lysis, or pancreatitis. Cause of hypocalcemia includes a combination of low albumin, hyperphosphatemia, tissue deposition of calcium, and impaired PTH secretion.

2468. Markers of poor prognosis in severe pancreatitis is?
Harrison's 20th Ed. Chapter 341 Page 2439

A. Elevated serum LDH levels (> 500 U/dL)
B. Azotemia
C. Hypoxemia (arterial PO_2 <=60 mm Hg)
D. All of the above

Azotemia is a significant risk factor for mortality.

2469. Serum amylase levels are elevated in all except?
Harrison's 20th Ed. Chapter 341 Page 2439

A. Pregnancy
B. Hypertriglyceridemia
C. Aortic aneurysm
D. Ruptured ectopic pregnancy

Serum amylase levels in patients with hypertriglyceridemia are often spuriously normal.

2470. Revised Atlanta criteria best relates to which of the following?
Harrison's 20th Ed. Chapter 341 Page 2440

A. Clinical features of acute pancreatitis
B. Morphologic features of acute pancreatitis on CT scan
C. Histopathologic features of acute pancreatitis
D. All of the above

Revised Atlanta criteria clearly outlines the morphologic features of acute pancreatitis on computed tomography (CT) scan.

2471. The Revised Atlanta Classification defines which of the following?
Harrison's 20th Ed. Chapter 341 Page 2440

A. Phases of acute pancreatitis
B. Severity of acute pancreatitis
C. Clarifies imaging definitions
D. All of the above

The Revised Atlanta Classification defines phases of acute pancreatitis, defines severity of acute pancreatitis and clarifies imaging definitions.

2472. Laboratory studies in acute pancreatitis may show?
Harrison's 20th Ed. Chapter 341 Page 2440

A. Leukocytosis
B. Hypocalcemia
C. Hyperglycemia
D. All of the above

2473. Risk factor for severity in acute pancreatitis is?
Harrison's 20th Ed. Chapter 341 Page 2441 Table 341-3

A. Age > 60 years
B. Obesity (BMI > 30)
C. Comorbid disease
D. All of the above

2474. Which of the following is a Comorbidity Index?
J Chronic Dis 1987;40(5):373-383

A. Andresen
B. Romano
C. Charlson
D. Grasso

The Charlson Comorbidity Index is a method of categorizing comorbidities of patients based on the International Classification of Diseases (ICD) diagnosis codes. It has 17 categories.

2475. Which of the following is not included in the bedside index of severity (BISAP) in acute pancreatitis?
Harrison's 20th Ed. Chapter 341 Page 2441 Table 341-3

A. PaO_2 < 60 mmHg
B. Blood urea nitrogen (BUN) > 25 mg%
C. Age > 60 years
D. Impaired mental status

BISAP or bedside index of severity in acute pancreatitis includes (B) Blood urea nitrogen (BUN) >25 mg%, (I) Impaired mental status, (S) SIRS: 2/4 present, (A) Age >60 years, (P) Pleural effusion

2476. Bedside Index of Severity in Acute Pancreatitis (BISAP) incorporates how many clinical and laboratory parameters?
Harrison's 20th Ed. Chapter 341 Page 2441 Table 341-3

A. 3
B. 5
C. 7
D. 9

Bedside Index of Severity in Acute Pancreatitis (BISAP), incorporates five clinical and laboratory parameters obtained within the first 24 hours of hospitalization. Presence of three or more of these factors is associated with substantially increased risk for in-hospital mortality in acute pancreatitis.

2477. Indicators of a severe attack of pancreatitis are all except?
Harrison's 20th Ed. Chapter 341 Page 2443

A. Age > 60 years
B. Body mass index (BMI) < 25
C. Hematocrit > 44%
D. Admission BUN (>22 mg/dL)

Indicators of a severe attack of pancreatitis are age > 60 years, BMI > 30, Hct > 44% & admission BUN (>22 mg/dL).

2478. Differential diagnosis of acute pancreatitis include?
Harrison's 20th Ed. Chapter 341 Page 2440

A. Perforated viscus
B. Dissecting aortic aneurysm
C. Connective tissue disorders with vasculitis
D. All of the above

Differential diagnosis of acute pancreatitis includes perforated viscus, acute cholecystitis, acute intestinal obstruction, mesenteric vascular occlusion, renal colic, myocardial infarction, dissecting aortic aneurysm, connective tissue disorders with vasculitis, pneumonia & diabetic ketoacidosis.

2479. Which of the following is true in diabetic ketoacidosis?
Harrison's 20th Ed. Chapter 341 Page 2440

A. Elevated total serum amylase levels
B. Pancreatic isoamylase levels not elevated

C. Serum lipase not elevated
D. All of the above

Diabetic ketoacidosis is accompanied by abdominal pain & elevated total serum amylase levels. Serum lipase level is not elevated in DKA.

2480. Which investigation is most helpful in differentiating acute cholecystitis from acute pancreatitis?
Harrison's 20th Ed. Chapter 341 Page 2440
A. Serum Lipase
B. Upper GI Endoscopy
C. Radionuclide scanning
D. FP abdomen

Pain of biliary tract origin is more right-sided or epigastric than periumbilical, ileus is usually absent. Sonography & radionuclide scanning are helpful in diagnosis of cholelithiasis & cholecystitis.

2481. Multiple factor scoring system for acute pancreatitis is?
Harrison's 20th Ed. Chapter 315 Page 2201
A. Ranson
B. Glasgow
C. APACHE II
D. All of the above

Ranson, Glasgow, Imrie & Apache II are multiple factor scoring systems for predicting outcome of acute pancreatitis.

2482. SOFA score stands for?
Lancet 2008; 371: 143-52
A. Septic organ failure assessment
B. Surgical organ failure assessment
C. Symptomatic organ failure assessment
D. Sequential organ failure assessment

2483. Test that is more specific for acute pancreatitis than serum amylase and lipase is?
N Engl J Med. 2006;354:2142-50
A. Urine Trypsinogen activation peptide (TAP)
B. Trypsinogen-2
C. Abdominal CT & MRI
D. All of the above

2484. Which of the following tests is more specific for the diagnosis of acute pancreatitis?
N Engl J Med. 2006;354:2142-50
A. Serum amylase
B. Serum lipase
C. Trypsinogen activation peptide
D. Trypsinogen-4

2485. At 24 hours after admission, the most sensitive & specific predictor of severe acute pancreatitis is?
N Engl J Med. 2006;354:2142-50
A. APACHE II score >=8
B. C-reactive protein level >150 mg/dl
C. PMN elastase >300 µg/liter
D. Urinary TAP >35 nmol/liter

2486. Pancreatic-duct disruption is suspected when?
N Engl J Med. 2006;354:2142-50
A. Fluid collections with very high levels of pancreatic enzymes
B. Pseudocysts
C. Ascites or pleural effusions
D. All of the above

2487. Recurrent pancreatitis in the absence of biliary disease, alcoholism, and toxic or metabolic causes suggests?
N Engl J Med. 2006;354:2142-50
A. Pancreas divisum
B. Duct-obstructing masses
C. Genetic susceptibility
D. Any of the above

2488. Test that identifies early pancreatic duct disruption is?
N Engl J Med. 2006;354:2142-50
A. CT abdomen
B. MRI abdomen
C. Transabdominal ultrasound
D. All of the above

2489. Biliary sludge is made up of?
Lancet 2008; 371: 143-52
A. Cholesterol crystals
B. Calcium bilirubinate granules
C. Gallbladder mucus
D. All of the above

Biliary sludge refers to a viscous bile suspension that contains cholesterol crystals and calcium bilirubinate granules embedded in strands of gallbladder mucus.

2490. Which test is more sensitive for identifying gallstones and sludge and for detecting bile-duct dilatation?
N Engl J Med. 2006;354:2142-50
A. Transabdominal ultrasonography
B. CT abdomen
C. MRI abdomen
D. ERCP

2491. Transabdominal ultrasonography is insensitive for detecting?
N Engl J Med. 2006;354:2142-50
A. Gallstones and sludge
B. Bile-duct dilatation
C. Stones in the distal bile duct
D. Stones in the proximal bile duct

2492. Which of the following genes may predict severity of acute pancreatitis?
N Engl J Med. 2006;354:2142-50
A. RET
B. MCP-1
C. MEN-1
D. VHL

2493. Recognized markers of risk of severe acute pancreatitis include all except?
N Engl J Med. 2006;354:2142-50

A. Elevated C-reactive protein
B. Ranson's & APACHE II scores
C. Obesity
D. High reticulocyte index

2494. Biliary sludge is associated with which of the following?
Lancet 2008; 371: 143-52

A. Total parenteral feeding
B. Long-lasting fast
C. Distal bile duct obstruction
D. All of the above

2495. Risk factors for post-ERCP pancreatitis include all except?
Lancet 2008; 371: 143-52

A. Old age
B. Female sex
C. Number of cannulation attempts of papilla
D. Poor emptying of pancreatic duct after opacification

Risk of acute pancreatitis is higher when ERCP is done to treat Oddi sphincter dysfunction than to remove bile duct stones. Other risk factors for post-ERCP pancreatitis include young age, female sex, number of cannulation attempts of papilla before success & poor emptying of pancreatic duct after opacification.

2496. The median prevalence of organ failure in necrotizing pancreatitis is?
Harrison's 20th Ed. Chapter 341 Page 2442

A. ~ 25%
B. ~ 50%
C. ~ 75%
D. ~ 95%

The median prevalence of organ failure is 54% in necrotizing pancreatitis.

2497. The mortality in acute pancreatitis with single organ system failure is?
Harrison's 20th Ed. Chapter 341 Page 2442

A. ~ 5%
B. ~ 10%
C. ~ 25%
D. ~ 50%

2498. The mortality in acute pancreatitis with multisystem organ system failure is?
Harrison's 20th Ed. Chapter 341 Page 2442

A. ~ 5%
B. ~ 10%
C. ~ 25%
D. ~ 50%

With single organ system failure, the mortality is 3–10% but increases to 47% with multisystem organ failure.

2499. What proportion of patients with acute pancreatitis have necrotizing pancreatitis?
Harrison's 20th Ed. Chapter 341 Page 2442

A. ~ 5%
B. ~ 10%
C. ~ 25%
D. ~ 50%

Necrotizing pancreatitis occurs in ~10% of all patients with acute pancreatitis.

2500. Necrosis is present in what percentage of patients with acute pancreatitis?
Harrison's 20th Ed. Chapter 341 Page 2442

A. 5 - 10%
B. 12 - 20%
C. 25 - 45%
D. 50 - 70%

Necrosis is present in 12 - 20% of patients with acute pancreatitis.

2501. In what proportion of acute pancreatitis, the disease is self-limited and subsides spontaneously?
Harrison's 20th Ed. Chapter 341 Page 2441

A. ~ 25%
B. ~ 50%
C. ~ 75%
D. ~ 90%

In most patients (85–90%) with acute pancreatitis, the disease is self-limited and subsides spontaneously, usually within three to seven days after treatment is instituted.

2502. In pancreatitis, oral intake is started by considering all of the following factors except?
Harrison's 20th Ed. Chapter 341 Page 2442

A. Resolution of abdominal pain
B. Patient is hungry
C. Organ dysfunction
D. Elevated levels of serum amylase / lipase

Inflammatory changes on CT scan or persistent elevations in serum amylase/lipase may not resolve for weeks to months & should not discourage feeding a hungry asymptomatic patient of pancreatitis.

2503. Which of the following is used in the management of pancreatitis?
Harrison's 20th Ed. Chapter 49 Page 309 Table 49-5

A. Nafamostat
B. Pentamidine
C. Tacrolimus
D. Aliskiren

Nafamostat, a protease inhibitor is utilized in the management of pancreatitis, disseminated intravascular coagulation, and extracorporeal circulation (ECC), such as during hemodialysis therapy (HD), plasmapheresis, and cardiopulmonary bypass. It inhibits aldosterone-induced proteases that activate ENaC by proteolytic cleavage. It may cause hyperkalemia.

2504. Preferred method of nutritional support in patients of necrotizing pancreatitis is?
Harrison's 20th Ed. Chapter 341 Page 2443

A. Total parenteral nutrition (TPN)
B. Feeding with a nasogastric tube
C. Enteral-feeding with a nasojejunal tube
D. PEG

Enteral-feeding with a nasojejunal tube has fewer infectious complications than with total parenteral nutrition (TPN) and is the preferred method of nutritional support. Also, enteral feeding helps to maintain integrity of the intestinal tract during severe acute pancreatitis.

2505. What proportion of patients of acute pancreatitis have a recurrence?
Harrison's 20th Ed. Chapter 341 Page 2444

A. ~ 25%
B. ~ 50%
C. ~ 75%
D. ~ 90%

~25% of patients who have had an attack of acute pancreatitis have a recurrence.

2506. Which of the following occult biliary tract diseases can lead to acute pancreatitis?
Harrison's 20th Ed. Chapter 341 Page 2444

A. Microlithiasis
B. Pancreatic cancer
C. Pancreas divisum
D. All of the above

If a cause could not be found in patients with recurrent pancreatitis, occult biliary tract disease should be looked at. These include microlithiasis, hypertriglyceridemia, drugs, pancreatic cancer, sphincter of Oddi dysfunction, pancreas divisum, cystic fibrosis, hereditary pancreatitis, choledochocele; ampullary tumors, pancreatic duct stones, stricture, and tumor.

2507. "Walled-off Necrosis" occurs how many weeks after necrotizing pancreatitis?
Harrison's 20th Ed. Chapter 341 Page 2440 Table 341-2

A. > 2 weeks
B. > 4 weeks
C. > 6 weeks
D. > 8 weeks

"Walled-off necrosis" or WON is a mature encapsulated collection of pancreatic and/or peripancreatic necrosis that has developed a well-defined inflammatory wall. WON usually occurs >4 weeks after onset of necrotizing pancreatitis.

2508. Which of the following is false about pancreatic pseudocysts?
Harrison's 20th Ed. Chapter 341 Page 2440 Table 341-2

A. Extrapancreatic
B. Minimal or no necrosis
C. Occurs >4 weeks after interstitial edematous pancreatitis
D. None of the above

An encapsulated collection of fluid with a well-defined inflammatory wall usually outside pancreas with minimal or no necrosis. It usually occurs >4 weeks after onset of interstitial edematous pancreatitis.

2509. After acute pancreatitis, pseudocysts of pancreas develop over a period of?
Harrison's 20th Ed. Chapter 341 Page 2440 Table 341-2

A. 1 - 2 weeks
B. 2 - 3 weeks
C. 3 - 4 weeks
D. 4 - 6 weeks

Pseudocysts of pancreas are collections of tissue, fluid, debris, pancreatic enzymes & blood that develop over 4-6 weeks after acute pancreatitis.

2510. Which of the following about pseudocysts of pancreas is false?
Harrison's 20th Ed. Chapter 341 Page 2440

A. Preceded by pancreatitis in 90% of cases
B. Mostly located in body or tail of pancreas
C. Abdominal pain is the usual presenting complaint
D. Serum amylase level is mostly normal

Serum amylase level is elevated in 75% of pseudocysts of pancreas at some point during their illness and may fluctuate markedly.

2511. Significant number of pancreatic pseudocysts resolve spontaneously how many weeks after their formation?
Harrison's 20th Ed. Chapter 341 Page 2443

A. > 1 week
B. > 2 weeks
C. > 4 weeks
D. > 6 weeks

Significant number of pancreatic pseudocysts resolve spontaneously >6 weeks after their formation.

2512. Which of the following statements is false for Purtscher's retinopathy?
Optom Vis Sci. 2014;91(2):e43-51

A. Due to occlusion of anterior retinal artery
B. Sudden and severe loss of vision
C. Cotton wool spots & hemorrhages in optical fundus
D. It is a complication of acute pancreatitis

Purtscher's retinopathy in acute pancreatitis is due to occlusion of posterior retinal artery with aggregated granulocytes. Optical fundus shows cotton-wool spots & hemorrhages confined to an area limited by optic disk & macula.

2513. Which of the following is a classification system for Chronic Pancreatitis and Pancreatic Exocrine Insufficiency?
Harrison's 20th Ed. Chapter 341 Page 2445 Table 341-5

A. RICOR
B. TEMNA
C. TIGAR-O
D. PROZE

TIGAR-O stands for toxic-metabolic, idiopathic, genetic, autoimmune, recurrent and obstructive.

2514. Complication of chronic pancreatitis is?
Harrison's 20th Ed. Chapter 341 Page 2445

A. Abdominal pain
B. Steatorrhea
C. Diabetes mellitus
D. All of the above

Complications of chronic pancreatitis are abdominal pain, steatorrhea, weight loss & diabetes mellitus.

2515. Which of the following is best related to chronic pancreatitis?
Harrison's 20th Ed. Chapter 341 Page 2445

A. Fluctuating symptomatology
B. Risk of malignancy
C. Irreversible damage to pancreas
D. All of the above

Chronic pancreatitis is characterized by irreversible damage to pancreas.

2516. There is a strong association of which of the following and chronic pancreatitis?
Harrison's 18th Ed. 2643

A. Smoking
B. Intravenous drug use

C. Prolonged fasting
D. Obesity

There is a strong independent, dose-dependent association of smoking and chronic and recurrent acute pancreatitis. Cigarette smoke leads to an increased susceptibility to pancreatic self-digestion and predisposes to dysregulation of duct cell CFTR function. It increases severity in alcohol-induced chronic pancreatitis.

2517. Which of the following plays a key role in the development of chronic pancreatitis?
Harrison's 20th Ed. Chapter 341 Page 2445

A. Islet cells of Langerhans
B. Pancreatic stellate cells (PSC)
C. Acinar epithelial cells
D. All of the above

Pancreatic stellate cells (PSC) play a role in maintaining normal pancreatic architecture that can shift toward fibrogenesis in the case of chronic pancreatitis.

2518. Which of the following hypothesis describes events in the pathogenesis of chronic pancreatitis?
Harrison's 20th Ed. Chapter 341 Page 2445

A. Sentinel acute pancreatitis event
B. Sentinel chronic pancreatitis event
C. Sequential acute pancreatitis event
D. Sequential chronic pancreatitis event

The sentinel acute pancreatitis event (SAPE) hypothesis uniformly describes the events in the pathogenesis of chronic pancreatitis.

2519. Which of the following induces pancreatic stellate cells (PSC) activity with subsequent new collagen synthesis?
Harrison's 20th Ed. Chapter 341 Page 2445

A. Proinflammatory cytokines
B. Oxidants
C. Growth factors
D. All of the above

Proinflammatory cytokines, tumor necrosis factor (TNF-α), interleukin 1 (IL-1), and interleukin 6 (IL-6) as well as oxidant complexes & growth factors are able to induce PSC activity with subsequent new collagen synthesis.

2520. Which of the following plays a role in self-activating autocrine pathways that lead to progression in chronic pancreatitis?
Harrison's 20th Ed. Chapter 341 Page 2445

A. Tumor necrosis factor (TNF-α)
B. Interleukin 1 (IL-1)
C. Interleukin 6 (IL-6)
D. Transforming growth factor (TGF-β)

PSCs also possess transforming growth factor (TGF-β)–mediated self-activating autocrine pathways that may explain disease progression in chronic pancreatitis even after removal of noxious stimuli.

2521. Which of the following is the most frequent cause of clinically apparent chronic pancreatitis in children?
Harrison's 20th Ed. Chapter 341 Page 2445

A. Cystic fibrosis
B. Hereditary pancreatitis
C. Isolated autoimmune chronic pancreatitis
D. Pancreas divisum

In United States, alcoholism is the most common cause of clinically apparent chronic pancreatitis in adults, while cystic fibrosis is the most frequent cause in children.

2522. In hereditary chronic pancreatitis, defect in gene encoding for which of the following is found?
Harrison's 20th Ed. Chapter 341 Page 2445

A. Pepsin
B. Chymotrypsin
C. Trypsinogen
D. All of the above

In hereditary chronic pancreatitis, a genetic defect that affects the gene encoding for trypsinogen was identified. The defect prevents the destruction of trypsinogen and allows it to be resistant to the effect of trypsin inhibitor, become spontaneously activated, and to remain activated leading to continual activation of digestive enzymes within the gland causing acute injury and eventually chronic pancreatitis.

2523. Which of the following mutation increases the risk of chronic pancreatitis?
Harrison's 20th Ed. Chapter 341 Page 2445

A. N32S SPINK1
B. N33S SPINK1
C. N34S SPINK1
D. N35S SPINK1

Presence of an N34S SPINK1 mutation increased the risk of chronic pancreatitis by twentyfold. A combination of two CFTR mutations and an N34S SPINK1 mutation increased the risk of chronic pancreatitis 900-fold.

2524. Autoimmune Pancreatitis (AIP) is which form of pancreatitis?
N Engl J Med. 2006;355:2670-6

A. Acute
B. Chronic
C. Recurrent
D. All of the above

2525. Autoimmune Pancreatitis (AIP) is also called?
N Engl J Med. 2006;355:2670-6

A. Sclerosing pancreatitis
B. Tumefactive pancreatitis
C. Nonalcoholic destructive pancreatitis
D. All of the above

AIP is also referred to as sclerosing pancreatitis, tumefactive pancreatitis and nonalcoholic destructive pancreatitis.

2526. Autoimmune pancreatitis is frequently associated with?
Harrison's 20th Ed. Chapter 341 Page 2446

A. Rheumatoid arthritis
B. Sjögren's syndrome
C. Ulcerative colitis
D. All of the above

AIP is associated with primary sclerosing cholangitis, primary biliary sclerosis, rheumatoid arthritis, Sjögren's syndrome, ulcerative colitis, mediastinal adenopathy, autoimmune thyroiditis, tubulointerstitial nephritis, and retroperitoneal fibrosis.

2527. Majority of patients with AIP present with?
Harrison's 20th Ed. Chapter 341 Page 2446

A. Obstructive jaundice
B. Acute pancreatitis

C. Recurrent pancreatitis
D. Malabsorption syndrome

In the United States, 50–75% of patients with AIP present with obstructive jaundice.

2528. Immunologic abnormalities in autoimmune pancreatitis include?

N Engl J Med. 2006;355:2670-6

A. Hypergammaglobulinemia
B. Autoantibodies against carbonic anhydrase
C. Autoantibodies against lactoferrin
D. All of the above

Autoimmune pancreatitis is characterized by the presence of increased serum gammaglobulin levels (IgG4), presence of autoantibodies (antinuclear antibodies, antilactoferrin antibodies, anticarbonic anhydrase antibodies & rheumatoid factor), pancreatic fibrosis with lymphocytic infiltration & an absence of pancreatic calcification, an association with other autoimmune diseases and response to steroid therapy.

2529. Serum levels of which of the following immunoglobulin is elevated in AIP?

Harrison's 20th Ed. Chapter 341 Page 2446

A. Immunoglobulin G1
B. Immunoglobulin G2
C. Immunoglobulin G3
D. Immunoglobulin G4

IgG constitutes ~75–85% of total serum immunoglobulin. The four IgG subclasses are numbered in order of their level in serum, IgG1 being found in greatest amounts and IgG4 the least. Serum IgG4 normally accounts for only 5–6% of the total IgG in healthy patients but is elevated at least twofold higher than 135 mg/dL in those with AIP.

2530. Which of the following syndrome is related to IgG4?

Harrison's 20th Ed. Chapter 341 Page 2446

A. IgG4-related immunologic disease
B. IgG4-related systemic disease
C. IgG4-related pulmonary disease
D. IgG4-related neuronal disease

IgG4-related systemic disease is a variety of acute tubulointerstitial disorder and a form of Acute Interstitial Nephritis (AIN). It is characterized by a dense inflammatory infiltrate containing IgG4-expressing plasma cells. Glucocorticoids lead to response.

2531. Which of the following syndrome is related to IgG4?

Harrison's 20th Ed. Chapter 341 Page 2446

A. Immunoglobulin G4–associated carditis
B. Immunoglobulin G4–associated neuritis
C. Immunoglobulin G4–associated pneumonitis
D. Immunoglobulin G4–associated cholangitis

Immunoglobulin G4–associated cholangitis is a biliary disease of unknown etiology with biochemical & cholangiographic features indistinguishable from PSC. It is associated with autoimmune pancreatitis and is characterized by elevated serum IgG4 and infiltration of IgG4-positive plasma cells in bile ducts and liver tissue. In contrast to PSC, it is not associated with inflammatory bowel disease.

2532. Which of the following is characteristic imaging finding in AIP?

Harrison's 20th Ed. Chapter 341 Page 2446

A. Enlargement at the head of pancreas
B. Strictures in bile duct
C. Narrowing of pancreatic bile duct
D. All of the above

2533. Which of the following drug is useful in AIP?

Harrison's 20th Ed. Chapter 341 Page 2446

A. Glucocorticoids
B. Azathioprine
C. 6-mercaptopurine
D. All of the above

Glucocorticoids, azathioprine, 6-mercaptapurine, rituximab, cyclosporine and cyclophosphamide are useful in AIP.

2534. Which of the following is false about chronic pancreatitis?

Harrison's 20th Ed. Chapter 341 Page 2446

A. Deficiencies of fat-soluble vitamins are uncommon
B. Serum amylase & lipase levels are raised
C. Best diagnostic test is secretin stimulation test
D. Vitamin B_{12} malabsorption is corrected by oral pancreatic enzymes

Serum amylase & lipase levels are normal.

2535. Which of the following tests is useful in identifying severe pancreatic exocrine insufficiency?

Harrison's 20th Ed. Chapter 341 Page 2446

A. D-xylose excretion test
B. Fecal elastase
C. Serum amylase
D. Serum lipase

Fecal elastase levels of < 100 μg per gram of stool strongly suggests severe pancreatic exocrine insufficiency.

2536. Severe pancreatic exocrine insufficiency is obvious when serum trypsinogen levels are?

Harrison's 19th Ed. 2099

A. < 20 mg/mL
B. < 40 mg/mL
C. < 60 mg/mL
D. < 80 mg/mL

Decrease of serum trypsinogen level to < 20 mg/mL strongly suggests severe pancreatic exocrine insufficiency.

2537. Absence of pancreatic calcification is a feature of?

Harrison's 20th Ed. Chapter 341 Page 2446, Gastroenterology 2007;132:1557-1573

A. Idiopathic chronic pancreatitis
B. Islet cell tumors
C. Autoimmune pancreatitis
D. Severe protein-calorie malnutrition

2538. In chronic pancreatitis, secretin stimulation test is abnormal when how much of pancreatic exocrine function is lost?

Harrison's 20th Ed. Chapter 341 Page 2446

A. 20%
B. 40%
C. 60%
D. 80%

In chronic pancreatitis, secretin stimulation test becomes abnormal when 60% of the pancreatic exocrine function has been lost. This correlates well with the onset of chronic abdominal pain.

2539. Most common cause of pancreatic calcification is?
Harrison's 20th Ed. Chapter 341 Page 2446

A. Idiopathic chronic pancreatitis
B. Hypercalcemic pancreatitis
C. Alcohol
D. Severe protein-calorie malnutrition

Alcohol is the most common cause of pancreatic calcification. Diffuse pancreatic calcifications on FP abdomen indicates ~80% damage to pancreas. Pancreatic calcification is also seen in severe protein-calorie malnutrition, hereditary pancreatitis, posttraumatic pancreatitis, hypercalcemic pancreatitis, islet cell tumors, idiopathic chronic pancreatitis and tropical pancreatitis.

2540. Tropical pancreatitis is characterized by all except?
Gastroenterology 2007;132:1557-1573

A. Early onset
B. Slow progression
C. Severe pancreatic damage
D. No history of alcohol abuse or biliary disease

Tropical pancreatitis is characterized by early onset, rapid progression & severe pancreatic damage in the absence of a history of alcohol abuse or biliary disease. Both exocrine & endocrine insufficiency is evident at very early stages, often at the time of presentation in majority (70%) of patients.

2541. Which of the following is an uncommon complication of chronic pancreatitis?
Harrison's 20th Ed. Chapter 341 Page 2447

A. Diabetic ketoacidosis
B. Pancreatic cancer
C. Gastrointestinal bleeding
D. Biliary cirrhosis

In chronic pancreatitis, most patients have impaired glucose tolerance, diabetic ketoacidosis and coma are uncommon.

2542. According to the American Diabetes Association, which of the following diabetes in found in chronic pancreatitis?
Gastroenterology 2007;132:1557-1573

A. Type I
B. Type II
C. Type IIIc
D. Any of the above

Diabetes of chronic pancreatitis is classified as type IIIc according to ADA & is characterized by destruction of both insulin & glucagon-producing cells.

2543. Hemosuccus pancreaticus best relates to?
Harrison's 20th Ed. Chapter 341 Page 2447

A. Pseudocyst eroding into the duodenum
B. Arterial bleeding into pancreatic duct
C. Ruptured varices secondary to splenic vein thrombosis
D. Pseudocyst eroding into the stomach

2544. Increased incidence of pancreatic carcinoma is seen in which of the following?
Harrison's 20th Ed. Chapter 341 Page 2447

A. Idiopathic chronic pancreatitis
B. Hypercalcemic pancreatitis
C. Hereditary pancreatitis
D. Severe protein-calorie malnutrition

Patients with hereditary pancreatitis develop pancreatic calcification, diabetes mellitus & steatorrhea. They have a tenfold higher risk of pancreatic carcinoma (40% by 70 years).

2545. Which of the following significantly relieves pain in severe refractory large-duct chronic pancreatitis?
Harrison's 20th Ed. Chapter 341 Page 2448

A. UDCA
B. Cholestyramine
C. Domperidone
D. Pregabalin

2546. The ideal pancreatic enzyme preparation is?
Harrison's 20th Ed. Chapter 341 Page 2448

A. Enteric-coated lipase & free proteases
B. Enteric-coated lipase & enteric-coated proteases
C. Free lipase & enteric-coated proteases
D. Free lipase & free proteases

Ideal pancreatic enzyme preparation is enteric-coated lipase & free proteases. Free proteases enter duodenum & evoke a positive feedback control mechanism & enteric-coated lipase open beyond duodenum & enhance fat absorption. Recent data suggests that dosages up to 80,000–100,000 units of lipase per meal may be necessary to normalize nutritional parameters in malnourished chronic pancreatitis patients.

2547. The major cause of death in alcoholic CP is?
Gastroenterology 2007;132:1557-1573

A. Cardiovascular disease
B. Severe infection
C. Malignancy
D. All of the above

Major causes of death in alcoholic CP are cardiovascular disease, infection & malignancy.

2548. The most common congenital anatomic variant of human pancreas is?
Harrison's 20th Ed. Chapter 341 Page 2449

A. Annular pancreas
B. Pancreas divisum
C. Sphincter of Oddi disorders
D. Pancreatic duct scars

Pancreas divisum is the most common congenital anatomic variant of the human pancreas.

2549. Which of the following does not predispose to the development of pancreatitis?
Harrison's 20th Ed. Chapter 341 Page 2449

A. Hereditary pancreatitis
B. Annular pancreas
C. Pancreas divisum
D. All of the above

Pancreas divisum does not predispose to the development of pancreatitis in the great majority of patients who harbor it.

2550. Macroamylasaemia is characterised by formation of large molecular complexes between amylase and?
Harrison's 20th Ed. Chapter 341 Page 2449

A. Urea
B. Haem
C. Clotting factors
D. Abnormal immunoglobulins

Macroamylasaemia is a syndrome characterised by formation of large molecular complexes between amylase & abnormal immunoglobulins.

2551. Paraduodenal pancreatitis is also called?

World J Gastrointest Pathophysiol. 2014;5(3):252-270

A. Ectopic pancreatitis
B. Groove pancreatitis
C. Minimal pancreatitis
D. Sentinel pancreatitis

Groove pancreatitis is a rare form of focal chronic pancreatitis involving the anatomic groove between the pancreatic head, duodenum and common bile duct.

2552. Which of the following about Tropical chronic pancreatitis (TCP) is false?

Indian J Pediatr 2006;73 (10):907-912

A. Juvenile form of chronic pancreatitis
B. Higher risk of pancreatic calculi, diabetes & pancreatic malignancy
C. Highly associated with SPINK1 N34S mutation
D. None of the above

Tropical chronic pancreatitis (TCP) is a juvenile form of chronic pancreatitis prevalent in tropical developing countries. TCP differs from temperate zone pancreatitis in its younger age of onset, more accelerated course, higher prevalence of pancreatic calculi and diabetes, and greater propensity to pancreatic malignancy. TCP involves the main pancreatic duct resulting in large ductal calculi & is highly associated with SPINK1 N34S mutation.

ANSWERS

1. D	46. D	91. D	136. A	181. D	226. D
2. B	47. D	92. A	137. D	182. B	227. C
3. C	48. A	93. D	138. C	183. D	228. D
4. C	49. D	94. D	139. A	184. D	229. B
5. D	50. A	95. D	140. C	185. D	230. A
6. C	51. D	96. D	141. C	186. C	231. D
7. C	52. D	97. B	142. D	187. B	232. B
8. C	53. A	98. D	143. A	188. D	233. A
9. B	54. D	99. D	144. D	189. C	234. A
10. D	55. D	100. D	145. B	190. C	235. B
11. D	56. D	101. D	146. B	191. D	236. A
12. D	57. A	102. D	147. D	192. D	237. B
13. D	58. D	103. A	148. B	193. A	238. D
14. D	59. B	104. C	149. D	194. D	239. D
15. A	60. D	105. B	150. B	195. B	240. D
16. D	61. D	106. D	151. A	196. D	241. D
17. A	62. D	107. D	152. A	197. A	242. D
18. B	63. D	108. B	153. A	198. C	243. D
19. A	64. B	109. B	154. D	199. C	244. D
20. A	65. D	110. D	155. C	200. D	245. D
21. C	66. C	111. D	156. D	201. A	246. D
22. D	67. D	112. D	157. A	202. A	247. D
23. D	68. D	113. B	158. C	203. A	248. A
24. C	69. A	114. C	159. A	204. D	249. B
25. B	70. D	115. C	160. D	205. D	250. D
26. C	71. C	116. D	161. D	206. B	251. D
27. D	72. D	117. C	162. D	207. D	252. D
28. D	73. A	118. C	163. D	208. D	253. C
29. A	74. B	119. D	164. C	209. C	254. A
30. D	75. C	120. D	165. C	210. D	255. B
31. C	76. C	121. A	166. D	211. D	256. D
32. D	77. B	122. D	167. C	212. D	257. B
33. D	78. A	123. A	168. C	213. B	258. C
34. D	79. D	124. D	169. B	214. C	259. A
35. D	80. D	125. D	170. A	215. D	260. D
36. A	81. A	126. D	171. B	216. D	261. A
37. D	82. A	127. A	172. D	217. B	262. D
38. D	83. D	128. C	173. C	218. A	263. D
39. D	84. D	129. D	174. D	219. D	264. C
40. D	85. B	130. D	175. B	220. B	265. A
41. A	86. B	131. A	176. A	221. D	266. C
42. C	87. B	132. B	177. D	222. A	267. D
43. C	88. B	133. D	178. B	223. A	268. D
44. D	89. D	134. C	179. B	224. B	269. A
45. C	90. B	135. B	180. D	225. B	270. D

ANSWERS

271. D	316. C	361. B	406. C	451. D	496. D
272. D	317. B	362. D	407. C	452. D	497. C
273. D	318. D	363. A	408. C	453. D	498. D
274. D	319. A	364. D	409. B	454. C	499. A
275. C	320. D	365. A	410. C	455. C	500. C
276. A	321. B	366. D	411. D	456. C	501. A
277. D	322. D	367. D	412. D	457. D	502. D
278. D	323. A	368. C	413. A	458. D	503. A
279. A	324. D	369. A	414. D	459. D	504. A
280. D	325. D	370. D	415. B	460. D	505. D
281. D	326. A	371. D	416. D	461. C	506. D
282. D	327. D	372. D	417. D	462. C	507. C
283. A	328. B	373. A	418. B	463. C	508. D
284. D	329. A	374. A	419. C	464. C	509. A
285. D	330. A	375. B	420. D	465. D	510. D
286. D	331. D	376. C	421. D	466. C	511. D
287. B	332. D	377. D	422. B	467. A	512. C
288. D	333. B	378. A	423. C	468. D	513. A
289. D	334. D	379. C	424. D	469. D	514. D
290. D	335. A	380. D	425. C	470. C	515. D
291. D	336. D	381. B	426. A	471. D	516. D
292. B	337. A	382. B	427. C	472. C	517. D
293. A	338. B	383. D	428. A	473. D	518. C
294. D	339. D	384. D	429. D	474. D	519. A
295. D	340. D	385. D	430. A	475. D	520. B
296. D	341. D	386. D	431. D	476. B	521. B
297. D	342. B	387. D	432. D	477. B	522. A
298. B	343. C	388. A	433. C	478. D	523. D
299. D	344. A	389. D	434. C	479. D	524. C
300. C	345. B	390. C	435. D	480. D	525. D
301. A	346. A	391. C	436. B	481. D	526. D
302. D	347. D	392. D	437. A	482. D	527. C
303. D	348. A	393. B	438. A	483. D	528. D
304. D	349. D	394. B	439. C	484. B	529. D
305. D	350. C	395. B	440. D	485. D	530. D
306. D	351. A	396. D	441. B	486. D	531. D
307. D	352. B	397. C	442. D	487. B	532. B
308. D	353. C	398. B	443. C	488. B	533. A
309. B	354. D	399. D	444. D	489. D	534. A
310. C	355. D	400. C	445. D	490. D	535. A
311. C	356. A	401. B	446. D	491. C	536. C
312. C	357. B	402. D	447. D	492. D	537. B
313. B	358. B	403. B	448. B	493. A	538. B
314. A	359. A	404. A	449. D	494. D	539. A
315. D	360. D	405. D	450. D	495. A	540. C

ANSWERS

541. D	586. C	631. D	676. D	721. B	766. D
542. D	587. B	632. D	677. A	722. C	767. D
543. B	588. C	633. C	678. D	723. C	768. D
544. B	589. D	634. C	679. A	724. A	769. D
545. C	590. C	635. C	680. D	725. C	770. D
546. C	591. D	636. D	681. C	726. A	771. A
547. D	592. B	637. A	682. A	727. D	772. D
548. D	593. C	638. C	683. A	728. A	773. B
549. D	594. D	639. B	684. B	729. D	774. D
550. C	595. D	640. B	685. B	730. A	775. D
551. B	596. B	641. C	686. B	731. D	776. B
552. D	597. D	642. C	687. B	732. D	777. B
553. D	598. B	643. C	688. D	733. A	778. C
554. D	599. B	644. C	689. A	734. D	779. A
555. A	600. B	645. A	690. D	735. C	780. B
556. B	601. C	646. C	691. D	736. D	781. D
557. B	602. D	647. D	692. B	737. B	782. A
558. C	603. B	648. A	693. D	738. C	783. D
559. C	604. D	649. B	694. D	739. A	784. D
560. B	605. C	650. A	695. C	740. D	785. A
561. C	606. B	651. C	696. A	741. C	786. B
562. D	607. D	652. D	697. A	742. C	787. A
563. B	608. B	653. D	698. D	743. A	788. D
564. C	609. D	654. C	699. D	744. A	789. A
565. B	610. D	655. A	700. C	745. D	790. C
566. B	611. D	656. C	701. B	746. B	791. C
567. D	612. A	657. C	702. A	747. C	792. D
568. B	613. C	658. D	703. C	748. B	793. A
569. B	614. D	659. A	704. C	749. D	794. C
570. B	615. D	660. D	705. A	750. B	795. B
571. D	616. C	661. A	706. A	751. B	796. D
572. D	617. A	662. B	707. A	752. A	797. B
573. D	618. B	663. D	708. A	753. D	798. B
574. D	619. D	664. D	709. D	754. D	799. D
575. B	620. B	665. C	710. D	755. B	800. C
576. D	621. B	666. C	711. C	756. C	801. A
577. C	622. D	667. D	712. D	757. A	802. D
578. C	623. D	668. A	713. A	758. B	803. A
579. B	624. D	669. D	714. B	759. D	804. A
580. C	625. C	670. B	715. D	760. B	805. C
581. D	626. C	671. A	716. A	761. D	806. C
582. A	627. B	672. A	717. C	762. D	807. B
583. D	628. A	673. C	718. D	763. B	808. D
584. D	629. D	674. C	719. C	764. D	809. D
585. A	630. A	675. C	720. D	765. D	810. C

ANSWERS

811. D	856. C	901. B	946. A	991. D	1036. D
812. A	857. B	902. D	947. B	992. D	1037. B
813. A	858. C	903. D	948. D	993. C	1038. C
814. D	859. B	904. D	949. D	994. C	1039. A
815. A	860. D	905. D	950. D	995. B	1040. D
816. A	861. C	906. C	951. D	996. B	1041. C
817. B	862. B	907. B	952. B	997. C	1042. A
818. D	863. C	908. B	953. A	998. B	1043. A
819. D	864. C	909. D	954. D	999. B	1044. D
820. D	865. B	910. B	955. C	1000. A	1045. D
821. D	866. B	911. C	956. D	1001. D	1046. D
822. D	867. A	912. C	957. D	1002. C	1047. D
823. D	868. D	913. D	958. C	1003. D	1048. C
824. D	869. C	914. D	959. D	1004. C	1049. D
825. C	870. A	915. D	960. B	1005. C	1050. A
826. B	871. D	916. B	961. C	1006. B	1051. A
827. B	872. D	917. D	962. C	1007. A	1052. A
828. C	873. D	918. B	963. C	1008. A	1053. D
829. C	874. D	919. D	964. C	1009. D	1054. D
830. A	875. D	920. A	965. B	1010. B	1055. D
831. D	876. B	921. B	966. B	1011. B	1056. A
832. D	877. D	922. C	967. B	1012. C	1057. D
833. B	878. D	923. D	968. C	1013. A	1058. D
834. D	879. D	924. C	969. A	1014. C	1059. A
835. A	880. D	925. D	970. D	1015. D	1060. D
836. D	881. D	926. D	971. C	1016. B	1061. A
837. C	882. D	927. B	972. B	1017. C	1062. D
838. D	883. D	928. C	973. C	1018. B	1063. B
839. D	884. D	929. D	974. B	1019. A	1064. C
840. B	885. C	930. C	975. D	1020. D	1065. C
841. C	886. D	931. D	976. C	1021. D	1066. B
842. D	887. A	932. A	977. A	1022. D	1067. D
843. D	888. C	933. A	978. C	1023. A	1068. D
844. D	889. B	934. C	979. A	1024. A	1069. D
845. A	890. D	935. D	980. A	1025. D	1070. D
846. A	891. C	936. B	981. B	1026. B	1071. D
847. A	892. A	937. D	982. D	1027. D	1072. D
848. B	893. A	938. B	983. B	1028. B	1073. D
849. C	894. D	939. A	984. A	1029. D	1074. B
850. B	895. A	940. D	985. B	1030. C	1075. D
851. D	896. A	941. D	986. D	1031. D	1076. D
852. C	897. B	942. C	987. B	1032. C	1077. B
853. B	898. C	943. D	988. D	1033. D	1078. B
854. D	899. D	944. A	989. A	1034. D	1079. A
855. A	900. D	945. D	990. C	1035. C	1080. A

ANSWERS

1081. A	1126. B,	1171. D	1216. C	1261. A	1306. D
1082. D	1127. C	1172. D	1217. C	1262. B	1307. B
1083. D	1128. C	1173. B	1218. C	1263. B	1308. D
1084. D	1129. C	1174. D	1219. D	1264. D	1309. D
1085. B	1130. B	1175. D	1220. C	1265. D	1310. D
1086. D	1131. D	1176. D	1221. D	1266. B	1311. D
1087. D	1132. D	1177. C	1222. B	1267. D	1312. D
1088. A	1133. C	1178. C	1223. D	1268. B	1313. A
1089. A	1134. D	1179. B	1224. D	1269. D	1314. C
1090. C	1135. B	1180. B	1225. D	1270. A	1315. D
1091. C	1136. D	1181. C	1226. D	1271. D	1316. D
1092. C	1137. D	1182. D	1227. A	1272. B	1317. A
1093. B	1138. B	1183. D	1228. D	1273. C	1318. C
1094. C	1139. A	1184. A	1229. A	1274. C	1319. D
1095. D	1140. D	1185. A	1230. B	1275. A	1320. A
1096. B	1141. D	1186. C	1231. C	1276. D	1321. B
1097. D	1142. C	1187. D	1232. B	1277. D	1322. D
1098. B	1143. B	1188. B	1233. B	1278. A	1323. A
1099. A	1144. C	1189. B	1234. C	1279. D	1324. D
1100. C	1145. D	1190. A	1235. B	1280. B	1325. A
1101. B	1146. D	1191. C	1236. B	1281. B	1326. B
1102. C	1147. A	1192. C	1237. A	1282. D	1327. C
1103. D	1148. D	1193. B	1238. A	1283. B	1328. A
1104. C	1149. D	1194. C	1239. D	1284. A	1329. D
1105. D	1150. C	1195. D	1240. A	1285. C	1330. A
1106. C	1151. C	1196. D	1241. C	1286. D	1331. A
1107. B	1152. D	1197. D	1242. D	1287. B	1332. B
1108. A	1153. C	1198. D	1243. B	1288. B	1333. B
1109. A	1154. B	1199. B	1244. C	1289. B	1334. C
1110. B	1155. C	1200. D	1245. C	1290. A	1335. D
1111. D	1156. B	1201. C	1246. D	1291. A	1336. D
1112. C	1157. A	1202. C	1247. C	1292. C	1337. B
1113. D	1158. D	1203. B	1248. B	1293. D	1338. D
1114. D	1159. C	1204. C	1249. B	1294. B	1339. C
1115. B	1160. B	1205. C	1250. B	1295. A	1340. D
1116. A	1161. B	1206. B	1251. D	1296. D	1341. D
1117. D	1162. D	1207. A	1252. D	1297. C	1342. D
1118. A	1163. B	1208. A	1253. C	1298. D	1343. D
1119. D	1164. B	1209. B	1254. B	1299. C	1344. D
1120. A	1165. C	1210. D	1255. D	1300. A	1345. D
1121. D	1166. D	1211. A	1256. D	1301. C	1346. A
1122. B	1167. D	1212. C	1257. D	1302. D	1347. A
1123. C	1168. D	1213. D	1258. B	1303. B	1348. C
1124. C	1169. C	1214. C	1259. D	1304. A	1349. A
1125. C	1170. A	1215. A	1260. D	1305. A	1350. B

ANSWERS

1351. D	1396. D	1441. B	1486. C	1531. D	1576. B
1352. C	1397. D	1442. D	1487. B	1532. A	1577. A
1353. D	1398. D	1443. C	1488. D	1533. C	1578. A
1354. A	1399. D	1444. C	1489. A	1534. D	1579. D
1355. D	1400. C	1445. C	1490. D	1535. D	1580. B
1356. D	1401. B	1446. D	1491. A	1536. A	1581. C
1357. D	1402. A	1447. B	1492. D	1537. A	1582. D
1358. A	1403. A	1448. D	1493. D	1538. B	1583. A
1359. C	1404. D	1449. D	1494. D	1539. B	1584. D
1360. D	1405. C	1450. C	1495. C	1540. C	1585. D
1361. D	1406. B	1451. A	1496. D	1541. C	1586. D
1362. D	1407. C	1452. C	1497. A	1542. A	1587. D
1363. D	1408. C	1453. D	1498. C	1543. B	1588. D
1364. B	1409. A	1454. B	1499. A	1544. D	1589. D
1365. D	1410. D	1455. D	1500. C	1545. C	1590. D
1366. C	1411. A	1456. D	1501. D	1546. D	1591. C
1367. A	1412. A	1457. A	1502. D	1547. D	1592. A
1368. A	1413. A	1458. B	1503. C	1548. C	1593. B
1369. D	1414. D	1459. D	1504. D	1549. B	1594. D
1370. D	1415. D	1460. D	1505. B	1550. D	1595. D
1371. D	1416. A	1461. D	1506. C	1551. C	1596. D
1372. D	1417. D	1462. D	1507. C	1552. A	1597. D
1373. B	1418. A	1463. D	1508. D	1553. B	1598. A
1374. C	1419. B	1464. B	1509. D	1554. C	1599. D
1375. D	1420. D	1465. B	1510. D	1555. D	1600. B
1376. C	1421. A	1466. C	1511. D	1556. A	1601. C
1377. D	1422. B	1467. D	1512. D	1557. B	1602. A
1378. A	1423. D	1468. D	1513. D	1558. C	1603. D
1379. D	1424. D	1469. A	1514. D	1559. D	1604. D
1380. B	1425. C	1470. A	1515. B	1560. C	1605. A
1381. C	1426. D	1471. B	1516. D	1561. C	1606. A
1382. C	1427. C	1472. C	1517. D	1562. A	1607. A
1383. B	1428. D	1473. D	1518. A	1563. D	1608. C
1384. D	1429. D	1474. D	1519. A	1564. A	1609. C
1385. D	1430. D	1475. B	1520. D	1565. C	1610. D
1386. A	1431. B	1476. D	1521. D	1566. D	1611. D
1387. C	1432. D	1477. D	1522. C	1567. D	1612. D
1388. B	1433. D	1478. D	1523. B	1568. A	1613. C
1389. D	1434. D	1479. D	1524. D	1569. C	1614. A
1390. A	1435. B	1480. D	1525. B	1570. A	1615. A
1391. D	1436. D	1481. C	1526. A	1571. D	1616. C
1392. D	1437. D	1482. D	1527. D	1572. D	1617. C
1393. D	1438. D	1483. D	1528. D	1573. D	1618. C
1394. D	1439. D	1484. B	1529. C	1574. D	1619. D
1395. A	1440. D	1485. D	1530. B	1575. D	1620. C

ANSWERS

1621. D	1666. B	1711. A	1756. B	1801. A	1846. A
1622. A	1667. D	1712. D	1757. A	1802. B	1847. D
1623. A	1668. B	1713. A	1758. C	1803. A	1848. D
1624. D	1669. D	1714. D	1759. C	1804. D	1849. D
1625. B	1670. C	1715. A	1760. B	1805. D	1850. B
1626. D	1671. D	1716. B	1761. D	1806. D	1851. D
1627. D	1672. A	1717. A	1762. B	1807. C	1852. C
1628. B	1673. B	1718. D	1763. A	1808. B	1853. A
1629. C	1674. D	1719. D	1764. D	1809. C	1854. D
1630. D	1675. D	1720. D	1765. D	1810. D	1855. D
1631. D	1676. D	1721. D	1766. A	1811. D	1856. C
1632. D	1677. A	1722. A	1767. C	1812. D	1857. C
1633. D	1678. A	1723. A	1768. A	1813. B	1858. A
1634. D	1679. D	1724. A	1769. A	1814. A	1859. C
1635. D	1680. D	1725. A	1770. A	1815. D	1860. D
1636. C	1681. A	1726. A	1771. D	1816. A	1861. A
1637. D	1682. D	1727. B	1772. A	1817. A	1862. A
1638. D	1683. C	1728. C	1773. C	1818. D	1863. D
1639. D	1684. B	1729. C	1774. D	1819. D	1864. A
1640. B	1685. D	1730. C	1775. A	1820. B	1865. C
1641. B	1686. C	1731. C	1776. A	1821. D	1866. C
1642. B	1687. D	1732. D	1777. C	1822. D	1867. B
1643. B	1688. B	1733. D	1778. D	1823. D	1868. C
1644. D	1689. B	1734. D	1779. C	1824. A	1869. B
1645. C	1690. B	1735. D	1780. B	1825. D	1870. D
1646. D	1691. D	1736. B	1781. C	1826. C	1871. C
1647. D	1692. B	1737. B	1782. A	1827. D	1872. D
1648. B	1693. D	1738. D	1783. C	1828. D	1873. A
1649. B	1694. D	1739. D	1784. A	1829. D	1874. B
1650. D	1695. D	1740. C	1785. D	1830. C	1875. B
1651. B	1696. B	1741. D	1786. D	1831. B	1876. D
1652. D	1697. A	1742. D	1787. D	1832. D	1877. B
1653. D	1698. C	1743. B	1788. B	1833. D	1878. D
1654. C	1699. A	1744. C	1789. C	1834. C	1879. C
1655. C	1700. A	1745. C	1790. A	1835. A	1880. C
1656. D	1701. D	1746. B	1791. D	1836. B	1881. B
1657. B	1702. A	1747. C	1792. A	1837. D	1882. B
1658. C	1703. D	1748. D	1793. D	1838. D	1883. C
1659. A	1704. D	1749. D	1794. D	1839. A	1884. B
1660. B	1705. D	1750. A	1795. D	1840. D	1885. A
1661. D	1706. C	1751. D	1796. D	1841. D	1886. D
1662. D	1707. D	1752. D	1797. C	1842. B	1887. A
1663. A	1708. D	1753. D	1798. C	1843. D	1888. D
1664. D	1709. B	1754. B	1799. D	1844. C	1889. B
1665. B	1710. D	1755. B	1800. C	1845. C,	1890. C

ANSWERS

1891. A	1936. D	1981. D	2026. C	2071. C	2116. D
1892. C	1937. C	1982. D	2027. B	2072. D	2117. D
1893. D	1938. C	1983. D	2028. D	2073. A	2118. D
1894. D	1939. D	1984. A	2029. D	2074. B	2119. D
1895. D	1940. A	1985. A	2030. D	2075. D	2120. D
1896. D	1941. B	1986. C	2031. D	2076. D	2121. B
1897. D	1942. C	1987. C	2032. D	2077. C	2122. C
1898. D	1943. D	1988. B	2033. B	2078. B	2123. C
1899. B	1944. D	1989. C	2034. C	2079. B	2124. D
1900. C	1945. C	1990. D	2035. A	2080. D	2125. C
1901. C	1946. D	1991. D	2036. A	2081. D	2126. B
1902. D	1947. D	1992. D	2037. C	2082. D	2127. D
1903. C	1948. D	1993. D	2038. D	2083. A	2128. C
1904. D	1949. B	1994. D	2039. D	2084. A	2129. D
1905. D	1950. A	1995. B	2040. D	2085. B	2130. C
1906. D	1951. D	1996. C	2041. D	2086. C	2131. B
1907. D	1952. A	1997. B	2042. D	2087. A	2132. B
1908. B	1953. D	1998. D	2043. D	2088. B	2133. D
1909. D	1954. D	1999. D	2044. A	2089. D	2134. D
1910. C	1955. D	2000. D	2045. D	2090. A	2135. A
1911. D	1956. C	2001. B	2046. D	2091. B	2136. A
1912. D	1957. C	2002. D	2047. B	2092. D	2137. C
1913. D	1958. D	2003. D	2048. D	2093. D	2138. D
1914. C	1959. D	2004. A	2049. C	2094. D	2139. A
1915. A	1960. D	2005. D	2050. C	2095. C	2140. D
1916. D	1961. D	2006. D	2051. A	2096. A	2141. D
1917. D	1962. D	2007. D	2052. D	2097. D	2142. B
1918. D	1963. D	2008. D	2053. D	2098. B	2143. B
1919. B	1964. D	2009. C	2054. C	2099. D	2144. D
1920. C	1965. D	2010. D	2055. C	2100. B	2145. D
1921. C	1966. C	2011. D	2056. A	2101. A	2146. B
1922. A	1967. C	2012. D	2057. C	2102. B	2147. D
1923. B	1968. D	2013. D	2058. A	2103. D	2148. D
1924. D	1969. B	2014. A	2059. A	2104. B	2149. D
1925. B	1970. B	2015. D	2060. D	2105. C	2150. A
1926. D	1971. C	2016. D	2061. A	2106. C	2151. D
1927. C	1972. D	2017. D	2062. C	2107. A	2152. D
1928. B	1973. D	2018. D	2063. A	2108. B	2153. B
1929. D	1974. A	2019. D	2064. D	2109. D	2154. D
1930. C	1975. B	2020. B	2065. D	2110. D	2155. D
1931. D	1976. D	2021. D	2066. D	2111. D	2156. C
1932. D	1977. D	2022. D	2067. D	2112. D	2157. D
1933. D	1978. D	2023. D	2068. A	2113. B	2158. D
1934. C	1979. D	2024. A	2069. D	2114. D	2159. B
1935. D	1980. D	2025. B	2070. D	2115. A	2160. D

ANSWERS

2161. D	2206. C	2251. B	2296. D	2341. D	2386. D
2162. A	2207. D	2252. A	2297. D	2342. A	2387. D
2163. A	2208. D	2253. A	2298. D	2343. D	2388. D
2164. A	2209. D	2254. D	2299. B	2344. D	2389. D
2165. A	2210. C	2255. C	2300. D	2345. D	2390. D
2166. D	2211. B	2256. B	2301. D	2346. D	2391. A
2167. B	2212. A	2257. A	2302. B	2347. D	2392. C
2168. B	2213. D	2258. D	2303. C	2348. C	2393. B
2169. B	2214. C	2259. A	2304. B	2349. B	2394. B
2170. C	2215. A	2260. D	2305. D	2350. D	2395. B
2171. A	2216. D	2261. C	2306. D	2351. D	2396. B
2172. B	2217. D	2262. D	2307. C	2352. A	2397. B
2173. A	2218. D	2263. C	2308. D	2353. D	2398. B
2174. C	2219. B	2264. D	2309. A	2354. C	2399. A
2175. C	2220. D	2265. D	2310. B	2355. D	2400. C
2176. D	2221. A	2266. D	2311. A	2356. D	2401. A
2177. B	2222. D	2267. B	2312. D	2357. A	2402. B
2178. A	2223. A	2268. B	2313. C	2358. B	2403. D
2179. D	2224. A	2269. C	2314. D	2359. B	2404. B
2180. A	2225. D	2270. C	2315. A	2360. A	2405. C
2181. B	2226. D	2271. C	2316. C	2361. D	2406. C
2182. D	2227. B	2272. D	2317. B	2362. C	2407. B
2183. D	2228. D	2273. D	2318. D	2363. C	2408. D
2184. C	2229. B	2274. B	2319. D	2364. D	2409. D
2185. C	2230. D	2275. B	2320. B	2365. A	2410. D
2186. C	2231. D	2276. A	2321. D	2366. A	2411. D
2187. D	2232. C	2277. A	2322. B	2367. B	2412. C
2188. D	2233. C	2278. D	2323. D	2368. C	2413. D
2189. A	2234. B	2279. D	2324. D	2369. D	2414. D
2190. C	2235. C	2280. C	2325. A	2370. D	2415. D
2191. B	2236. D	2281. C	2326. A	2371. D	2416. D
2192. B	2237. D	2282. D	2327. B	2372. D	2417. D
2193. D	2238. D	2283. D	2328. D	2373. D	2418. A
2194. B	2239. C	2284. D	2329. D	2374. D	2419. C
2195. D	2240. A	2285. B	2330. D	2375. A	2420. B
2196. C	2241. B	2286. C	2331. B	2376. D	2421. A
2197. D	2242. D	2287. B	2332. D	2377. B	2422. B
2198. C	2243. C	2288. A	2333. D	2378. D	2423. D
2199. C	2244. D	2289. D	2334. D	2379. B	2424. A
2200. D	2245. D	2290. A	2335. C	2380. D	2425. A
2201. D	2246. D	2291. D	2336. C	2381. D	2426. C
2202. D	2247. A	2292. D	2337. D	2382. D	2427. D
2203. A	2248. B	2293. C	2338. D	2383. D	2428. D
2204. C	2249. C	2294. C	2339. B	2384. D	2429. C
2205. D	2250. B	2295. D	2340. D	2385. C	2430. D

ANSWERS

2431. D	2451. D	2471. D	2491. C	2511. D	2531. D
2432. A	2452. D	2472. D	2492. B	2512. A	2532. D
2433. C	2453. A	2473. D	2493. D	2513. C	2533. D
2434. B	2454. D	2474. C	2494. D	2514. D	2534. B
2435. B	2455. D	2475. A	2495. A	2515. C	2535. B
2436. D	2456. A	2476. B	2496. B	2516. A	2536. A
2437. A	2457. B	2477. B	2497. A	2517. B	2537. C
2438. D	2458. D	2478. D	2498. D	2518. A	2538. C
2439. D	2459. D	2479. D	2499. B	2519. D	2539. C
2440. D	2460. A	2480. C	2500. B	2520. D	2540. B
2441. A	2461. D	2481. D	2501. D	2521. A	2541. A
2442. D	2462. D	2482. D	2502. D	2522. C	2542. C
2443. A	2463. D	2483. D	2503. A	2523. C	2543. B
2444. A	2464. A	2484. C	2504. C	2524. B	2544. C
2445. D	2465. A	2485. C	2505. A	2525. D	2545. D
2446. D	2466. D	2486. A	2506. D	2526. D	2546. A
2447. D	2467. D	2487. D	2507. B	2527. A	2547. D
2448. B	2468. D	2488. B	2508. D	2528. D	2548. B
2449. C	2469. B	2489. D	2509. D	2529. D	2549. C
2450. D	2470. B	2490. A	2510. D	2530. B	2550. D
					2551. B
					2552. D

EU GSPR Authorised Reprsentative
Logos Europe, 9 rue Nicolas Poussin
1700, La Rochelle, France
Phone: +33 (0) 6 67 93 73 78
E-mail: contact@logoseurope.eu

www.ingramcontent.com/pod-product-compliance
Ingram Content Group UK Ltd.
Pitfield, Milton Keynes, MK11 3LW, UK
UKHW050458150426
5217IPUK00025B/1749